Health Education and Community Pharmacy

A Comprehensive Textbook for Diploma and Degree Students in Pharmacy

Health Education and Community Pharmacy

A Comprehensive Textbook for Diploma and Degree Students in Pharmacy

NS Parmar
MPharm (Pharmacol) MSc (Med.) PhD
Principal and Professor of Pharmacology
BN College of Pharmaceutical Sciences, Udaipur
Formerly
Principal, AR College of Pharmacy and
Dean, Faculty of Pharmaceutical Sciences
Sardar Patel University, Vallabh Vidyanagar, and
Assistant Professor of Clinical Pharmacy
College of Pharmacy, King Saud University, Riyadh
Saudi Arabia

CBSPD

CBS Publishers & Distributors Pvt Ltd

New Delhi • Bengaluru • Chennai • Kochi • Kolkata • Lucknow • Mumbai
Hyderabad • Jharkhand • Nagpur • Patna • Pune • Uttarakhand

Disclaimer

Science and technology are constantly changing fields. New research and experience broaden the scope of information and knowledge. The author has tried her best in giving information available to her while preparing the material for this book. Although all efforts have been made to ensure optimum accuracy of the material, yet it is quite possible some errors might have been left uncorrected. The publisher, the printer and the author will not be held responsible for any inadvertent errors, omissions or inaccuracies.

Health Education and Community Pharmacy

ISBN: 978-81-239-0407-8

First Edition: 1995

Reprint: 1996, 1998, 1999, 2001, 2002, 2004, 2005, 2006, 2007, 2008, 2009, 2010, 2011, 2012, 2013, 2014, 2015, 2016, 2017, 2018, 2019, 2020, 2022, 2023, **2024** 2025 **2026**

Published by **Satish Kumar Jain** and produced by **Varun Jain** for

CBS Publishers & Distributors Pvt Ltd

4819/XI Prahlad Street, 24 Ansari Road, Daryaganj, New Delhi 110 002, India.
Ph: 011-23266838, 23289259 Website: www.cbspd.com
e-mail: delhi@cbspd.com

Corporate Office: 204 FIE, Industrial Area, Patparganj, Delhi 110 092
Ph: 011-4934 4934 Fax: 011-4934 4935
e-mail: publishing@cbspd.com; publicity@cbspd.com

Branches

- **Bengaluru:** Seema House 2975, 17th Cross, KR Road, Banasankari 2nd Stage, Bengaluru 560 070, Karnataka, India
  Ph: +91-80-26771678/79 Fax: +91-80-26771680 e-mail: bangalore@cbspd.com
- **Chennai:** 7, Subbaraya Street, Shenoy Nagar, Chennai 600 030, Tamil Nadu, India
  Ph: +91-44-26680620, 26681266 Fax: +91-44-42032115 e-mail: chennai@cbspd.com
- **Kochi:** 42/1325, 1326, Power House Road, Opp KSEB, Power House, Ernakulum Kochi 682 018, Kerala, India
  Ph: +91-484-4059061-65,67 Fax: +91-484-4059065 e-mail: kochi@cbspd.com
- **Kolkata:** 147, Hind Ceramics Compound, 1st Floor, Nilgunj Road, Belghoria, Kolkata-700056, West Bengal, India
  Ph: +033-25633055, 033-25633056 e-mail: kolkata@cbspd.com
- **Lucknow:** Basement, Khushnuma Complex, 7 Meerabai Marg (Behind Jawahar Bhawan), Lucknow-226001, UP, India
  Ph: +0522-4000032 e-mail: tiwari.lucknow@cbspd.com
- **Mumbai:** PWD Shed, Gala no 25/26, Ramchandra Bhatt Marg, Next to JJ Hospital Gate no. 2, Opp. Union Bank of India, Noorbaug, Mumbai-400009, Maharashtra, India
  Ph: 022-66661880/89 e-mail: mumbai@cbspd.com

Representatives

- Hyderabad 0-9885175004
- Patna 0-9334159340
- Jharkhand 0-9811541605
- Pune 0-9664372571
- Nagpur 0-8692091830
- Uttarakhand 0-9716462459

Printed at Glorious Printers, Jhilmil Industrial Area, Delhi, India

Dedicated to
My Dear Wife Usha
and Loving
Children
Pragya
and Pankaj

FOREWORD

I take great pleasure in writing the foreword for this comprehensive textbook on Health Education and Community Pharmacy written by Prof. N.S. Parmar for the students of diploma and degree courses in Pharmacy. There is dearth of standard books giving adequate coverage of all the topics included in the syllabus of this newly introduced subject which may be referred to, by the students and teachers alike. Having gone through the manuscript, I feel that Prof. Parmar's book fulfils this need. He has done full justice to every topic emphasizing the role of pharmacist in different areas of Health Education and Community Pharmacy. He has also dealt the topics of communicable and noncommunicable diseases more extensively which may appear heavy to some colleagues but these chapters provide proper understanding of the etiology, signs and symptoms, complications, prevention, management and prognosis of important diseases like tuberculosis, AIDs, malaria, cancers, diabetes, hypertension, and epilepsy. This knowledge is essential for a community pharmacist and it will also prepare a strong background for grasping the subjects of Pharmacology and Clinical Pharmacy in the later year(s). Prof. Parmar, with his long experience of teaching the subjects of Pharmacology and Clinical Pharmacy to the students of medicine and pharmacy in reputed institutions, has made commendable efforts in dealing with the subject in a lucid manner. Other impressive features of the book are the many diagrammatic illustrations which will be very helpful to the students in having a clear understanding of the subject and a number of tables which summarize the text material for a quick glance and revision. I am sure this textbook will be useful to the students, not only for studying the subject as a part of their curriculum but also for the practice and promotion of community pharmacy as professional pharmacists in future.

C.K. KOKATE
M. Pharm., Ph.D.
Vice-President, Pharmacy Council of India,
Ex - Dean, University College of
Pharmaceutical Sciences, Kakatiya University,
Warangal-506009

ABOUT THE AUTHOR

Professor N.S. Parmar is presently functioning as Principal & Professor of Pharmacology, B.N. College of Pharmaceutical Sciences, Udaipur. Having passed his M. Pharm. in Pharmacology from S.M.S. Medical College, Jaipur in 1966, he joined as Senior Demonstrator of Pharmacology, J.L.N. Medical College, Ajmer in 1967, completed his M.Sc. (Medicine) in 1970 and became a Lecturer at the Jawaharlal Institute of Postgraduate Medical Education and Research, Pondicherry. He obtained his Ph.D. in Pharmacology in 1978 and became Assistant Professor of Clinical Pharmacy at the King Saud University, Riyadh Saudi Arabia in 1982. He joined as the Principal of the A.R. College of Pharmacy, Vallabh Vidyanagar in 1987. Before joining his present assignment in 1993, he served the B.V. Patel Pharmaceutical Education and Research Development Centre, Ahemdabad for a spell of two years as Assistant Director and Professor of Pharmacology.

Prof. Parmar has teaching experience of over 27 years. He has authored 85 research papers most of which have been published in international journals. His research interests include pharmacology of peptic ulcer disease and inflammation. He is specially interested in the promotion and development of professional pharmacy. He has been awarded for his published research work-the B. Mukerji Prize and B. Uvnas Prize of the Indian Pharmacological Society, C.L. Malhotra Prize of the Association of Physiologists and Pharmacologists of India and the Hari Om Ashram Prize of the Sardar Patel University.

Currently he is a Member of the Pharmacy Council of India and also a Member of the All India Board of Pharmaceutical Education of the A.I.C.T.E. He has also been awarded the membership of the New York Academy of Sciences very recently.

PREFACE

The Pharmacy Council of India has undertaken a much desired step of revising and updating the curriculum of Diploma in Pharmacy course and implementing the Education Regulations 1991 in letter and spirit. The addition of new subjects of Health Education and Community Pharmacy and Hospital and Clinical Pharmacy which have become the backbone of professional pharmacy services in the developed countries, would go a long way in enhancing the prestige of this professional course till such time as we are able to raise the minimum qualification of our professional pharmacist to a degree level. Recently, many universities of our country have also introduced the components of health education, community pharmacy, pathophysiology and clinical pharmacy in the curriculum of their degree and postgraduate courses which is again a welcome step towards the enhancement of professional pharmacy and making the training of our students more patient oriented.

This book encompasses the syllabi of Health Education and Community Pharmacy for the Diploma in Pharmacy course in accordance with the ER-91 and also the B. Pharm. course of the University of Rajasthan. The matter has been presented in some detail in order to prepare the students for the better understanding of the course on Clinical Pharmacy in the latter year(s). I am sanguine that the book will be equally useful to the students of diploma and degree courses in Pharmacy and also to the teachers for a thorough understanding and effective teaching of this newly introduced subject.

In preparing the subject matter, I have freely consulted a number of text books and monographs mentioned at the end of this book. I humbly apologise for inadvertently quoting some textual matter from these titles in order to make certain points clear for the ultimate benefit of our students.

I am highly thankful to my colleague Dr. O.P. Katare and my daughter Dr. (Miss) Pragya Parmar for their constant help and suggestions in preparing the text of some chapters and to my wife Mrs. Usha Parmar for the correction of galley proofs. I also thankfully acknowledge the help rendered by my colleague Shri Gaurang B. Shah in the preparation of the glossary of medical terms. I appreciate the efforts of my students Mr. Pankaj Jain and Mr. Kamal Singh Rathore in designing the cover page and some illustrations of this book respectively. I am also thankful to Mr. Vikram Singh Ranawat for doing all the typing work and for bearing with my repeated last minute corrections at various stages. Last but not the least, the co-operation of the publishers M/s CBS Publishers & Distributors is very much appreciated for bringing out the book in a record time.

UDAIPUR **N.S. Parmar**
Ist June, 1995

CONTENTS

1

HEALTH EDUCATION AND COMMUNITY PHARMACY, AN INTRODUCTION

Health education is a process that informs, motivates and helps people to adopt and maintain healthy practices and life styles, advocates environmental changes as needed to facilitate this goal and conducts professional training and research to the same end.

According to this definition the three main objectives of health education are:

(i) **Informing the people:** This involves providing the information to the people and thus disseminating scientific knowledge about the prevention of disease and promotion of health. Exposure to knowledge will remove the barriers of ignorance, prejudices, misconceptions and superstitions which people may have about health and disease.

(ii) **Motivation of the people:** This objective is concerned with the motivation of the people to change their habits and ways of living. The commonly adopted health practices which are detrimental to health have to be changed e.g. out-door defecation, use of polluted water, indulgence in drinking and smoking, abuse of drugs, physical inactivity, and not limiting the family size etc. Health education should motivate the people for adopting healthy practices which may keep them free of avoidable diseases and improve the quaity of life.

(iii) **Guidance of the people:** Health education should be provided by a variety of well trained health, education and communication personnel starting with the physician. People in general need help to adopt and maintain healthy practices and life styles. People should be encouraged and guided to use judiciously the health services available to them e.g. timely immunization, adoption of suitable methods of family planning, use of safe drinking water and rehabilitation of alcoholics and drug addicts etc.

Components of Health Education:

Health education envisages a number of effective areas which are briefly outlined below:

(a) Knowledge about the human body, its structure and functions.
(b) Nutrition and balanced diet.
(c) Personal and environmental hygiene.
(d) Family health: Care of the mother and the child, family planning, immunization and the care of elderly.
(e) Control of communicable and noncommunicable diseases.
(f) Mental and social health.
(g) Prevention of accidents and utilization of first aid measures.
(h) Proper use of available health services.

Pharmacist and Public Health

With the rise of population world wide during the last few decades, it has been realized that the traditional medical and health services now play a limited role in the overall improvement of health status. This fact has driven all health professionals to the common goal of disease prevention and health promotion. In the developed countries the clinical direction of pharmacy has de-emphasized the manipulatve product oriented and distributive skills and focussed more on the public health awareness. Today, the pharmacist's attention is directed towards the patient, his environment and his state of general well-being. The following areas have now emerged wherein the pharmacist can be actively involved in the delivery of health care to the community.

(a) **All the drug related problems:** The pharmacist's involvement in this area amounts to performing disease preventing and health promoting activities, which include counselling on proper use of OTC and prescribed medications, taking drug and medical problem histories, referring patients to specific health care provisions, obtaining immunization schedules from health centres and advise parents about the importance of adhering to the times recommended therein.
(b) **Pharmacoepidemiology:** Recently a specific area of epidemiology has emerged which is referred to as pharmacoepidemiology. It is concerned with the safety or risk assessment of a new drug which starts with its early use and continues with its longer and widespread use. It generates infomation about pharmaceutical outcomes and monitors associated risks and adverse drug reactions in the postmarketing phase.
(c) **Communicable diseases:** While a number of serious communi-

cable diseases have been practically eradicated, some like tuberculosis, syphilis and gonorrhea are still common, and certain viral diseases like herpes genitalis and acquired immune deficiency syndrome (AIDs) have been recognized as very serious. The recent spread of AIDs has catapulted this sexually transmitted disease into critical dimensions. The life threatening nature of AIDs has caused it to take precedence over all others in the group. The pharmacist can be involved in educational programmes promoting safe sexual practices, particularly where the use of condoms is essential.

The role of the pharmacist in the control of communicable diseases consists of an awareness of the natural history of these diseases in both the individual and the community, referral of patients to proper medical care facilities when so required and public education of an informed type at all times. It is in this aspect of community disease control that the pharmacist can play a very important role.

(d) **Chronic disease control:** A community pharmacist can encourage his/her clients to avail themselves of the few proven techniques in chronic disease prevention.Good living habits and moderate exercise have been recommended as methods of preventing cardiovascular diseases. The prevention of strokes is concerned with the control of high blood pressure. The pharmacist can take client's blood pressure and refer him/her to a proper physician for treatment and encourage the patients compliance with the prescribed regimens. He can promote measures as quitting smoking, controlling high blood pressure, lowering cholesterol intake, increasing physical activity and good overall health consciousness.

(e) **Health education:** In the developed countries many professional pharmacies now participate in patient health education through the use of pamphlets and bulletins freely available on display racks. These cover every important major disease, drug classes, drugs of abuse, drug and food interactions, sexually transmitted diseases, immunizations, family planning, health promotion, fluoridation, poison prevention, quackery, disaster preparedness, environmental protection and work place safety. More than this the pharmacist can actively promote good health by reaching out to impart professional information to the public whom he or she serves. Formal methods of health education have their place in public health and preventive medicine but in the pharmacy the informed direction and guidance of members of the public are much more realistic. The participation of pharmacists in community health education should be in the every day person to person contact with the people whom they can serve most effectively.

(f) **Maternal and child health:** No public health programme has proved its worth more than the care of the mother and child. The basic idea behind the maternal and the child health is to take adequate care of the mother and her child through the time they are exposed to the greatest risks of disease and death i.e., during pregnancy, the puerperium and the first year of life. The early diagnosis of pregnancy with informed supervsion of its progress through the delivery and the immediate postpartum period constitutes the bulwark of care in maternal and child health programmes. The earlier the prenatal care is given, the more beneficial is the effect not only to the mother but also to the child as the health of the infant is directly influenced by the care it receives while *in utero*. Thus, the pharmacist, who understands the normal course of pregnancy and infancy is at a distinct advantage as he or she can guide the mother in simple matters of hygiene and management of her pregnancy and of her infant. This is more beneficial to those women who through lack of education, have an incomplete understanding of how important it is to have early professional prenatal care. The pharmacist must encourage breast feeding of the child after it is born as the mother's milk is the best food designed for it. Later on the pharmacist can play another major role by guiding the mother for the protection of her child against the diseases of childhood by following proper immunization schedules against polio, diphtheria, tetanus, pertussis, mumps and typhoid etc.

(g) **Nutrition:** The pharmacist can make significant contributions in assuring adequate nutrition by advising his patients about basic food needs, helping to correct improper food habits in children, advising on special requirements for nutrients during prenatal and maternal periods in females, suggesting special diet instructions for diabetic patients and people with food allergies and participating in supporting school lunch programs and schemes like mid-day meals etc. in rural areas.

(h) **Environmental health:** The pharmacist's role in environmental health is one of alertness to the conditions prevailing in his community and towards the control of any hazards. This is especially true of air and water pollution which require concerted community action for their control but pharmacist can also play a much more important role in the control of food borne diseases.

The first indication of an outbreak of food borne disease is the unusually large number of people falling sick and seeking relief from nausea, vomiting and diarrhoea more so if they are concerted within a short period of time. If this type of epidemic results in an increase in over the counter sales of anti-nauseant and antidiarrhoeal drugs, the local health authority should be notified immediately. The pharmacist should also be aware of local occupations and their hazards and alert to the first symptom of disease. For example all occupations in which the workers are exposed to dust are hazardous depending upon the size of dust particles and their ability to penetrate into lungs. The workers of an asbestos industry are prone to lung cancer. The pharmacist's continuing education should include watching local pattern of society and its diseases and changing his or her emphasis towards the evolving patterns of diseases and their control.

(i) **Alcoholism and drug abuse:** The diseases of alcoholism and drug abuse also come under the purview of the community pharmacist. The pharmacist will have many opportunities to help individuals who become dependent upon alcohol. Drug abuse is similar to alcoholism yet different because it has been gaining more acceptance among young people on the campuses of educational

AREAS OF PHARMACIST'S INVOLVEMENT IN PUBLIC HEALTH THROUGH COMMUNITY PHARMACY

1. Drug and Nutrition Counselling.
2. Proper use of Prescribed and OTC Drugs.
3. Family Planning.
4. Pregnancy and Infant Care.
5. Immunizations.
6. Sexually Transmitted Diseases.
7. Control of Toxic Agents.
8. Occupaitonal Health and Safety.
9. Control of Accidental Injuries.
10. Fluoridation of Community Water Supplies.
11. Smoking Cessation.
12. Reduction of Misuse of Alcohol and Drugs.
13. Improved Nutrition.
14. Environmental Protection.
15. Programmes on Weight Control.
16. Poisoning and Cancer Signals.

institutions. Here again the pharmacist is in the unparalleled position of being professionally a competent member of the community to advise local agencies about drugs and their harmful effects. The participation of pharmacist in the prevention of alcoholism and drug abuse will add to his or her credit both professionally and financially as the contacts, publicity and recognition from such interest will also reflect in his business returns.

Unfortunately in our country, the involvement of pharmacists in these areas of health education and public health is minimal. With the upgradation of the educational level of the professional pharmacist and greater awareness of the public in due course, it is expected that our professional and community pharmacists shall play a very significant role in the prevention of many communicable and noncommunicable diseases, their treatment and rehabilitation wherever necessary. The important areas of pharmacist's involvement in public health through community pharmacy services have been listed in the adjoining box.

2

CONCEPT OF HEALTH AND DISEASE

Concept of health—Definition of physical health • mental health • social health • spiritual health • concept of disease • natural history of disease • the disease agents • concept of prevention of diseases.

Definition of Health

The widely accepted definition of health is that given by World Health Organization (1948) in the preamble to its constitution, which is as follows:

"Health is a state of complete physical, mental and social well-being and not merely as absence of disease or infirmity".

In recent years this statement has been expanded to include the ability to lead a "socially and economically productive life".

OPERATIONAL DEFINITION OF HEALTH

The WHO definition of health cannot be considered as an operational definition because it does not lend itself to direct measurement. Epidemiological studies of health have been hampered because of our inability to measure health and well being directly.

In order to overcome this lacuna a WHO group has devised an operational definition of health. According to this definition the concept of health is viewed as being of two orders. In a broad sense health can be defined as "a condition or quality of the human organism expressing the adequate functioning of the organism in given conditions, generic or environmental".

In a narrow sense, which is more suitable for measurement, health means:

(a) There is no obvious evidence of disease and that a person is functioning normally, i.e., confirming within normal limits of variation to the standards of health criteria generally accepted for one's age, sex, community and geographic region, and

(b) The several organs of the body are functioning adequately in themselves and in relation to one-another, which means a kind of equilibrium or homeostasis, a condition relatively stable but which may vary as human beings adopt to internal and external stimuli.

DIMENSIONS OF HEALTH

As evident from above-mentioned definitions, health is multidimensional. The WHO definition envisages three specific dimensions—the physical, the mental and the social. Some other dimensions may also be considered as more knowledge is acquired on them in due course of time. They include spiritual, emotional and vocational dimensions. Although these dimensions function and interact with one another, each has its own nature and characteristics and they will be dealt separately for descriptive purposes.

1. Physical Dimension:

The state of physical health implies the notion of perfect functioning of the body. Physical health is conceptualized as a biological state in which every cell and every organ is functioning at optimum capacity, and in perfect harmony with the rest of the body.

The signs of physical health in an individual are, a good complexion, a clean and healthy skin, bright eyes, lustrous hair with a body well clothed with firm flesh, not too fat or obese, a sweet breath, a good appetite, sound sleep, regular activity of bowels and bladder, and smooth, easy and well co-ordinated bodily movements. All the organs of the body are of unexceptional size and function normaly, all the special senses are intact and the resting pulse rate, blood pressure and exercise tolerance are within the normal range for the individual's age and sex.

2. Mental Dimensions:

Mental health is not merely the absence of mental illness. Good mental health is reflected by the ability to respond to the many varied experiences of life with flexibility and a sense of purpose. Mental health has been recently defined as "a state of balance between the individual and the surrounding world, a state of harmony between oneself and others, a co-existence between the realities of the self and that of other people and that of the environment". Psychologists have mentioned the following characteristics of a mentally healthy person:

(a) a mentally healthy person is free from internal conflicts, he is not at 'war with himself.'

(b) he is well adjusted i.e., he is able to get along well with others. He accepts criticism and is not easily upset.
(c) he searches for identity.
(d) he has a strong sense of self esteem.
(e) he knows himself, his needs, problems and goals.
(f) he has good self-control, balances, rationality and emotionality.
(g) he faces problems and tries to solve them intelligently, i.e., he is able to cope well with stress and anxiety.

3. Social Dimension:

Social well-being implies harmony and integration within the individual, between the individual and other members of the society and between the individuals and the world in which they live. It is the quantity and quality of an individual's interpersonal ties and the extent of involvement with the community.

The social dimension of health also includes the levels of social skills and interaction one possesses, social functioning and the ability to see oneself as a member of a larger society. Social health also takes into account that every individual is part of a family and of wider community and focusses on social and economic conditions and well being of the "whole person" in the context of his social network.Social health originates from "positive material environment" (focusing on financial and residential matters) and "positive human environment" which is concerned with the social network of the individual.

4. Spiritual Dimension:

According to the proponents of holistic health concept, spiritual dimension plays a significant role in health and disease. Spiritual health refers to that component of individual's thinking which reaches out and strives for meaning and purpose in life. It includes integrity, principles, ethics, the purpose in life, commitment to some higher being and belief in concepts that are not subject to "state of the art" explanation.

DETERMINATION OF HEALTH

The factors that influence health lie both within the individual and externally in the environment in which he or she lives. It is a well recognised fact that what a man is and to what disease he may fall a victim depends on the combination of two sets of factors—his **genetic factors** and the **environmental factors** to which he is exposed. Some such important factors that may determine the health status of an individual are described below:

1. **Heredity:** The physical and mental traits of every human being are to some extent determined by the nature of his genes at the moment of conception. A number of diseases are now known to be of genetic origin e.g. epilepsy, mental retardation, diabetes, cancers, chromosomal abnormalities and errors of metabolism etc. Genetic factors are also responsible for certain abnormal types of responses to drugs or different metabolic patterns like succinylcholine apnea, acetylation of isoniazid, hemolysis caused by antimalarials and hepatic porphyrias caused by barbiturates. The state of health, therefore, depends partly on the genetic constitution of man.
2. **Environment:** Hippocrates first related diseases to the environment e.g. climatc, water and air etc. This concept of disease environment association stands true even today. It is an established fact now that environment directly influences the physical, mental and social well-being of the human population. The environmental factors range from housing, water supply, air, noise, psychological stress and family structure through social and economic support system, to the organization of health and social welfare services in the community.
3. **Life Style:** Life style denotes the way people live, reflecting the social values, attitudes and activities. It consists of cultural and behavioural patterns and life-long personal habits like smoking and alcoholism. Life styles are adopted through social interaction with parents, peer groups, friends and siblings and through schools and mass media. There is definite association between health and life styles of individuals. Many health problems encountered today, especially in the developed countries like coronary heart disease, obesity, lung cancer and drug addiction, are associated with the life styles. However, certain life style factors also promote health. Examples include adequate nutrition, enough sleep, and sufficient physical activity.
4. **Socio-economic conditions:** Socio-economic conditions significantly influence the health of human beings. The health status of a given population is primarily determined by per capita GNP, education, nutrition, employment, housing and the political system of the country. Some of the important factors are:

(a) **Economic Status:** The per capita GNP is an accepted index of the general economic status of any country. Economic progress has been a major factor in reducing morbidity, increasing life expectancy and improving the quality of life. Economic status determines purchasing power, standard of living, quality of life, family size, and attention towards health care. On the contrary affluence can also be a contributory cause of illness as exemplified by the high incidence of coronary heart disease, obesity and diabetes etc in upper socio-economic groups.

(b) **Education:** Education greatly influences the health care status. Illiteracy closely coincides with poverty, malnutrition, ill health and high infant mortality rates. Education remarkably compensates the effect of poverty on health irrespective of availability of health facilities. In the Indian state of Kerala, a major factor in the low mortaility rate is its highest female literacy rate of about 66 per cent as compared to about 25% of the country as a whole.

(c) **Occupation:** Suitable employment in productive work promotes health. Job satisfaction is an important factor contributing to mental health and well-being. Proper employment generates income and raises economic status which in turn promotes health and education of the family.

(d) **Political System:** Political decision and political will concerning resource allocation, man power policy, choice of technology, environment protection and the extent to which health services are made available and accessible to the different segments of the society are the means through which the political system can shape the health of the people in any country.

5. **Health Services:** The purpose of effective health services is to improve the health status of population. For example; provision of safe water and healthy environment, general screening programs for infective diseases and propensity to blindness and cancers, immunization of prospective mothers, infants and children, and nutritional care of pregnant women and children can contribute to the health status of any segment of the population. All these components taken together, now form the concept of primry health care which promotes better health for the people.

INDICATORS OF HEALTH

Indicators of health are required not only for measuring the health status of a community but also for comparing the health status of one country with another, for the estimation of health care requirements, for the allocation of resources and for the monitoring and evaluation of health services, activities and programmes. Indicators are also necessary for measuring the extent to which the objectives and targets of a health programme have been achieved.

As the indicators have to be scientifically relevant and dependable for the measurement of the health status of a given community, they should be valid, reliable, sensitive and specific for a given situation. However, there are only a few indicators which fit into these requirements. Further, a complete status of health cannot be assessed using any single indicator and hence it must be evaluated using a profile employing many indicators. These may be classified and explained as under:

1. Mortality Indicators:

(a) **Crude Death Rate:** It is defined as number of deaths per 1000 population per year in a given community. It is a fair indicator of the comparative health of the people. When used for international comparison, the usefulness of the crude death rate is restricted because it is influenced by the age sex composition of the population. Though it is not a perfect measure of health status, a decrease in crude death rate provides a good tool for assessing the overall health improvement in a population.

(b) **Expectation of Life:** Life expectancy at birth is defined as the average number of years that will be lived by those born alive into a population if the current age-specific mortality rates persist. Life expectancy is good indicator of socio-economic development and it has been adopted as a global health indicator. A minimum life expectancy at birth of 60 years is the goal of **Health for all by the 2000 AD.**

(c) **Infant Mortality Rate:** It is the ratio of deaths under 1 year of age in a given year to the live number of births in the same year. It is usually expressed as a rate per 1000 live births. It is one of the most universally accepted indicators of health status not only of infants, but also of the whole populations and of their socio-economic conditions. It is also a sensitive indicator of the availability, utilization and effectiveness of health care, in particular the perinatal care. A maximum infant mortality rate of 50 per 1000 live births is the goal of **Health for all by 2000 AD.**

(d) **Child Mortality Rate:** This is another indicator related to overall health status which takes note of early childhood (1-4 years) mortality rate. It is defined as the number of deaths at ages 1-4 years in given year per 1000 children in that age group at the midpoint of the year concerned. Whereas the Infant Mortality Rate may be more than 10 times higher in the least developed countries than in the developed countries, the Child Mortality Rate may be as much as 250 times higher. This highlights the magnitude of the gap and scope for improvement.

(e) **Under-5 Proportionate Mortality Rate:** This indicates the proportion of total deaths occurring under-5 age group and thus incorporates both Infant Mortality Rate and Child Mortality Rate. In communities with poor hygiene this rate may exceed 60% which indicates high birth rate, high child mortality rate and shorter life expectancy.

(f) **Maternal Mortality Rate:** Maternal mortality is responsible for the greatest proportions of deaths among women of reproductive age in most of the developing countries. Maternal mortality rates vary according to socio-economic status of any country.

(g) **Disease specific Mortality:** Mortality rates can be worked out for specific diseases. For example the mortality rates due to communicable diseases have been brought down following the discoveries of chemotherapeutic agents but the increase in mortality rates due to cancers, diabetes and cardiovascular diseases have posed greater problems in the recent years.

(h) **Proportional Mortaility Rate:** The simplest measure of estimating the burden of disease in a community is proportional mortality rate, i.e., the proportion of all deaths currently attributed to it.

2. Morbidity Indicators:

As mortality indicators do not reveal the burden of ill health in a community in certain instances like those of mental illness, rheumatoid arthritis, asthma and epilepsy etc., the morbidity indicators are used to supplement the mortality data for describing the health status of a population.

The following morbitidy rates are used for assessing ill health in the community:

(a) Incidence and prevalence.
(b) Attendance rates at outpatient departments and health centres.
(c) Admission, re-admission and discharge rates.
(d) Duration of stay in the hospital.
(e) Spell of sickness or absence from work or school.
(f) Notification rates.

3. Disability rates:

Since death rates due to many chronic diseases have not changed markedly in recent years, despite the extensive health care facilities made available, disability rates related to different types of illnesses and injuries have come into use to supplement mortality and morbidity indicators. These are mainly the **event type indicators** like numbers of days of restricted activity and confinement to bed or loss of work/school days, or the **person type indicators** like limitations of mobility and normal activities.

Sullivan's index which indicates expectation of life free of disability is computed by subtracting from the life expectancy the probable period of bed disability and inability to perform major activities. It is considered to be one of the most advanced indicators of disability currently used.

4. Nutritional Status Indicators:

Nutrition status is an useful indicator of health status. The following nutritional status indicators are currently used:

(a) Anthropometric measurements of preschool children: e.g., weight, height and mid-arm circumference.
(b) Height and weight of children at school entry.
(c) Prevalence of low birth weight (less than 2.5 kg).

5. Health Care Delivery Indicators:

The most commonly used indicators of health care delivery include:

(a) Doctor : Population ratio.
(b) Doctor : Nurse ratio.
(c) Population : Hospital bed ratio.
(d) Population covered by a health centre.
(e) Population per traditional birth attendent.

These indicators highlight the equity of distribution of health resources in different parts of the country and of the provision of health care.

6. Utilization Rates:

A definite relationship exists between utilization of health care services and health need and status. Health care utilization is also influenced by the availability and accessibility of health services and the attitude of an individual towards the health and health care system. Some examples of utilization rates are given as under:

(a) Proportion of infants fully immunized against the six diseases under **Extended Programme on Immunization** namely diphtheria, whooping cough, tetanus, polio, tuberculosis and measles.
(b) Proportion of pregnant women who receive proper antenatal care.
(c) Percentage of the population using various methods of family planning.
(d) Bed occupancy rate in hospitals.

7. Indicators of Social and Mental Health:

These include the incidences of suicides, homicides, juvenile delinquency, alcohol or drug abuse, smoking, road traffic accidents,family violence, battered-baby and battered-wife syndromes. These indicators provide required guidance for social action and improving the health of the people.

8. Environment Indicators:

These indicators reflect the quality of physical and biological environment in which diseases occur and in which the people live. They include indicators relating to pollution of air and water, radiation, solid wastes, noise, exposure to toxic substances in food and drinks etc.

9. Socio-economic Indicators:

These indicators cannot be used for directly measuring the health status. However, they are important in the interpretation of the indicators of health care. These include

(a) Rate of increase in the population.
(b) Per capita GNP.
(c) Level of unemployment.
(d) Dependency ratio.
(e) Literacy rate.
(f) Family size.
(g) Housing, (number of persons per room).
(h) Per capita calorie availability.

10. Health Policy Indicators:

Allocation of adequate resources by a Government for health care is the most important health policy indicator. The determinants of this indicator include the proportion of GNP spent on health services, health related activities (e.g. water supply, sanitation, housing, nutrition) and on primary health care.

11. Health for all Indicators:

For monitoring the progress towards the goal of **"Health for all by 2000 AD"** the WHO has listed the following four categories of indicators which have been discussed in the preceding paragraphs under different headings.

(a) Health policy indicators.
(b) Social and economic indicators related to health.
(c) Indicators for provision of health care.
(d) Health status indicators.

CONCEPT OF DISEASE

It has been a difficult proposition to define disease. The Oxford English Dictionary defines disease as "a condition of the body or some part or organ of the body, in which its functions are disrupted or deranged". From an ecological point of view disease is defined as a maladjustment of the human organism to the environment. In a very simple way disease can be defined as just the opposite of health i.e. any deviation from normal functioning or state of complete physical or mental well being since health and disease are mutually exclusive. These definitions are however considered inadequate because they do not give a criterion by which to decide when a disease state begins, nor do they lend themselves to the measurement of disease.

Diseases manifest in different ways which may range from an inapparent form (subclinical) to severe symptoms. Some diseases commence acutely (asthma) and some insidiously (rheumatism). A carrier state occurs in some diseases during which the individual is apparently healthy but is able to infect others (amoebiasis, typhoid). In some cases the same organism (streptococcus) can cause more than one manifestation and on the other hand the same disease (diarrhoea) can be caused by more than one organism. In most of the diseases the signs and symptoms are clearly manifested but in some the difference between normal and abnormal is quite indistinct as in diabetes and hypertension. The final outcome of diseases are also variable ranging from complete recovery, or disability to the death of the patient.

CAUSATION

There are a number of factors which may be responsible for the causation of any disease. They can be summarized as under:

(a) Germ-theory of disease:

The concept of cause embodied in the germ theory of disease is generally referred to as one to one relationship between the causative agent and disease. It is now realized that a disease is rarely caused by a single agent alone but depends upon a number of factors which simultaneously contribute to its occurrence.

(b) Epidemiological triad:

The epidemiological triad conceptualizes the role of the causative agent, host factors and the environment in the causation of diseases, particularly the infectious ones. For example not everyone exposed to tuberculosis develops the disease. The same exposure in an undernourished or otherwise susceptible person living in unhygienic conditions may result in clinical disease.

(c) Multifactorial Causation:

As a result of advances in public health, chemotherapy, and vector control measures the incidence of communicable diseases has considerably declined. However, these diseases have now been replaced by the modern diseases of civilization which include lung cancer, coronary heart disease, chronic bronchitis and mental illness etc. These diseases can neither be attributed to the infective causative organisms, nor they can be prevented by traditional methods of isolation or immunization. This led to the establishment of the role of other factors in the etiology of diseases which include smoking, excess fat intake, lack of physical exrcise, obesity and drugs etc. Most of these factors are linked to the life style and different patterns of human behavior.

NATURAL HISTORY OF DISEASE

As outlined above, disease results from a complex interaction between man, a causative agent and the environment. The natural history of disease is a very important concept of epidemiology. It unfolds the way in which a disease evolves over time from the earliest stage of its pre-pathogenesis to its full-blown development, the occurrence of signs and symptoms due to its pathogenicity and finally its temination as recovery, disability or death in the absence of treatment or prevention or at times in spite of them. The events occurring in the natural history of an infectious disease can be summarized in the following two phases.

(i) Prepathogenesis Phase:

It refers to the period preliminary to the onset of disease in man. Though the causative agent has not yet entered the human body, the factors which favour its interaction with the human host are already existing in the environment. This is clearly the situation when the man is exposed to the risk of a disease. An interaction between the epidemiological triad is then necessary to initiate the disease process. These factors combinely operate not only to initiate the disease which may range from a single case to an epidemic, but also cause the distribution of the disease in the community.

(ii) Pathogenesis Phase:

This phase begins with the entry of the causative agent in the susceptible human host. In case of the infectious diseases it multiplies and induces tissue and physiological changes. The disease progresses through a period of incubation and later through early and late pathogenesis. The pathogenesis phase can be modified by intervention measures such as immunization and chemotherapy.

In non-infective chronic diseases (e.g. coronary heart disease, hypertension,) the early pathogenesis phase is less dramatic and is referred to as presymptomatic phase. The clinical stage begins when recognizable signs and symptoms appear and by this time the disease is already well advanced into the late pathogenesis phase. In many chronic diseases the role of epidemiological triad and their interactions have not been clearly delineated.

THE DISEASE AGENTS

Disease agent is the first link in the process of disease transmission. It is defined as a substance living or nonliving or a force tangible or intangible, the excessive presence or relative lack of which may initiate or perpetuate a disease process. Disease agents can be classified into the following groups:

1. Biological Agents:

These are living agents responsible for the causation of infections and/or communicable diseases. They include bacteria, viruses, fungi, protozoa, metazoa and rickettsiae. They exhibit host related biological properties such as infectivity, pathogenicity and virulence.

2. Nutritional Agents:

These agents include carbohydrates, fats, proteins, vitamins and minerals. They are generally responsible for deficiency diseases like malnutrition, anemia and scurvy etc. However, excess intake of some of these nutrients can initiate diseases like hypercholesterolemia, obesity and goitre.

3. Physical Agents:

These include heat, cold, humidity, pressure, radiation etc. and excessive exposure to any one of them may result in illness.

4. Chemical Agents:

Chemical agents leading to disease production can be divided in two broad groups; a) **Endogenous** : Chemicals produced in the body as a derangement of some metabolic processes like-urea, bilirubin, ketones, uric acid or calcium carbonate can be responsible for diseases like uremia, jaundice, ketosis and renal stones etc. **b) Exogenous:** Disease agents acquired from the environment like allergens, metals, fumes, dusts, gases and insecticides can cause various acute and chronic diseases.

5. Mechanical Agents (factors):

Excessive exposure to chronic friction and other mechanical forces like vibrations may result in injury, sprains, tearing, dislocation and stress and at times some of these factors can even cause fatality.

6. Social Agents:

These agents include poverty, smoking, abuse of drugs and alcohol, unhealthy life styles, social isolation and maternal deprivation etc.

CONCEPT OF PREVENTION OF DISEASES

Successful prevention of any disease depends on the knowledge of its causation, mode of its transmission, identification of risk factors and risk groups, availability of prophylactic measures and facilities for early detection and treatment, an organization for applying these measures to appropriate persons or groups and continuous evaluation and development of the procedures.

The objective of preventive medicine is to intercept or oppose the "cause" and thereby the disease process. However, the epidemiological concept permits the inclusion of treatment as one of the methods of intervention. It is now customary to deal with prevention at three levels.

1. Primary Prevention :

It is defined as the measures taken prior to the onset of disease which ensure that the disease will never occur. Primary prevention may be achieved through measures designed to promote general health and well being and the quality of the life of people by specific protective measures. The concept of primary prevention is now being applied to the prevention of chronic diseases, like hypertension, coronary heart disease and cancers based on the elimination of risk factors of disease or their modification. The following approaches for the primary prevention of chronic diseases have been recommended by WHO where the risk factors have been adequately identified.

(a) **Primordial Prevention :** This is primary prevention in true sense. It deals with the prevention of the emergence or development of risk factors in population groups in which they have not yet appeared. Many adult health problems like obesity and hypertension have their early origin in childhood as during this time life styles are formed, for example eating patterns, physical exercise and smoking. In primordial prevention, efforts are made to discourage children from adopting such harmful life styles.

(b) **Population Strategy:** It is directed at the whole population irrespective of individual risk levels. For example even a small reduction of the average B.P. or serum cholesterol of a population may lead to a large reduction in the incidence of cardiovascular diseases.

(c) **High Risk Strategy:** It aims to provide preventive care to individuals at high risk. Such individuals are detected by the optimum use of clinical and diagnostic methods.

Primary prevention utilizes the knowledge of prepathogenesis phase of disease, embracing the agent, host and environment. The safety and negligible cost of primary prevention justify its wider application and it has now become synonymous with health education.

2. Secondary Prevention:

Secondary prevention halts the progress of a disease at its incipient stage and prevents complications. The specific interventions are early diagnosis and adequate treatment. The secondary preventive measures thus arrest the disease process, restore health by seeking out unrecognized disease and treating it before irreversible pathological changes occur and reverse the communicability of infective diseases. It is largely the domain of clinical medicine. It is often more expensive and less effective as compared to primary prevention.

3. Tertiary Prevention:

Tertiary prevention signifies the intervention in the late pathogenesis phase. It includes all measures available to reduce or limit impairments and disabilities, minimizes suffering caused by the disease and promotes patient's adjustment to untreatable conditions. Tertiary prevention also extends the concept of prevention into the arena of rehabilitation.

3

EPIDEMIOLOGY

Scope of epidemiology • methods • uses • dynamics of disease transmission • immunity and immunization • immunological products and their dose schedule • principles of disease control and prevention • hospital acquired infections • prevention and control. Disinfection • types of disinfectants • disinfection procedures for faeces • urine• sputum • room • linen • instruments and dead bodies.

Epidemiology is derived from epidemic (epi = among; demos = people; logos = study) which is a very old word dating back to the 3rd Century B.C. The foundations of epidemiology were laid in the 19th Century when a few classic studies made major contribution to the saving of life. In the past epidemiology was equated with the study of epidemics. Modern epidemiology has taken within its scope all diseases (whether acute or chronic, communicable or noncommunicable) and health related states and events occurring in man. Epidemiology has been defined in a number of ways by various epidemiologists and although there is no single definition to which all of them subscribe, three important components are common to most of them. They are (i) Studies of disease frequency, (ii) Studies of distribution of disease and (iii) Studies of the determinants of disease. These components are being described briefly in the following paragraphs.

(a) **Disease frequency :** The measurement of frequency of disease, disability or death and summarizing this information in the form of rates and ratios (prevalence rate, incidence rate, death rate etc.) are inherent in the definition and scope of epidemiology. The basic measure of disease frequency is a rate or ratio. These rates are essential for comparing disease frequency in different populations in relation to suspected causal factors. Such comparisons yield important clues to the etiology of a disease.

(b) **Distribution of disease :** This component involves the determination of the patten of distribution of disease in relation to time, place and person. Epidemiologists examine whether there has been an increase or decrease of disease over a given time span, whether there is a higher incidence of disease in a particular geographic area, whether the disease occurs more often in men or women or in a particular age group and whether the host characteristic or behavior of those affected are different from those who are not affected. This study may contribute to the formulation of an etiological hypothesis. This aspect of epidemiology is also known as "descriptive epidemiology".

(c) **Determinants of disease :** This aspect is concerned with the testing of etiological hypotheses and identification of underlying causes or risk factors of a disease. This requires the application of epidemiological principles and methods and is described as "analytical epidemiology". Analytical strategies help in developing scientifically sound health programmes, interventions and policies.

AIMS OF EPIDEMIOLOGY

According to the International Epidemiological Association, epidemiology has three main aims:

(i) to describe the distribution and size of disease problems in human populations.

(ii) to identify etiological factors in the pathogenesis of disease, and

(iii) to provide the data essential to the planning, implementation and evaluation of services for the prevention, control and treatment of disease and to the setting up of priority among these services.

EPIDEMIOLOGICAL METHODS

The most important task of an epidemiologist is to study disease occurrence in people, who during the course of their lives are exposed to numerous factors and circumstances, some of which may have role in disease etiology. Whereas the clinician or laboratory investigator is able to study disease conditions more precisely, the epidemiologist employs carefully designed research strategies to explore disease etiology. These strategies are of three main types:

(a) Descriptive epidemiology.

(b) Analytical epidemiology.

(c) Experimental epidemiology.

These studies compliment one another in order to fulfil the aims of epidemiology.

(a) Descriptive epidemiology

Descriptive studies are concerned with the distribution of disease or health related characteristics in human populations and identifying the characteristics with which the disease in question appears to be associated. The procedures involved in such studies include:

(i) defining the population to be studied.

(ii) defining the disease under study.

(iii) describing the distribution of the disease in relation to a) time, b) place and c) person.

(iv) measurement of disease in terms of mortality, morbidity and disability etc.

(v) formulation of an etiological hypothesis.

Descriptive studies provide the following important information:

(i) data regarding the magnitude and type of disease problems in a community in terms of morbidity and mortality rates and ratios.

(ii) clues to the aetiology of a disease and a possible causal association between a factor and disease e.g. smoking and lung cancer.

(iii) background data for planning, organizing and evaluating preventive and curative services.

(b) Analytical Epidemiology

Analytical studies comprise of two distinct types of observational studies:

(a) Case control study.

(b) Cohort study.

From both the study designs one can determine whether a statistically significant association exists between a disease and a suspected factor and if one exists, the strength of the association.

Case Control Study

Case control studies are also referred to as retrospective studies and they serve as first approach to test any causal hypothesis. Case control study has three distinct features:

(i) both the exposure and outcome (in the form of a disease) have occurred before the study is taken up.

(ii) the study proceeds backwards from effect to cause.

(iii) it uses a control group to support or refute an inference.

Cohort Study

Cohort study is generally undertaken to obtain additional evidence to refute or support the existence of an association between suspected cause and disease. It is also known as prospective study. The distinguishing features of cohort study are:

(i) the cohorts are identified prior to the appearance of disease under investigation.

(ii) the study groups are observed over a period of time to determine the frequency of diseases among them.

(iii) the study proceeds forwards from cause to effect.

In epidemiology the term cohort is defined as group of people who share a common characteristic or experience within defined time period (e.g. age, occupation, exposure to a drug or vaccine, pregnancy etc.)

(c) Experimental Epidemiology

Experimental studies are aimed to—

(i) provide scientific proof of etiological factors which may permit the modification or control of disease in question and

(ii) provide a method of measuring the effectiveness and efficiency of health services for the prevention, control and treatment of disease and improve the health of the community.

Experimental studies have become a major area of epidemiological studies. They are of two types:

(a) Randomized controlled trials (i.e., those involving a process of random allocation); and

(b) Non-randomized or non-experimental trials (i.e., those departing from strict randomization for practical purposes, but in such a manner that non-randomization does not seriously affect the theoretical basis of conclusions).

USES OF EPIDEMIOLOGY

Whereas epidemiology is mainly concerned with the distribution of diseases and their causation, the techniques used in the study of epidemiology have wider applications. They cover more important areas of health and health services. Applications of epidemiology extend beyond the search for causes of disease and bring it nearer to the day to day concerns of modern medicine. These include:

1. Study of the history of disease pattern in the population

The first use of epidemiology refers to the history of disease in human population. There are fluctuations in the disease patterns both over short and long time. As old diseases are conquered and eradicated (e.g. small pox) new ones are identified (e.g. AIDs). Epidemiology plays significant role as it provides a means to study the disease profiles and thus identify health problems of the future.

2. Community diagnosis

Community diagnosis comprises of identification and quantification of health problems in a community in terms of mortality and morbidity rates and ratios and identification of other factors for the purpose of defining those individuals or groups at risk or those in need of health care. It helps in laying down priorities in disease control and prevention, serves as an indicator for the evaluation of health services retrospectively and provides new knowledge about disease distribution, causation and prevention.

3. Planning and evaluation

Epidemiological studies about the distribution of health problems over time and place provide the fundamental basis for planning and developing the heath services required for a community. Further, epidemiology also helps in the evaluation of the effectiveness of such measures undertaken by telling us whether they have been responsible for reducing the frequency of the disease.

4. Evaluation of Individual's risks

Evaluation studies also help in the prediction of the degree of risk in a population. Any causal association between a risk factor and disease can evaluate individual's risk and chances. The risk assessment for smokers of developing lung cancer and for hypertensive patients of developing congestive heart failure are wellknown examples.

5. Identification of syndromes

A number of medical syndromes have been identified by frequently associated findings in individual patients. Epidemiological investigations are used to correctly define such syndromes.

6. Completing the natural history of disease

As the epidemiologist is concerned with all the cases in a defined population regardless of severity or the source of medical care, his perspective of disease is the broadest. By studying the disease pattern in the community in relation to an agent (risk factor), host and other environmental factors, he is in a better position to fill up the gaps in the natural history of disease than the clinician.

7. Search for risk factors

Epidemiology has made significant contribution by searching and establishing the causes and risk factors involved in the etiology of many chronic and acute diseases. It is due to epidemiological studies that we know about the role of thalidomide in teratogenicity, stilboestrol in the genesis of adenocarcinoma of vaginal tract at puberty, rubella as the cause of congenital defects in the new born and smoking as the cause of lung cancer.

DYNAMICS OF DISEASE TRANSMISSION

The starting point of the spread of a communicable disease is the existence of a reservoir or source of infection. The source of infection may be a person, an animal, an object or a substance from which an infectious agent is disseminated to the host.

Reservoir is defined as any person, animal, arthropod, plant, soil or substance (or a combination of these) in which an infectious agent survives and multiplies in such a manner that it can be transmitted to a susceptible host. The terms source and reservoir may not always be synonymous. For example in typhoid fever the reservoir of infection may be a patient or a carrier but the source of infection may be feces, wine or contaminated food item. The reservoirs are of three kinds.

1. Human reservoir

The most important source or reservoir of infection is man himself. The human reservoir may be a case or a carrier. A case is defined as a person having the particular disease, health disorder or the condition under investigation. Case is generally identified by the signs and symptoms of a disease which in many instances is confirmed by biochemical, hematological, radiological or other diagnostic methods.

A carrier is defined as an infected person that harbors a specific infectious agent in the absence of discernible clinical disease and serves as a potential source of infection for others. The important characteristics of a carrier state are

(i) presence of an infective agent in the body.
(ii) absence of the recognizable signs and symptoms of disease.
(iii) shedding of the infectious agent in the discharges or excretions which can infect other persons.

2. Animal reservoir

The animals and birds also serve as source of infections. The diseases and infections which are transmitted to man from vertebrates are known as zoonotic diseases. The best known examples of such diseases are rabies, yellow fever and influenza.

3. Non-living reservoir

The soil and other inanimate matters can also act as reservoirs of infection. Soil may harbour infectious agents which may cause tetanus and anthrax. It may also be source of certain helminithic infections. Rust is also a known source of tetanus.

ROUTES OF TRANSMISSION

Infectious diseases are transmitted from the reservoir or source of infection to a susceptible individual in a number of ways depending on the infectious agent, portal of entry and the local ecological conditions. Most of the infectious diseases are transmitted only by one route e.g. typhoid fever by vehicle transmission or common cold by direct contact but there are some which are transmitted by more than one route, e.g. hepatitis B, salmonellosis, brucellosis and AIDs etc. The modes of transmission of communicable diseases can be either direct or indirect.

Direct Transmission

(i) Direct Contact : It leads to direct and essentially immediate transfer of an infectious agent from the source or reservoir to a susceptible person e.g. skin to skin contact as by touching, kissing or sexual intercourse. Example of direct transmission include syphilis, gonorrhoea, AIDs, leprosy, conjunctivitis and skin infections.

(ii) Droplet Infection : Minute droplets of saliva and nasopharyngeal secretions are spread into the surrounding atmosphere during sneezing coughing, spitting, singing or talking. The droplet spread is usually limited to a distance of 30-60 cm between the source and host. When a person comes within the range of these infectious droplets, he is likely to inhale some of them and get infected. Droplet infections include common cold, diphtheria, whooping cough, tuberculosis, and meningococcus meningitis etc.

Potential of droplet infection is increased in conditions of close proximity, overcrowding or lack of proper ventilation.

(iii) Contact with soil : Direct exposure of susceptible tissue to an infectious agent in the soil, compost or decaying vegetable matter can lead to infections like hookworm, tetanus and mycosis etc.

(iv) Bite of an animal : It can lead to direct transmission of a disease. The best example is that of rabies.

(v) Transplacental transmission: Certain infectious agents can be transmitted through the placenta. Example of this type include syphilis, hepatitis B and AIDs.

INDIRECT TRANSMISSION

For indirect transmission the infectious agent must be capable of surviving outside the human host in the external environment and retain its basic characteristic of pathogenesis and virulence till it finds a new host.

(i) Vehicle-borne transmission

It implies the transmission of an infectious agent through the agency of water, food, ice, blood, serum, plasma or other biological products. Water and food are the most frequent vehicles of transmission. Diseases transmitted by water and food include acute diarrhoeas, typhoid, cholera, hepatitis A, food poisoning and intestinal parasites.

(ii) Vector-borne transmission

In epidemiology vector is arthropod or any living carrier that transports an infectious agent to a susceptible individual. Examples of vector-borne transmission include malaria, plague, filariasis, schistosomiasis and encephalitis.

(iii) Air-borne transmission

It can be affected by "droplet nuclei" or dust. Droplet nuclei are tiny particles (1-10 micron) that represent the dried residue of droplets. They are formed by the evaporation of droplets coughed or sneezed into the air. They remain air-borne for considerable period of time and retain their virulence. Tuberculosis, influenza, chickenpox and measles may be spread by air-borne transmission through droplet nuclei. Some of the larger droplets expelled during coughing, sneezing or talking settle down on the floor, carpet, furniture and clothes. A variety of infectious agents have been found in the dust of hospital wards and living rooms. Diseases carried by dust include pneumonia, tuberculosis, Q fever, streptococcal and staphylococcal infections. This type of transmission is most common in hospital acquired (nosocomial) infections.

(iv) Fomite-borne transmission

Fomites are the articles and substances capable of transmitting an infectious agent. They get contaminated by pathogenic organisms and transmit the diseases like typhoid, diphtheria, bacillary dysentery, hepatitis A, eye and ear infections. Fomites include soiled clothes, towels, linen, handkerchiefs, cups, spoons, pencils, books, toys, drinking glasses, taps, lavatory chains and door handles etc.

(v) Uncleaned hands and fingers

Hands and fingers are the most common medium which transfer pathogenic agents from skin, nose, bowel and food items both directly and indirectly. Examples include staphylococcal and streptococcal infections, typhoid, dysentery, hepatitis and intestinal parasites. Unclean hands and fingers imply lack of personal hygiene which coupled with poor sanitation favours person to person transmission of infection.

IMMUNITY

The term immunity refers to the resistance exhibited by the host towards injury caused by microorganisms and their products. Protection against infectious diseases is only one of the consequences of the immune response, which in its entirety is concerned with the reaction of the body against any foreign antigen.

The science of immunology is concerned with the specific mechanisms by which living tissues react to foreign biological materials including invading microorganisms so that resistance or immunity develops. The integrity of the defense system of the host, and its ability to react to and overcome invasion by microorganisms, is of vital importance for the survival of the individual.

Immunity against infectious diseases is of different types:

1. Innate immunity:

(a) Nonspecific	Species
(b) Specific	Racial
	Individual

2. Acquired immunity

(a) Active	Natural
	Artificial
(b) Passive	Natural
	Artificial

Innate Immunity

Innate immunity is characterized by the resistance to infections which an individual possesses by virtue of his genetic and constitutional make-up. It does not depend on a prior contact with microorganism or immunization. It is considered nonspecific, when it shows a degree of resistance to infections in general and specific when resistance is confined to particular pathogen. It is further subdivided on the basis of species, race or individual.

Species immunity refers to the refractoriness to a pathogen shown by all members of a species. For instance human beings are totally insusceptible to plant pathogens. Species immunity may be due to the physiological and biochemical differences between the tissues of the different host species which determine whether or not a pathogen can multiply in them. Racial immunity is said to occur when within a species, different races show differences in susceptibility to infections. An interesting example of genetic resistance to **Plasmodium falciparum** malaria has been reported from some parts of Africa and the Mediterranean coast. A hereditary abnormality of red cells prevalent in the area confers immunity to infection by the malarial parasite.

The differences in innate immunity exhibited by different individuals in a race is known as individual immunity. The genetic basis of individual immunity is evident from studies on the incidence of infectious diseases in twins. It has been well documented that homozygous twins exhibit similar degrees of resistance or susceptibility to lepromatous leprosy and tuberculosis. Such correlations are not seen in cases of heterozygous twins. The factors which may influence the level of innate immunity in an individual include age, hormonal influences and nutritional status.

ACQUIRED IMMUNITY

The resistance that an individual acquires during life is acquired immunity. It is thus different from the inborn innate immunity. Acquired immunity is of two types, active and passive.

Active Immunity

The resistance that an individual acquires, as a result of infection or by specific immunization and is usually associated with the presence of antibodies or cells having a specific action on the microorganism responsible for causing a particular infectious disease or on its toxin, is referred to as active immunity. The active immunity thus depends upon the humoral and cellular response of the host. The immunity produced is specific for a particular disease i.e., the individual in most cases becomes immune to further infection with the same organism or antigenically related organism for varying periods depending upon the disease.

Active immunity sets in only after a latent period which is required for the immunological mechanism to set in and function. During the development of active immunity, there is often a negative phase during which the level of measurable immunity may be lower than before the antigenic stimulus. This is due to the antigen combining with any pre-existing antibody and lowering its level in circulation. Once developed, the active immunity is long lasting and may persist for several years. If an individual who has been, actively immunized against an antigen, is exposed to the same antigen subsequently, the immune response occurs more quickly and abundantly than during the first exposure. This is known as secondary response. Besides the development of humoral and cellular immunity, active immunity is associated with "immunological memory'. This implies that the immune system is able to retain for long period the memory of a previous antigenic exposure and to produce a secondary response when it is exposed to the same antigen again. Active immunization is more effective and confers better protection than passive immunization.

Active immunity may be natural or artificial. Natural active immunity results from either a clinical or a subclinical (inapparent) infection with a pathogenic organism. A person who recovers from an attack of measles develops natural active immunity. A large number of adults in the developing countries exhibit natural active immunity to poliomyelitis due to repeated inapparent infections with the polio viruses during their childhood. Such immunity is usually long lasting but the duration varies with the types of pathogen. The immunity may be lifelong following chicken pox or measles whereas the immunity following influenza or common cold may be short-lived. The immunity following bacterial infection is generally shortlived as compared to that following viral infections.

Artificial active immunity is the resistance induced by vaccines. Vaccines are the preparations of live or killed microorganisms or their products used for immunization. Some important examples of vaccines are as follows:

(a) Bacterial Vaccines

(i) Live —	BCG for tuberculosis.
(ii) Killed —	Salk for enteric fever

(b) Viral Vaccines

(i) Live —	Oral poliomyelitis.
(ii) killed —	Salk vaccine for poliomyelitis.

(c) Bacterial Products — toxoids for diphtheria and tetanus.

Live vaccines initiate an infection without causing any injury or disease. The immunity following live vaccine administration is therefore similar to that caused by natural infection, though it may not be as profound. The immunity lasts for several years but booster doses may be necessary. Live vaccines may be administered orally (e.g. Sabin vaccine for poliomyelitis) or parenterally (e.g. measles vaccine). Killed vaccines are generally less immunogenic than live vaccines and the protection lasts only for a short period. They have, therefore, to be administered repeatedly, generally at least two doses being required for the production of immunity. The first is known as the primary dose and the subsequent ones as the booster doses.

Passive Immunity

It implies the resistance that is transmitted to a recipient in a 'ready-made' form. In passive immunity the recipient's immune system plays no active role. There is no antigenic stimulus, instead, preformed antibodies are administered. There is no latent period in passive immunity and the protection becomes effective immediately after passive immunization. There is no negative phase. The immunity is transient, lasting only for days or weeks until the transmitted antibodies are metabolized and eliminated. No secondary response occurs in passive immunity. On the contrary passive immunity decreases in effect with repetition because when a foreign body is administered a second time it is eliminated more rapidly. Following the first administration of an antibody e.g. immune horse serum, the elimination is only by metabolic breakdown but during subsequent injections of horse serum its elimination becomes much quicker as it combines with antibodies to horse serum, which are generated following its initial injection. This factor of "immune elimination" limits the usefulness of repeated passive immunization. Thus passive immunization is less effective and it provides an immunity which is inferior to that produced by the active process. The main advantage of passive immunization is that it is immediate in onset and it can therefore be employed when "instant" immunity is desired. The important features of active and passive immunization have been compared in Table-3.1.

Table 3.1. Comparison between active and passive immunity

Active Immunity	Passive Immunity
It is produced actively by the host's immune system	Passively transferred to the host. Host's immune system does not participate.
It is induced by infectious diseases or by immunogens like vaccines (toxoids) and allergens.	It is conferred by the antibodies present in the hyperimmune sera or gamma globulin.
It affords long lasting and effective protection.	It produces transient and less effective protection.
Immunity effectively develops after a lag period (time required for the generation of antibodies)	Immunity becomes effective immediately after the injection.
Immunological memory present; subsequent challenge more effective (booster effect)	Immunological memory absent. Subsequent administration less effective due to "immune elimination".
Negative phase can occur during the latent period.	No negative phase.
It is not applicable in immunodeficient host.	Applicable and effective in immunodeficient hosts.

Natural passive immunity is the resistance passively transferred from the mother to the body. In human infants maternal antibodies are transmitted predominantly through the placenta. However, human colostrum, which is also rich in lgA antibodies and is resistant to intestinal digestion, confers protection to the neonate. It is only about the age of 3 months that the infant acquires a satisfactory level of immunological independence. Till then the maternal antibodies give passive protection against infectious diseases to the infant. It is for this reason that most pediatric infections are more common after the age of 3 months than in younger infants. By active immunization of mothers during pregnancy, it is, therefore, possible to improve the quality of passive immunity in infants. Immunization of pregnant women with tetanus toxoid is recommended for this purpose in communities in which neonatal tetanus is common.

Artificial passive immunity is the resistance passively transferred to a recipient by administration of antibodies. Hyperimmune sera of animal or human origin, convalescent sera and pooled human gamma globulin are used for the induction of artificial passive immunity. The oldest and most common method is to employ hyperimmune horse sera. They are prepared by active hyperimmunization of horses using the appropriate antigen. For instant, anti-tetanus serum (ATS) used for passive immunization against tetanus is prepared by administering a series of doses of tetanus toxoid to horses, bleeding them and separating the serum. ATS is administered subcutaneously for prophylaxis and intravenously for the treatment of tetanus. ATS provides an immediate supply of the antitoxin in the recipient's circulation. However, ATS from horse, being a foreign protein can cause severe hypersensitivity reactions. Recently, human ATS, prepared by hyperimmunization of adult human volunteers with tetanus toxoid, has been employed to overcome this complication of hypersensitivity. With human ATS the protection lasts longer as no immune elimination of human globulins takes place.

Sera collected from patients who are convalescing from infectious diseases contain high levels of specific antibody. Convalescent sera have been employed for passive immunization against measles and rubella viruses.

Sera of healthy adults contain antibodies against the common infectious agents prevalent in the community. The antibody fraction (gamma globulin) from pooled sera of healthy persons is used for passive immunization of common infectious diseases. The placenta provides an excellent source of human gamma globulin.

Passive immunization is indicated for providing immediate and temporary protection in nonimmune host, faced with the threat of an acute and serious infection when there is insufficient time for active immunization to take effect, it is also employed for the suppression active immunity when it may be injurious, for example, the Rh immune globulin is used during delivery to prevent immune response to the Rheus factor in Rh-negative mothers with Rh-positive babies.

On certain occasions a combination of active and passive methods of immunization is employed simultaneously. This is described as combined immunization. In the treatment of tetanus, ATS is injected in one arm and the first dose of tetanus toxoid in the other. This is followed by the full course of phased tetanus toxoid injections. In this method ATS provides the necessary protection initially and in the mean time adequate immunity develops in response to the tetanus toxoid.

Herd Immunity

It is the level of resistance of a community or group of people to a particular disease. When a large proportion of individuals in a community (herd) are immune to a pathogen, the herd immunity to the pathogen is considered satisfactory. If the herd immunity is sufficiently high, the occurrence of an epidemic is regarded as highly unlikely. If that high level of immunity is maintained and stepped up by an ongoing immunization programme, it may gradually lead to complete eradication of disease in due course. This has been achieved in such diseases as diphtheria and poliomyelitis.

IMMUNIZATION

Providing immunity by using an immunizing agent (biological or immunobiologic) is referred to as immunization. The immunizing agents may be classified as Biologicals for active immunization (vaccines and toxoids) and Biologicals for passive immunization (antisera and immunoglobulins). The currently used immunizing agents are summarized in Table-3.2.

Vaccines :

Vaccine is an immunobiological substance designed to produce specific protection against a given infectious disease. It stimulates, the production of protective antibody and also other immune mechanisms.

(a) Live vaccines : Live vaccines such as BCG, measles and oral polio are prepared from live, generally attenuated organisms. They are more potent than the killed vaccines because (i) Live organisms multiply in the host and thus the resulting antigenic dose is larger than what is injected (ii) Live vaccines have all major and minor antigenic components, (iii) Live vaccine harbour certain tissues of the body e.g., intestinal tissue by oral polio vaccine. Live vaccine should not be administered to persons with immune deficiency diseases or with suppressed immune response due to other reasons.

In case of live vaccine, immunization is generally achieved with a single dose. The polio vaccine is however an exception and it needs three or more doses to be given at spaced intervals to produce effective immunity. Live vaccines usually produce a long lasting state of immunity. They need proper storage to retain effectiveness. The manufacturer's instructions for storage must be adhered to very strictly.

Table-3.2 Biologicals used for immunization
(Immunization agents, Immunobiologicals)

Vaccines		
Live attenuated vaccines		
	Bacterial :	BCG
	Viral :	Measles, Mumps Polio, Rubella Yellow fever, MMR
Inactivated or killed vaccines		
	Bacterial :	Cholera, Pertussis, Plague, Typhoid
	Viral :	Hepatitis B, Influenza, Polio, Rabies
Toxoids		
Diphtheria		
Tetanus		
Mixed toxoid DT or DTP		
Human Immune Sera		
Immune Globulin		
Hepatitis B Immune Globulin		
Rabies Immune Globulin		
Tetanus Immune Globulin		
Animal Immune Sera (Equine)		
Tetanus Antitoxin		
Botulinum Antitoxin, Diphtheria Antitoxin		
Antirabies Serum, Antivenins		

Killed or Inactivated Vaccines

Microorganisms killed by heat or chemicals, when injected into the body produce active immunization. Killed vaccines are generally less effective than the live ones. Killed vaccines usually require the administration of 2 or 3 consecuitive doses at defined intervals in order to produce adequate immunity and in most of the cases a booster injection is also necessary. The period of effective immunity may vary from months to years. Inactivated polio vaccine has been quite effective and in certain countries it has been responsible for the elimination of the disease. Killed vaccines are administered by subcutaneous or intramuscular route.

Toxoids

Toxoids are considered highly effective and safe immunizing agents. They are modified bacterial toxins that have been rendered nontoxic (detoxified) but retain the ability to stimulate the formation of antitoxin and thus prevent bacterial toxicities.

Tetanus toxoid and Diphtheria toxoid are the examples of most commonly used effective immunizing agents from this class.

Cellular fractions :

Certain vaccines are prepared from extracted cellular fractions, for example meningococcal vaccine from the polysaccharide antigen of the cell wall and the peneumococcal vaccine from the polysaccharide contained in the capsule of the organism. Though, there is limited experience with these vaccines they appear to be highly effective and safe.

Combinations

When more than one kind of immunizing agent are incorporated in a vaccine it is called a mixed or combined vaccine.

The aim of combined vaccines is to simplify administration, reduce the cost and minimize the number of visits of the patients to the health care centre or hospital.

Some of the commonly used mixed vaccines include.

(i) Measles, Mumps and Rubella Virus Vaccine live (MMR Vaccine).

(ii) Diphtheria and Tetanus Toxoids and Pertusis Vaccine Adsorbed (Tri-immunal)

Polyvalent Vaccines

The vaccines prepared from two or more strains of the same species are known as polyvalent vaccines, e.g., Pneumococcal Vaccine Poly Valent (Pneumovax 23), Poliovirus Vaccine.

Immunoglobulins

The human immunoglobulin system consists of five major classes (lgG, lgM, lgA, lgD and IgE) and their subclasses, which represent different functional groups that are required to meet different types of antigenic challenges.

IgG : This is the major serum immunoglobulin, comprising about 75% of the total. Because of its low molecular weight (1,60,000) it can diffuse into the interstitial fluid. It is distributed approximately equally between the intravascular and extravascular compartments. IgG is the only maternal immunoglobulin that is normally transported across the placenta and provides natural passive immunity in the new born. It is protective against those infective agents which are active in blood and tissues. Antibodies to gram-positive pyogenic bacteria, anti-viral and anti-toxic antibodies are found exclusively amongst IgG globulins.

IgA : It is the second most abundant class constituting about 15 percent of total serum immunoglobulins. IgA is found in relatively large quantities in body secretions like the saliva, milk, colostrum, tears, bronchial secretions, nasal mucosa, prostatic fluid, vaginal secretions and mucus secretions of the small intestine. It provides the primary defence mechanism at the mucous membranes against local infections. It may function by inhibiting the adherence of microorganisms to the surface of mucosal cells by covering the organisms and thereby preventing their entry into body tissues. It also promotes phagocytosis and intracellular killing of microorganisms.

IgM : IgM constitutes about 8-10 percent of serum immunoglobulins. Its presence is indicative of recent infection being largely confined to the intravascular space. IgM is believed to be responsible for protection against blood invasion by microorganisms. Its deficiency is often associated with septicemias.

IgD : It resembles IgM structurally and is mostly intravascular. Its function has not been clearly determined as yet.

IgE : It resembles IgG structurally. It is heat stable and it shows unique affinity for the surface of most cells. Its levels are increased during atopic conditions like asthma, hay fever and eczema, and also in children with severe helminthiasis IgE is considered responsible for the anaphylactic type of hypersensitivity.

Immunoglobulin Preparations

Two types of immunoglobulin preparations are available for general use

(i) Normal human immunoglobulin

(ii) Specific (hyperimmune) human immunoglobulin.

Immunoglobulins are used in the prophylaxis of viral and bacterial infections.

Normal human Ig is an antibody rich fraction obtained from a pool of at least 1000 donors. The specific human Ig should contain at least 5 times the antibody potential of the standard preparation per unit volume. Immunoglobulins are generally administered by intramuscular injections. The advantages of immunoglobulins include a) freedom from hepatitis B,b) antibodies are concentrated in small volumes for intramuscular use, and c) on proper storage the antibody contents are stable. The uses of immunoglobulins have been summarized in Table-3.3.

Table-3.3 Important Immunoglobulins in the Prevention/Treatment of Infections Diseases

Infective Agents	Conditions for use	Preparation and dose
Hepatitis A	Contact through family members	Ig 0.02 ml/kg body weight for prevention
Hepatitis B	Percutaneous or mucosal exposure	HBIG 0.05-0.07 ml/kg body weight for prevention Repeated after one month
Measles	Infants less than 1 year old or contacts of acute cases within 6 days of exposure	Ig 0.25 to 0.50 ml/kg body weight for prevention.
Rabies	Subjects exposed to rabid animals	RIG 20 IU/kg body weight for prevention.
Tetanus	Following significant exposure or immediately after the diagnosis of infection.	TIG 250 units for prevention 3000-6000 units for treatment.

Ig : Human Immunoglobulin, **HBIG** : Hepatitis B immunoglobulin, **RIG** : Rabies immune gobulin **TIG**: Tetanus immune globulin.

PRINCIPLES OF DISEASE PREVENTION AND CONTROL

As outlined earlier the three most important factors forming the chain of disease transmission are :

(a) The reservoir or source of infection.

(b) The routes of transmission.

(c) The susceptible host (population at risk)

It is important to take necessary measures to prevent the transmission of infective diseases at one or more of these levels. It may often be necessary to use more than one method of control simultaneously.

Controlling the reservoir:

The general measures of controlling the reservoir comprise of early diagnosis, notification, isolation, treatment, quarantine, surveillance and disinfection. All these measures which ultimately reduce the quantum of infectious agent available for dissemination are briefly described in the following paragraphs.

(i) Early Diagnosis : Rapid identification of an infectious disease is the first step in its control. It is necessary for

(a) treatment of the infected population
(b) epidemiological investigations and
(c) for the institution of preventive control measures.

(ii) Notification

After the detection or even suspicion of an infected disease, it must be notified to the local health authority, who is responsible for initiating health control measures. Some diseases are statutorily notifiable. However, they may differ from country to country. Notification is an important source of epidemiological information about such diseases. Generally notification is made by the attending physician or head of the family. Under international Health Regulations important infectious diseases like cholera, plague, yellow fever, louse-borne typhus fever, relapsing fever, paralytic polio, malaria and viral influenza are notifiable.

(iii) Epidemiological Investigations

After any disease outbreak, the epidemiological investigations become necessary. They include the identification of source of infection and the factors which may be responsible for its spread in the community.

(iv) Isolation

Isolation has been defined as separation of infected persons for the period during which the disease remains communicable, in order to prevent the direct or indirect transmission of the infectious agent to those who are susceptible. The main purpose of isolation is to protect the community by preventing transfer of infection from the reservoir to the possible susceptible hosts. Isolation has been well established as a very effective measure in the control of certain highly infectious diseases like diphtheria, cholera, plague and chicken pox etc.

(v) Treatment

Treatment is directed to kill the infectious agent when it is still in the reservoir. It reduces the communicability of disease, cuts short the duration of illness and prevents development of secondary cases. Early diagnosis and treatment of diseases like syphilis, gonorrhoea, tuberculosis and leprosy is of primary importance in interrupting their transmission.

Blocking the routes of transfer

By changing certain components of man's environment a number of communicable diseases can be controlled. Adequate treatment of water can eliminate diseases like typhoid, dysentery, hepatitis A, cholera and gastroenteritis. Clean practices like washing of hands, adequate cooking of food, prompt refrigeration of prepared food and disposal of contaminated food can prevent food borne diseases. Similarly proper vector control can prevent a number of vector borne diseases.

Protection of susceptible host

The susceptible host can be protected by immunization against the disease(s), chemoprophylaxis and by using certain non-specific measures. These strategies are summarized under the following headings:

(i) Active Immunization

Strengthening the natural host defenses against infective diseases is a very effective method of controlling them. Active immunization is one of the most commonly used and highly effective method of increasing the host's immunity.

Immunization is planned according to the need of the situation. Following characteristics are important in designing an effective immunization schedule.

(a) it must be **Epidemiologically relevant :** Immunization should be done only against such diseases which are public health problems in the region and against which an effective vaccine exists.

(b) It should be **Immunologically effective.** The age of child and the interval between the doses of any vaccine are important in the formation of host defenses.

(c) It should be **operationally feasible** considering the cost effectiveness and a high degree of coverage in the given population.

Universal Immunization Programme

The World Health Organization launched a global immunization programme which is generally referred to as Expanded Programme on Immunization (EPI). It has been designed to protect the children all the world over against six diseases which can be effectively prevented by proper vaccination. These include **diphtheria, whooping cough, tetanus, polio, tuberculosis and measles.** EPI has been further strengthened through its adoption by the UNICEF in 1985 and it is now known as Universal Child Immunization 1990. These programmes aim to protect all the children of the world against the six diseases by the year 2000.

IMMUNIZATION SCHEDULES

(a) National Immunization Schedule :

The National Immunization Schedule has been summarized in Table-3.4

Table-3.4 National Immunization Schedule

State of immunization	Age	Immunizing Agent	No. of doses and route of administration
Infants	6 weeks to 9 months	DPT	3, i.m.
		Polio	3, p.o.
		BCG	1, i.d.
	9-12 months	Measles	1, s.c.
Children	16-24 months	DPT	1*, i.m.
		Polio	1*. p.o.
	5-6 years	DT	1, i.m.
		Typhoid	2; s.c.
	10 years	TT	1, i.m.
		Typhoid	1. s.c.
	16 years	TT	1, i.m.
		Typhoid	1, s.c.
Pregnant women	16-36 weeks of pregnancy	TT	1, i.m.

* Booster dose

N.B. : Interval between 2 doses should not be less than one month.
: BCG is administered at birth in case of institutional deliveries.

The first immunization is made when the infant is 6 weeks old. Subsequent visits are made at intervals of 1-2 months. Oral polio vaccine is given concurrently with DPT. BCG vaccination can be given with any of the three doses. The schedule also includes the immunization of pregnant women against tetanus.

(b) WHO EPI Immunization Schedule :

This schedule has been summarized in Table 3.5. Under this schedule BCG and Polio are either administered at birth or at first contact in developing countries where these diseases have not been controlled. Minor illness should not be taken as contraindication for immunization and the schedule should not be postponed if the child is suffering from low grade fever, mild respiratory infection or diarrhoea.

Table-3.5 WHO EPI Immunization Schedule

Age of the Child	Immunizing Agent
At Birth	BCG and Oral Polio
6 Weeks	DPT and Oral Polio
10 Weeks	DPT and Oral Polio
14 Weeks	DPT and Oral Polio
9 Weeks	Measles

(ii) Passive Immunization

The preparations used for inducing passive immunity include normal human immunoglobulin, specific or hyperimmune human immunoglobulin and antisera/antitoxins.

The duration of immunity produced by these measures is short and variable (1-6 weeks). It is useful only when an individual is likely to be exposed to it within the next few days. Passive immunization, thus, has a limited value in the prevention and control of infective diseases. Since human immunoglobulin preparations are available only for a small number of diseases, antitoxins prepared from non-human sources are generally used for passive immunization. The diseases treated by passive immunization include diphtheria, tetanus, gas-gangrene, rabies and botulism.

(iii) Chemoprophylaxis

Chemoprophylaxis with drugs is useful in the protection from or prevention of an infective disease. It is particularly useful in the close contacts of patients suffering from diseases like cholera, diphtheria, meningococcal meningitis, plague and conjunctivitis etc.

HOSPITAL-ACQUIRED INFECTIONS

Hospital surroundings have been responsible for causing certain infections to their inpatients. The term hospital infection, hospital-acquired infection or nosocomial infection are used for infections developing in hospitalized patients, which were neither present nor under incubation at the time of their admission. Such infections generally become evident during their stay in the hospital or sometimes after their discharge. The source of hospital infections may be any part of the hospital ecosystem including people, objects, food, water and air in the hospital.

There are number of factors which contribute to the occurrence and severity of hospital acquired infections

(i) Many inpatients have impaired defence mechanisms due to their disease or the therapy administered to them. They are highly susceptible and prone to infection.

(ii) The hospital environment is heavily laden with a wide variety of pathogenic microorganisms. Patients shed them from their bodies and hospital personnel spread them through their hands and clothes. Beddings, linens and utensils serve as formites and even equipments may be contaminated. The hospital air, dust, routine medicaments, surgical dressings, contaminated food and water, all may cause outbreaks of infections.

(iii) Slight lapse in maintaining aseptic conditions during major invasive procedures can lead to infection.

(iv) Hospital-acquired infections are generally more serious and refractory to antibiotics treatment as the causative organisms become resistant to most antibiotics in common use.

(v) Advanced surgical procedures employed for the treatment of cancers, organ transplantation, implanted prosthesis and other sophisticated techniques enhance the risk of infection to the inpatients.

Common hospital-acquired microbes

The pathogens which are able to survive in the hospital environment for long periods and develop resistance to commonly used antibiotics and disinfectants are of greater significance in causing the nosocomial infections. The most important amongst them include:

(a) **Staphylococcus aureus strains,** resistant to multiple antibiotics spread globally in the 1950s and 1960s, colonizing hospitals and causing hospital infections with such frequency that they became wellknown as 'hospital staphylococci"

(b) **Gram negative bacilli** : Recently, the gram negative bacilli E. coli, Klebsiella, Enterobacter, Proteus and Serratia have become the most important group of hospital pathogens. A multidrug resistant salmonellae **S. typhimurium** has also become a prominent source of nosocomial infection since the late 1970s.

(c) **Pseudomonas : Ps aeruginosa** and other species of pseudomonas have been responsible for causing serious and fatal hospital infections because of their intrinsic resistance to most antibiotics and their ability to survive and even multiply at low temperatures and in disinfectant solutions.

(d) **Tetanus** : Tetanus spores survive in dust for long and can contaminate cotton suture materials, plaster of Paris and other routine items used in hospitals. Inadequate sterilization and other lapses in the maintenance of asepsis are also responsible for tetanus incidences of hospital origin.

(e) **Viruses** : Hepatitis B is perhaps the most important and life threatening virus infection in a hospital. It is transmitted by blood transfusion and other procedures involving transfer and administration of blood, plasma or body fluids. Viral diarrhoea, chicken pox, cytomegalovirus, herpes virus, influenza, enteroviruses and arenavirus are also involved in nosocomial infections.

(f) **Other infections :** Hospital-acquired infections can also be due to yeasts (mainly **Candida albicans),** moulds (Aspergillus, Mucor) and protozoa **(Entamoeba histolytica, Pneumocystis carinii and Toxoplasma gondii).**

Common types of nosocomial infections

The above-mentioned microorganisms can cause different types of infections in the patients. The following four types are characterized by their frequent occurrence in any hospital.

(a) **Wound infections** : Post-operative wound infections at times manifest within a week of surgery inspite of routine post-operative antibiotics treatment. The commonly involved organisms include

Staph. epidermidis, Strep. pyogens and clostridium species. Nonsurgical sites of wound infection include injections, umbilical stumps, ulcers and burns. **Ps aeruginosa** is the most frequent and important cause of infection in patients of burns. Neonatal tetanus has been reported due to the use of contaminated umbilical cord ties.

(b) **Urinary tract infections** : UTIs generally occur in hospitalized patients following catheterization more so with the use of indwelling catheters. **E coli, Ps. aeruginosa, Proteus** and other gram negative bacilli are the frequently encountered causative agents and mixed infection is often seen.

(c) **Respiratory infections** : Nosocomial pneumonia secondary to aspiration in unconscious patients or following pulmonary ventilation or instrumentation can be attributed to **Staph aureus** or gram negative pathogens.

(d) **Bacteraemia and Septicaemia** : These are commonly associated with infected intravenous cannulae. The longer the cannulae are kept in situ, the greater the risk of infections. "Cut-downs" on the leg veins in infants and children with diarrhoea, generally get left in place for long periods, the site being bathed in diarrheal stools. Phlebitis sets in with consequent bacteraemia. Many children admitted with diarrhoea thus die of septicaemia. Gram negative bacilli are the common pathogens. Infections can be prevented by proper skin wash before "cut-down" and the use of stainless steel needles instead of plastic cannulae.

Prevention and Control of Nosocomial Infections

Nosocomial infections may occur sporadically or as outbreaks. Etiological diagnosis is made by the routine bacteriological methods of smear, culture, identification and sensitivity testing. In the event of an outbreak, the source has to be identified and eliminated as early as possible. This requires sampling of possible sources of infection such as hospital personnel, water, air, food, surgical dressings, and inanimate objects. Typical examples of sources of outbreaks are nasal carriage of staphylococci by surgeons or pseudomonas growing in hand lotion. Carriers should be adequately treated, sterilization techniques used in the hospital must be tested. It may be a defective autoclave or improper technique such as boiling of an infusion set in ward sterilizer that may be responsible for the outbreak.

The control of hospital infection should be a permanent ongoing activity in a large hospital. An infection control team consisting of microbiologists, medical and nursing staff and hospital administrators should take this responsibility. Apart from controlling any sudden outbreak, they should formulate guidelines for admission, nursing and treatment of infectious patients, surveillance on sterilization and education of patients and hospital staff on infection control. Such meansures are very helpful in reducing the incidence and severity of nosocomial infection to a great extent. Antibiotics should not be indiscriminately used for the prevention and control of infections in a hospital. This may be harmful by encouraging selective colonization by antibiotic resistant pathogens.

DISINFECTION

Definitions

Disinfection can be defined as a process that removes infections potential by destroying microorganisms but not ordinarily bacterial spores. The term usually is used to designate the results of the application of chemical agents to inanimate objects.

Sterilization is a process by which all viable forms of microorganisms including bacterial spores are destroyed.

Antiseptic is a substance that arrests or prevents the growth of microorganisms by inhibiting their activity without necessarily destroying them. Antiseptics are suitable for application to living tissues. A disinfectant can act as an antiseptic in low concentrations or dilutions.

TYPES OF DISINFECTIONS

(a) Concurrent disinfection

In concurrent disinfection the microorganisms are destroyed as soon as they are released from the body and in this way the further spread of the disease is stopped. It generally consists of the disinfection of urine, faeces, vomitus, contaminated linen, clothes, dressings, gloves, aprons, hands etc. throughout the course of an illness.

(b) Terminal disinfection

It consists of the application of disinfective measures after the patient has been removed by death or shifted to another hospital or has ceased to be a source of infection. Terminal disinfection is now scarcely practised as terminal cleaning is considered adequate enough alongwith the proper airing and exposure to sunlight.

(c) Precurrent or prophylactic disinfection

It is achieved by disinfection of water, using chlorine, pasteurization of milk and washing of hands etc.

DISINFECTANTS

The various agents used for disinfection can be classified as follows:

(a) Physical Agents:

1. Sunlight
2. Burning
3. Hot air
4. Boiling
5. Autoclaving
6. Radiation

(b) Chemical Agents :

1. Alcohols
2. Phenols and related compounds
3. Surface active compounds
4. Halogens
5. Dyes
6. Gases

PHYSICAL AGENTS

Sunlight : Sunlight possesses appreciable bactericidal activity and plays an important role in the spontaneous sterilization that occurs under natural conditions. The ultraviolet rays of sunlight are particularly lethal to bacteria and some viruses. Articles like linen, bedding and furniture may be disinfected by exposure to sunlight for several hours.

Burning : Burning and particularly incineration are excellent methods of disinfection. Discarded articles like contaminated dressings, rags and swabs can be disposed of by burning. It is desirable that burning should not be done in open air and it is now best done in an incinerator.

Hot Air : Hot air sterilization is done in a hot air oven where temperature can be raised upto 160-180°C. It is particularly useful for the sterilization of glass wares, glass syringes, swabs, dressings and sharp instruments. It has no penetrating power and hence it is not suitable for bulky articles.

Boiling : Boiling provides temperature above 90°C alongwith the atmosphere of steam. It is suitable for the sterilization of small instruments and tools, which are not used for surgical procedures e.g., linen and rubber goods like gloves etc. In cases where boiling is considered adequate, the material should be immersed in the water and boiled for 10-30 minutes. Addition of 2% sodium bicarbonate to water promotes sterilization.

Autoclaving : Water boils when its vapour pressure equals that of surrounding atmosphere. When pressure inside a closed vessel increases, the temperature at which water boils also increases. Autoclaves thus generate steam under pressure and this saturated steam has greater penetration power and is considered a highly effective sterilizing agent. Sterilization by steam under pressure is carried out at temperatures between 108°C and 147°C. By using appropriate temperature and time a variety of materials such as dressings, gloves, instruments, culture media, syringes, glasswares and pharmaceutical products can be sterilized.

Radiation : Gamma radiation is now being increasingly used in the large commercial plants for the sterilization of most bandages, dressings, catguts, swabs, catheters, syringes, culture plates, surgical instruments and commonly used plastics and rubber items. The objects to be sterilized are placed in plastic bags before radiation and they remain sterile until opened. The method is most effective but expensive and requires special packing and equipment.

CHEMICAL AGENTS

Alcohols

Ethylalcohol and isopropyl alcohol are frequently used antiseptics and disinfectants. They are used mainly as skin antiseptics and act by denaturing bacterial proteins. They have no action on spores and viruses. To be effective, they must be used at a concentration of 60-70 % in water. Ethylalcohol in the form of industrial methylated spirit is the most commonly used alcohol for skin disinfection and hand washing. However, isopropylalcohol should be preferred to ethylalcohol as it is a better fat solvent, more bactericidal and less volatile. It is used for the disinfection of clinical thermometers.

Phenols and related compounds

Phenols are obtained by distillation of coal tar between the temperatures of 170°C and 270°C. Lister, the father of antiseptic surgery, first introduced their use in surgery in 1865. Thereafter, a wide range of phenolic compounds have been developed as disinfectants. The lethal effect of phenols has been attributed to cell membrane damage, thus releasing cell contents and causing lysis. Low concentrations of phenol precipitate proteins, and the membrane bound oxidases and dehydrogenases are irreversibly inactivated by the concentrations of phenol that are rapidly bactericidal for the organism. Phenol (carbolic acid) is a powerful bactericidal agent. It is not readily inactivated by organic matter but its effect is weakened by dilution. It is used for the disinfection of faeces in not less than 10 percent strength. In 5 per cent strength it is used for the mopping of floors and for cleaning the drains.

Cresol is another excellent all purpose coal tar disinfectant. It is 3 to 10 times more effective than phenol but not more toxic. Cresol (5-10 percent) is used as a disinfectant for faeces and urine. Cresol emulsified with soap is known as saponified cresol or Lysol and it contains 50-60 percent cresol. A 2 percent solution of Lysol is used for disinfection of faeces. Chlorhexidine (Hibitane) is a relatively nontoxic skin antiseptic most active against Gram positive organisms and fairly effective against Gram negative ones. Creams and lotions containing 1 percent chlorhexidine are used for burns and hand disinfection. Aqueous solutions are used in the treatment of wounds. It is inactivated by soaps and detergents. Hexachlorophene is potentially toxic and should be used with care. It is highly effective against Gram positive organisms but less effective against Gram negative organisms. It is slow in action and shows a cumulative effect on skin and is compatible with soaps.

Chloroxylenol (Dettol) is a relatively nontoxic antiseptic. It can be used safely in high concentrations. It is more easily inactivated by organic matter than other phenolic antiseptics. It is used in 5 percent concentration for disinfection of instruments and plastic equipments.

Surface active agents

Substances which alter energy relationships at interfaces, producing a reduction of surface or interfacial tension are known as surface active agents. They can be classified in four main groups, viz. anionic, cationic, nonionic and amphoteric. Amongst them cationic surface active agents are most effective as antiseptic and disinfectants. They act on the phosphate groups of the cell membrane and also enter the cell. The semipermeability of the cell membranes is lost and the cell proteins are denatured. The cationic compound in the form of quaternary ammonium compounds are markedly bactericidal against gram positive organisms but much less so against the gram negative organisms. The commonly used compounds are cetavalon or cetrimide and benzalkonium chloride. Their activity is reduced by organic matter and anionic surface active agents like ordinary soap inactivate them.

Savlon which is a combination of cetavalon and chlorhexidine, is generally used as an all purpose antiseptic and for the disinfection of clinical thermometers and plastic appliances.

Halogens

Iodine in alcoholic solution of 1-2% is one of the most effective skin antiseptics but it stains the skin and occasionally produces sensitivity reactions in some people. It is bactericidal with a moderate activity against spores. It is also effective against tubercle bacillus and a number of viruses. Compounds of iodine with nonionic wetting or surface active agents known as iodophors are claimed to be more active than the aqueous or alcoholic solutions of iodine. Povidone-iodine (Betadine) is claimed to be as effective as iodine but nonirritant and it does not stain the skin.

Chlorine and its compounds have been used as disinfectants for many decades. Bleaching powder, sodium hypochlorite and halazone have been used for disinfection of water supplies, swimming pools and in the food and dairy industry. The organic chloramines are used for the dressing of wounds.

Aldehydes

Formaldehyde : Generally known in solution as formalin, formaldehyde is a highly toxic and irritant gas which precipitates and destroys proteins. In aqueous solutions it is markedly bactericidal, fungicidal, sporicidal and has a lethal effect on viruses. It is used to preserve anatomical specimens and for destroying anthrax spores in hair and wool. Ten percent formalin containing 0.5% tetraborate is used for sterilizing clean metal instruments.

Formaldehyde gas is used for sterilizing instruments and heat sensitive catheters. It is also used for fumigating wards, sick rooms and laboratories. Under properly controlled conditions formaldehyde can be used for the disinfection of clothing, bedding, blankets, books, furniture and other valuable articles. The gas is irritant and toxic when inhaled. Surfaces and articles disinfected by formaldehyde may emanate an irritant vapour for sometime after its use and this can be overcome by exposure to ammonia vapour when disinfection has been completed.

Glutaraldehyde : Its action and uses are similar to formaldehyde. It is particularly effective against tubercle bacilli, fungi and viruses. It is comparatively less toxic and irritant to eyes and skin than formaldehyde. It has no deleterious effect on the cement or lenses of instruments such as cystoscopes and bronchoscopes. It can be safely used for the sterilization of corrugated rubber anaesthetic tubes and face masks, plastic endotracheal tubes, metal instruments and polythene tubing.

Dyes

The aniline and acridine dyes are extensively used as skin and wound antiseptics. They are bacteriostatic in high dilution but are not so effective as bactericidal agents.

The aniline dyes in use are brilliant green, malachite green and crystal violet. They are more active against gram positive than gram negative organisms. Though they are nonirritant to the tissues and nontoxic, they are considerably inhibited by organic material such as pus. They are believed to be effective as bacteriostatic due to their reaction with the acid groups in the cell.

The acridine dyes include proflavine, acriflavine, euflavine and aminacrine. They have similar bacteriostatic spectrum as aniline dyes but they are little affected by the presence of pus. If impregnated in gauze, they are slowly released in a moist environment and are thus useful as antiseptic against wounds. They impair the DNA complex of the oranisms and thus kill or destroy the reproductive capacity of the cell.

Gases

Ethylene Oxide : Its a highly inflammable gas and in concentrations of more than 3 percent in air it is highly explosive. By mixing it with inert gases like carbon dioxide or nitrogen, its explosive potential is compromised. Its bactericidal action is due to its power of alkylating the amino, carboxyl, hydroxyl and sulphydryl groups in the protein molecule. It also reacts with the DNA and RNA inside the cell. It is effective against all types of microorganisms including the viruses and spores. However, its use as disinfectant is not very popular as it presents some potential hazards of toxicity to man including mutagenicity and carcinogenicity. It has been used for the sterilization of wide range of materials such as glass. metal and paper surfaces, clothing, plastics, soil, foodstuffs, sutures and books. It is specially used for the sterilization of heart-lung machines, respirators and dental equipments. It is an irritant and the personnel handling it, have to take strict precautions.

Formaldehyde gas : As described above it is widely employed for the fumigation of operation theatres and laboratories. After sealing the windows and other outlets, formaldehyde gas is generated by the addition of 150 g of potassium permangnate to 280 ml of formalin for every 1000 cu ft (28.3 Cu metre) of room volume. The reaction produces considerable heat and hence only heat resistant vessels must be used. After starting the generation of formaldehyde gas the doors should be sealed and left closed for 48 hours.

DISINFECTION PROCEDURES

Faeces and urine

Faeces and urine are collected in impervious containers and disinfected by adding an equal volume of one of the disinfectant listed below :

Bleaching power	:	5 percent
Crude phenol	:	10 percent
Cresol	:	5 percent
Formalin	:	10 percent

In the absence of these disinfectants 10-20 percent aqueous suspension of lime can be mixed in an equal volume and left for 2 hours. After disintection the excretal matter is either emptied into water closet or buried in the ground. Bedpans and urinals should ideally be steam disinfected. They can also be disinfected with 2.5 percent cresol for an hour after cleaning.

Sputum

Sputum is taken out on a piece of gauze or paper handkerchief and destroyed by burning. In case the amount of sputum is considerable as in the patients of tuberculosis, it can be collected in a sputum cup half filled with 5 percent cresol. When the cup is full, it is allowed to stand for an hour and the contents are then disposed off.

Rooms

Generally thorough cleaning, proper ventilation, and exposure to sunlight for long hours are enough to keep any room disinfected. If necessary floors and hard surfaces in the room should be washed with soap suds and hot water. For chemical disinfection floors and hard surfaces should be sprayed or mopped with one of the following disinfectants: Phenolic disinfectants like 2.5 percent cresol, formalin 1 percent or more, or chlorine preparations like bleaching powder or chlorinated lime that leave 25 ppm of free chlorine. Chemical disinfectants should remain in contact with the surfaces for 4 hours before final washing.

Under rare circumstance, when fumigation is required, the most commonly used gas is formaldehyde. The process of room sterilization with formaldehyde gas has been described earlier.

Linen and instruments

These are best sterilized by autoclaving for routine use. Sterilization for 15 minutes at a temperature of 122^{0}C (which reaches at 15 lbs/sq. inch pressure) is adequate for this purpose. Surgical instruments can also be effectively sterilized by radiation and also by chemical disinfectants like formaldehyde, hexachlorophene, iodophors, surface active agents and alcohols etc. Whenever instruments are to be sterilized or disinfected, it is mandatory that they first be scrubbed thoroughly and then washed with soap and water prior to being treated to remove any residual organic debris. They are usually placed in an ultrasonic cleaner for removing the organic debris.

Dead bodies

Dead bodies are preserved in formalin for the purpose of dissection by students for the learning of anatomy in medical colleges. Bodies of patients who have died of serious infectious diseases may be cleaned with a suitable disinfectant and stored in a mortuary till they are cremated. All dead bodies must be cremated or buried at the earliest possible after the death. The mortuary has to be kept clean and properly disinfected from time to time.

4

ENVIRONMENT AND HEALTH

Sources of water supply • water pollution • purification of water • health and air • noise • light • solid wastes-disposal and control. Medical Entomology- Arthropod borne diseases and their control • rodents • other animals and diseases.

The health status of an individual is determined by the integration of the internal environment of man himself and the external environment which surrounds him. According to modern concept diseases are due to disturbances in the delicate balance between man and his environment.

In India much of the ill-health of the country is due to the defective environment. The first and most important step in any health programme is the elimination through environmental control of those factors which are detrimental to health. The environmental factors which are basic and fundamental to individual and community health are described below :

WATER

An important cause of the ill health in underdeveloped countries is the lack of safe drinking water. Water intended for human consumption should not only be safe but also wholesome. It should be free from pathogenic agents and harmful chemical substances, pleasant to taste and usable for domestic purposes. Water containing infective and parasitic agents, poisonous chemical substances, industrial or other wastes or sewage is said to be contaminated or polluted.

From public health point of view, water should be provided in adequate quantity. An average daily supply of 150-200 liters per head is considered the optimum quantity. However, the consumption of water depends upon climatic conditions, standard of living and habits of the people.

Sources of Water Supply

The selection of source for any given population needs professional advice. The two important considerations for selecting a proper source are : a) the quality of water must be acceptable, and b) the quantity must be enough to meet the present and the future requirements. The three main sources of water are :

1. Rain Water.
2. Surface Water and
3. Ground Water.

1. RAIN WATER

Rain is the prime source of all water. Rain water that sinks into the ground forms ground water, and that runs off to form streams, rivers and tanks, constitutes the surface water. Rain as a direct source of water, is rarely utilized except the rare example of Gibralter.

2. SURFACE WATER

As described above surface water originates mostly from rain water. The surface water sources include.

(a) Impounding Reservoirs

These are artificial lakes constructed usually of earthwork or masonry in which large quantities of surface water is stored. Dams built across rivers and mountain stream also provide large reserves of surface water. Impounding reservoirs usually furnish a fairly good quality of water. It is clear, palatable and reasonably pure. It is soft and considered to be free from pathogenic organisms. The upland surface water derives its impurities from the catchment area, the sources being human habitations and animal keeping or grazing.

(b) Rivers

Many rivers provide a dependable source of water. The main drawback of river water is that it is often grossly polluted due to dissolved and suspended impurities of all kinds. The bacterial count including the human intestinal organisms may be quite high. River water needs purification before it can be used for human consumption.

(c) Tanks

These are large excavations which store surface water and form important source of drinking water in our villages. Tank water is highly contaminated due to the presence of sill colloidal water and aquatic vegetation. It is quite dangerous as a source of drinking water and is responsible for spreading a number of diseases. The sanitary quality of tank water can be considerably improved by, a) elevating the edges of tank to prevent entry of surface washings, b) putting a fence around to prevent access to animals, c) making an elevated platform to draw water from the tank, d) periodically removing the weeds, e) cleaning the tank at the end of dry season and f) adding chlorine from time to time. Recently, a process of sand filtration has been adopted to render the tank water safe for drinking.

3. GROUND WATER

It is the cheapest and comparatively safer means of providing water to communities in villages and small towns. It is superior to surface water as ground itself provides an effective filtering medium. It is likely to be free from pathogenic contaminants and generally it does not require treatment with disinfectants. Its supply can be maintained during the dry season. However, it has a high content of minerals in the form of calcium and magnesium salts which render it hard and it needs pumping or lifting from the source for routine use. The usual ground water sources are wells and springs.

(a) Wells

Wells are the most common source of water in rural areas and small townships. They are of two types, shallow and deep. A shallow well taps water from above the first impervious layer in the ground whereas deep well penetrates the first impervious layer in the ground and taps the water lying beneath the impervious layer. The water from the shallow wells is moderately hard and often grossly contaminated and they often go dry in summer. On the other hand the water from deep wells is much hard but purer as compared to that of shallow well and they provide a source of constant supply.

(b) Sanitary Wells

Sanitary wells are well planned, properly located, well constructed and adequately protected against contamination in order to yield a constant supply of safe water. However, strict cleanliness should be enforced in the vicinity of the well to maintain the quality of water from these wells.

(c) Tube Wells

Tube wells serve as a source of drinking water in many parts of the country. They provide bacteriologically safe water and are cheap as compared to other sources of water supply. Shallow tube wells have now become the largest individual source of water supply to the rural population of India. The tube well consists of a galvanized iron pipe sunk into the water bearing stratum and fitted with a strainer at the bottom and a handpump at the top. Deep tube wells are sunk by drilling through successive substrate of gravel until a suitable supply of water is located and they are several hundred feet deep. The yield is very high and does not depend upon direct rainfall in the immediate vicinity.

WATER POLLUTION

Water may contain impurities of different kinds. These impurities can be considered under three important headings :

1. **Dissolved Impurities:** These include dissolved gases (e.g. hydrogen sulphide, ammonia, carbon dioxide and nitrogen) and dissolved minerals (e.g., salts of sodium, calcium and magnesium).
2. **Suspended impurities:** These include fine clay silt, sand and mud, and microscopic plants and animals.
3. **Water pollution caused by human activity** : Urbanization and industrialization are responsible for water pollution to a great extent which is generally caused by
   - (a) **Sewage**—as it contains decomposable organic matter and pathogenic agents.
   - (b) **Industrial and trade wastes** which contain toxic substances ranging from metal salts to complex synthetic organic chemicals.
   - (c) **Agricultural pollutants** which consist of pesticides and fertilizers and
   - (d) **Physical pollutants** like heat (thermal pollution) and radioactive substances.

HAZARDS OF WATER POLLUTION

Contaminated water can adversely affect the health of man either directly or through the food and by its use for personal hygiene or recreation. The hazards of water pollution can be discussed under two broad groups.

(a) Biological hazards: These consists of water-borne diseases caused by the presence of an infective agent or an aquatic host in water. Typical examples include viral hepatitis, poliomyelitis, cholera, typhoid, bacillary dysentery, amoebiasis, giardiasis and helminthic infections like round worm, thread worm and whipworm. On the other hand schistosomiasis and guinea worm infestations are due to the presence of an aquatic host.

(b) **Chemical hazards**: These are caused by the chemical pollutants derived from industrial or agricultural wastes which find their way into public water supplies. These pollutants comprise of detergent solvents, heavy metals, cyanides, heavy metals, minerals, organic acids, nitrogenous substances, bleaching agents, pigments, dyes, sulphide, ammonia, and other toxic and biocidal compounds. The long term toxic effects of these pollutants are matter of serious concern.

PURIFICATION OF WATER

Purification of water plays an important role in community medicine as polluted or contaminated water is responsible for the spread of a number of infectious diseases and health hazards. Purification of water can be considered under two headings.

1. Large Scale Purification of Water : Purification of water on large scale such as in urban water supply systems is done in three stages:

(a) **Storage** : Storage of water obtained from proper source excludes further pollution and causes automatic purification during an optimum period. Quality of water improves on storage as suspended impurities settle down and water becomes clearer thus allowing penetration of light and reducing the work of filters. The aerobic bacteria oxidize the organic matter present in water with the aid of dissolved oxygen. Also, the bacterial count of water shows a highly significant decrease on storage.

(b) **Filtration** : It is the second stage in the purification of water. Filtration removes 98-99% of bacteria apart from the other impurities. Two types of filters are in current use, the 'slow sand' or 'biological' filters and the 'rapid sand' or 'mechanical' filters.

Slow sand filters

The elements of slow sand filter include the supernatant water, a bed of graded sand, an under drainage system and a system of filter control valves. The most important part of this filter is the sand bed. As the operation of this system starts the surface of sand bed gets covered with a slimy growth known as vital layer which is gelatinous form of life including plankton, diatoms and bacteria. The formation of vital layer is described as the 'ripening' of the filter. It removes organic matter, holds back bacteria and oxidizes ammoniacal nitrogen into nitrates and helps yielding a bacteria free water. At the bottom of the filter bed is the under drainage system which consists of porous or perforated pipes which provide an outlet for filtered water.

Slow sand filters are simple to construct and operate. They are more economical as compared to rapid sand filters and the physical, chemical and bacteriological quality of water is quite high. Under ideal working conditions they reduce total bacterial counts by 90.90 to 99.99 percent.

Rapid Sand Filters

These filters include the components for coagulation, rapid mixing, flocculation, sedimentation and filtration operating in the same order. The raw water is first treated with alum which is a chemical coagulant. The treated water is then subjected to violent agitation for rapid mixing which allows a quick and thorough dissemination of alum throughout the bulk of water. The next phase involves a slow and gentle stirring of treated water in a flocculation chamber for 30 min which results in the formation of thick, copious, white flocculent precipitate of aluminium hydroxide. This coagulated water is then led to sedimentation tank where it is allowed to stand for 2-6 hours during which the flocculent precipitate settles down along with the other impurities and bacteria. The precipitate or sludge which settles down is removed from time to time. The partly clarified water is then subjected to rapid sand filtration in the filter beds.

The rapid sand filters can deal with the raw water directly and no preliminary storage is necessary. The filter beds occupy less space, filtration is rapid, the washing of the filter is easy and the operation is more flexible.

The rapid sand filters can deal with the raw water directly and no preliminary storage is necessary. The filter beds occupy less space. filtration is rapid, the washing of the filter is easy and the operation is more flexible.

(c) Chlorination

Chlorination is one of the most effective methods of water purification. It supplements sand filtration by killing pathogenic bacteria. Chlorine also oxidizes iron, manganese and hydrogen sulphide, destroys certain constituent which produce bad taste and unpleasant odour, controls algae and slime organisms and aids in the process of coagulation.

When chlorine is added to water, it leads to formation of hydrochoric and hypochlorous acids. The HCl is neutralized by the alkalinity of water. The hypochlorous acid ionizes to form hydrogen and hypochlorite ions.

$$H_2O + Cl_2 \rightarrow HCl + HOCl$$
$$HOCl \rightarrow H^+ + OCl^-$$

The hypochlorous acid is mainly responsible for the disinfectant action of chlorine as it is the most effective form of chlorine for disinfection of water. Chlorine produces its maximum disinfectant action when the pH of water is around 7 because of the predominance of hypochlorous acid. When the pH value exceeds 8.5. about 90% of hypochlorous acid gets ionized to hypochlorite ion which retains only marginal disinfectant activity.

The disinfectant action of chlorine is based on the following principles:

1. It is important that the water to be chlorinated should be clear and free from turbidity.

2. The chlorine demand of the water should be estimated prior to large scale chlorination. Chlorine demand has been defined as the difference between the amount of chlorine added to water and the amount of residual chlorine remaining at the end of a specific period of contact which is usually one hour at a given temperature and pH of water. The point, at which the chlorine demand of the water is met, is called the break-point. If further chlorine is added beyond the breakpoint, free chlorine begins to appear in the water. The free residual chlorine provides a margin of safety against subsequent microbial contamination. The sum of chlorine demand of the specific water plus the free residual chlorine of 0.5 mg/l consitutes the optimum dose of chlorine to be used.

For disinfecting large volumes of water, chlorine is used as chlorine gas, chloramine or perchloron. Amongst them chlorine gas is the first choice as it is quick in action, efficient, easy to apply and economical for large scale disinfection. Since chlorine gas produces irritation of eyes and it is poisonous, a special chlorinating equipment known as Paterson's chloronome is used for measuring, regulating and administrating chlorine to water supplies. Chloramine and perchloron have certain advantages over chlorine gas but they are not used for large scale chlorination of urban water supplies.

2. Small Scale Purification of Water :

(a) For household purification of water, three methods are most commonly used. They are boiling of water, chemical purification and filtration. Boiling the water for 5-10 minutes is satisfactory for household purpose. It kills bacteria, spores, cysts and ova and yields sterilized water. It also removes temporary hardness by driving off carbon dioxide and precipitating calcium carbonate. It slightly alters the taste of water. However, it offers no residual protection against subsequent microbial contamination.

Chemical purification of water can be achieved by using different preparations which act by liberating chlorine in the water. They include bleaching powder, chlorine solution, high test hypochlorite or chlorine tablets.

Filtration of water for domestic use can be effectively achieved by filtering the water through ceramic filters such as Pasteur Chamberland filter, Berkefield filter and Kayadyn filter. The essential part of the filter is a candle made of porcelain in the Chamberland type and of Kieselguhr in the Berkefield filter. In the Katadyn filter the surface of the filter is coated with a silver catalyst so that the bacteria coming in contact with the surface are killed by the oligodynamic action of silver ions liberated in the water. Filter candles usually remove bacteria found in the drinking water but not the viruses. They also get clogged with impurities and bacteria and must be cleaned by scrubbing with a hard brush under running water and sterilized by boiling once in a week. Only clean water should be used with ceramic filters.

(b) Disinfection of Wells

Wells are the most common source of water supply in villages and small towns. The most effective and economical method of disinfecting wells is by bleaching powder.

HEALTH AND AIR

All forms of life depend on air which constitutes the immediate environment of man. In addition to the supply of life-giving oxygen, air and atmospheric conditions serve many other functions. The human body is cooled by the contact with air, and the special senses of hearing and smelling function through air transmitted stimuli. On the other hand the disease producing agents and micro-organisms are also carried by the air.

Pollution of air by dust, smoke, toxic gases and chemical vapours can result in sickness and death. The term air pollution is applied when there is an excessive concentration of foreign matter in the outdoor atmosphere which is harmful to man or his environment.

Air pollution sources are generally classified into four broad categories. They include:

(a) **Industrial outlets**: Chemical industries, textile industries, metallurgical industries, oil refineries and fertilizer factories etc. contribute to air pollution.

(b) **Combustion**: Industrial and domestic combustion of coal, oil and other fuel is the source of smoke, dust and sulphur dioxide.

(c) **Motor Vehicles**: Both heavy and light motor vehicles, trucks, air crafts and trains and other forms of transport contribute to air pollution by emitting hydrocarbons, carbon monoxide, lead, nitrogen oxides and particulate matter. Strong sunlight converts some of these hydrocarbons and nitrogen oxides into photochemical pollutant of oxidizing nature.

(d) **Miscellaneous** : Agricultural activities like crop spraying and pest control, burning of refuse and nuclear energy programmes also contribute to air pollution.

The important chemical pollutants include, carbon dioxide, carbon monoxide, sulphur dioxide, hydrogen sulphide, and organic sulphides, fluorine compounds, oxides of nitrogen and ammonia, aldehydes, beryllium and carcinogenic agents like benzpyrenes and radioactive substances etc. Amongst them, the best indicators of air pollution are:

1. **Sulphur dioxide**: It is a major contaminant in most urban and industrial areas. Its concentration is measured in all air pollution surveys.
2. **Smoke Index**: It is measured by filtering the air through a paper tape and measuring the intensity by a photoelectric meter.
3. **Suspended Particles:** Particulate matter such as dust and soot from domestic and industrial sources is another useful indicator of air pollution.

Other important parameters of air pollution include carbon monoxide, oxidants, nitrogen oxides and lead.

EFFECTS OF AIR POLLUTION ON HEALTH

(a) **Immediate effects:** According to epidemiological studies a sudden increase in air pollution has often been associated with immediate increase in mortality and morbidity. The Bhopal MIC gas tragedy and the Chernobyl disaster of U.S.S.R. are the most recent examples. The symptoms usually involve the respiratory system and lead to definite increase in mortality and morbidity.

(b) **Delayed effects:** The diseases which are generally attributed to air pollution are chronic bronchitis and primary lung cancer.

LIGHT

Adequate lighting is essential for an efficient vision. When subjected to inadequate lighting conditions, the human visual apparatus is put to strain which leads to general fatigue and loss of efficiency. For an efficient vision the following criteria of light is usually applied.

(a) Sufficient light: The lighting should be sufficient for the eye to easily discern the object and surrounding without any strain. An illumination of 15-20 foot candles is accepted as basic minimum for satisfactory vision.

(b) Distribution: The light should be uniformly distributed having the same intensity over the whole field of work.

(c) Absence of Glare: Glare is harsh dazzling light. It is best exemplified by the automobile head lights at night due to excessive contrast. The eye does not tolerate glare as it causes acute discomfort and reduces critical vision.

(d) Absence of sharp shadows: Shadows should not be present in the field of vision as they cause confusion to the eye.

(e) Steadiness: Light should be projected constantly without any interruption. Flickering of light causes strain to the eye and may lead to accidents.

(f) Surroundings: For efficient vision, the color schemes in the rooms and halls is important. Ceilings and roofs should ideally have a reflection factor of 80 percent; walls 50 to 60 percent and furniture 30 to 40 percent. Reflection from floor should be minimum-not more than 15-20 percent.

Natural Lighting:

Natural lighting is obtained partly from the visible sky and partly from reflection. Considerable amount of light comes to rooms by reflection from light coloured objects. Perfect utilization of natural light depends on careful design, location and orientation of buildings. Natural lighting varies with the time of the day. Proper orientation of buildings, removal of obstructions in the way of lighting, placement and size of windows and interior designing of rooms can improve the daylight illumination.

Artificial Lighting :

Day light may not meet the adequate requirement of illumination during all the hours and on cloudy days. On many occasions, it has to be supplemented by artificial lighting for adequate illumination, which should be as close as possible to daylight in composition. There are five systems of artificial lighting.

(a) **Direct Lighting**: In this system 99-100 percent of light is directly projected towards working area. It is economical and efficient but it casts sharp shadows which are not desirable.

(b) **Semi Direct**: In this system 10-40 percent of the light is projected upwards which in turn is reflected back by the ceiling on the object.

(c) **Indirect**: It does not strike a surface directly because 90-100 percent of the light is projected towards the ceiling and walls. It produces general illumination of the whole room.

(d) **Semi-indirect**: Here 60-90 percent of light is directed upwards and the rest towards the working area.

(e) **Direct-Indirect**: In this system light is distributed equally towards the ceiling and the working area.

Methods of Artificial Lighting:

Filament lamps are most widely used source of artificial lighting. The electric current heats up the tungsten filament and the light emitted depends upon the temperature. The hotter filaments produce bluer light. Fluorescent lamps are the better source of artificial light. They are economical in the consumption of electricity, cool, efficient and the light emitted by fluorescent lamps simulates natural light. These lamps are made of glass tube filled with mercury vapor and an electrode fitted at each end. The inside of the tube is coated with fluorescent chemicals which absorb practically all ultraviolet radiation and emit radiation in the visible range.

Lighting Standards:

The human eyes respond to a range of illumination ranging from 0.1 lux (full moonlight night) to 1,00,000 lux (bright sunshine). The visual efficiency increases with the increase of illumination but the curve flattens out at higher levels. A practical rule is that the illumination level should be 30 times higher than the level at which the task can just be done.

Biological Effects of Light:

Light has been shown to produce interesting biological effects. The observation that daylight could cause the in vitro degradation of bilirubin has been used as therapeutic measure for controlling the hyperbilirubinemia in premature infants. Other biological effects of light include the effect on biological rhythms of body temperature, physical activity, stimulation of melanin synthesis, activation of precursors in the biosynthesis of vitamin D, adrenocortical secretion and food consumption.

NOISE

Noise can be defined as loud, confused and senseless shouting or a sound that lacks agreeable quality and is noticeably unpleasant. The term noise pollution has recently been coined to signify the vast cacophony of sounds that are annoying, harmful and lead to health hazards and environmental pollution.

Sources:

There are a number of sources of noise which can produce environmental pollution. These include factories, automobiles, industries, air crafts and the domestic appliances like radios, transistors, televisions and stereo systems of high wattage and also the public address systems and loudspeakers etc.

Properties:

Noise has two important properties, loudness (intensity) and frequency. Loudness or intensity signifies the amplitude of vibrations which initiate the noise. Intensity of sound is measured in terms of decibels (dB). One decibel (dB) is defined as the smallest distinguishable noise or the 'reference' sound pressure which is equal to 0.0002 microbar or dynes/cm^2. A dyne is 1/10,00,000 of atmospheric pressure. Normal conversation ranges in the between 60-65 dB; whispering 20-30 dB and heavy street traffic 60-80 dB. A boiler factory may generate noise level of 120 dB. Most of the people can tolerate a daily exposure of noise upto 85 dB without any substantial damage to their auditory functions.

Frequency :

Frequency is measured in Hertz (Hz). One Hz is equal to one wave per second. The human ear can hear frequencies from 20 to 20,000 Hz. This range reduces with age and other subjective factors. Many animals like dogs can hear sounds inaudible to human ears.

Sometimes noise is expressed in psycho-acoustic terms the 'phon' which is an index taking into account both the intensity and frequency of sounds. Three basic instruments are used in studies on noise. 1. The Sound Level Meter which measures the intensity of sound in dB. 2. The Octave Band Frequency Analyzer which measures sound in octave bands, and 3. The Audiometer which measures the hearing ability.

Effects of Noise:

The effects of noise exposures are of two types, auditory and non-auditory.

Auditory Effect :

Auditory Fatigue : It is characterized by side effects such as whistling and buzzing in the ears. It generally appears in the 90 dB region and is maximum at 4000 Hz.

Deafness : There may be temporary or permanent hearing loss. Mostly temporary hearing loss occurs following an exposure to 4000-6000 Hz and it disappears within 24 hours. However, repeated or continuous exposure to noise around 100 dB may result in permanent hearing loss which is generally due to inner ear damage.

Nonauditory Effects:

Nonauditory effects of noise are characterized by interference with speech and efficiency, and certain physiological changes of temporary nature. Frequencies causing maximum interference with speech lie in the 300-500 Hz. Such frequencies are commonly present in noise [illegible] by road and air traffic. Other temporary physiological changes induced by noise include the increases in heart rate, blood pressure and intracranial pressure, and sweating. Noise also interferes with sleep and causes nausea, giddiness and fatigue.

NOISE CONTROL

The important measures which can be undertaken for controlling noise include:

(a) **Control of noise at source:** This can be achieved by segregating noise producing machines, application of muffers and other noise reducers to machines.

(b) **Control of transmission of noise**: This can be done by building enclosures and covering the walls of the rooms with sound absorbing material.

(c) **Protection of exposed persons**: Hearing protection is necessary for all workers who are constantly exposed to noise louder than 85 dB in the frequency bands above 150 Hz.

(d) **Education:** The education of public through mass communication media is also required to highlight the importance of noise as health hazard.

SOLID WASTES DISPOSAL AND CONTROL

Solid wastes refer to discarded waste material from houses, street sweeping, commercial, industrial and agricultural operations. It comprises of dust, ash, vegetables and putrescible matter, paper and packings of all kinds, rags and other fabrics, glass and other combustible and noncombustible debris. In cities it is called refuse, in the country side, it is called litter and in general it is known as solid wastes.

The accumulation of solid wastes in man's surroundings constitutes a positive health hazard because:

(i) The organic matter of solid wastes ferments and favours the breeding of flies.

(ii) The garbage in the refuse attracts rats and pigs.

(iii) Pathogens from refuse may be carried to man through house flies and dust.

(iv) There is risk of air and water pollution through combustion and fermentation of refuse.

(v) From aesthetic point of view accumulation of refuse is a nuisance.

Therefore efficient collection, removal and disposal of refuse are essential components of environmental health service which reflect the social development of a community.

Sources of Refuse :

People at large are primarily concerned with the domestic refuse. It consists of ash, rubbish and garbage. Residue from fire used for cooking and heating forms the ash. Rubbish comprises of paper, clothing, bits of wood, metals, glass, dust and dirt. Garbage is the waste matter which comes from the preparation, cooking and consumption of food items. It mainly comprises of peelings of vegetables and fruits, waste food, egg shells, left overs of chicken and meat and other organic matter. Quick removal and disposal of garbage is essential as it ferments rapidly on storage.

Storage:

Proper storage of refuse is important before it is collected for disposal. A galvanized steel dustbin or a plastic dustbin with close fitting cover is suitable for a household purpose. For a family of 5-6 members a dustbin of 2 cubic feet capacity would be adequate if the collection is made once in three days. Public bins cater for a larger community. They are kept on concrete platform which is raised 2-3 inches above the ground to prevent the entry of rain water. In bigger municipalities the bins are emptied mechanically by lorries fitted with cranes.

A recent innovation for the storage of refuse is the polythene sack. Once the sack is full of refuse it is removed with the contents for disposal and replaced by a new sack.

COLLECTION

House to house collection is the best method for the collection of refuse. In our country, people are expected to dump the refuse in the nearest public dustbin. The refuse is then transported to the ultimate place for disposal by collection vehicles. However, the collection methods practised in most of our cities need considerable improvement.

METHODS OF DISPOSAL

There are a number of methods available for the disposal of refuse. The choice of a particular method depends upon the local factors such as cost and availability of land and labour. The most common methods of refuse disposal include:

(a) Dumping:

Dumping of refuse in low lying areas is an easy method of disposal of dry refuse. It also adds to the reclamation of such land. Due to the bacterial decomposition refuse decreases in volume and is converted gradually into humus. The reclaimed land is then leased for cultivation.

However, there are a number of draw-backs of this method. The refuse is exposed to flies and rodents and causes nuisance due to its smell and unsightly appearance. It can pollute the air and also contaminate the surface and ground water. According to a WHO Expert Committee dumping is most in-sanitary method that creates public health hazards, nuisance and severe pollution of the environment.

(b) Controlled tipping:

If suitable land is available, controlled tipping or sanitary landfill is considered the most satisfactory method of refuse disposal. In this method the material is placed in a trench or other prepared area, adequately compacted and covered with earth at the end of the working day. In this process chemical, bacteriological and physiological changes occur in buried refuse. The temperature, which may rise to more than 60^0C within a weeks' time, kills all the pathogenic organisms and hastens the process of decomposition. Then it cools down within 2 to 3 weeks. It may take 4 to 6 months for complete decomposition of organic matter into an innocuous mass.

(c) Incineration:

Another very hygienic method of refuse disposal is by burning or incineration. It is very suitable for cities where adequate land is not available for controlled tipping. Hospital refuse which is highly infectious is best disposed by incineration. However, disposal by burning is not economical as it leads to total loss of the much needed manure. In our country burning has a limited application in the disposal of refuse.

(d) Composting:

It is a method used for the disposal of refuse along with the night soil or sludge. It is a natural process during which the organic matter breaks down under bacterial action resulting in the formation of a relatively stable humus like material called the compost which has considerable value as manure for agricultural purpose. The main by-products of composting are carbon dioxide, water and heat. The heat produced during composting, which may be well above 60°C over a period of several days destroys eggs and larvae of flies, weeds, seeds and pathogenic agents. The compost formed at the end contains major plant nutrients such as nitrates and phosphates. It is odourless, innocuous material of high manurial value.

(e) Manure pits:

It is one of the most practical and effective methods of refuse disposal in rural areas of our country. The garbage, cattle dung, straw and leaves are dumped into the manure pits and covered with earth after each day's dumping. In 5-6 months time the refuse is converted into manure which can be used in the fields.

MEDICAL ENTOMOLOGY

1. ARTHROPOD BORNE DISEASES AND THEIR CONTROL

A study of the arthropods of medical importance is known as medical entomology, which is an important branch of preventive medicine. Majority of arthropods are either of no use to man or his dreaded enemies. They destroy the crops and food reserves and many of them live close to man and act as vectors or carriers of different diseases.

Arthropods may be responsible for disease in four ways. They may act as vectors of infectious agents; they may envenomate through strings or bites; they may infest or even infect the human body directly: and they may cause allergic dermatitis. Arthropod borne diseases consitute a major health problem in India. Malaria is the most widely prevalent vector-borne disease with an annual morbidity of 4 to 5 million cases. Filaria and guinea worm disease are other arthropod borne diseases which are endemic. Scabies is another widespread disease particularly in rural areas. Dengue, hemorrhagic fever, Japanese encephalitis and Kyasanur forest disease (KFD) are among the important virus diseases which are spread by arthropods. Trachoma, which is a major cause of blindness has a prevalence rate of 0.5 percent in West Bengal to 70 percent in Haryana and Punjab.

Arthropods of medical importance can be classified in three important groups

1. **Class insecta**: it includes mosquitoes, flies, human lice, fleas and winged bugs.
2. **Class arachnida**: it includes ticks and mites.
3. **Class crustacea**: it is represented by cyclops.

The distinctive characters of the arthropods have been summarized in Table-4.1

Table-4.1 Distinctive Characteristics of Arthropods

Characteristics		Insecta	Arachnida	Crustacea
(a)	Divisions of the body	Head, thorax and abdomen	Cephalothorax and abdomen	Cephalothorax and abdomen
(b)	Legs	3 pairs	4 pairs	5 pairs
(c)	Antennae	1 pair	None	2 pairs
(d)	Wings	One or two pairs, some are wingless	None	None
(e)	Habitat	on land	on land	in water
(f)	Examples	Mosquito, Housefly, Human lice, Rat fleas and Winged bugs	Hard ticks, Soft ticks, Mites	Cyclops

Transmission of arthropod-borne diseases.

Three types of transmission processes are responsible for the spread of arthropod-borne diseases. They are through:

(i) **Direct contract :** In this process arthropods are directly transferred from man to man through close contact, e.g. scabies and pediculosis (lice).

(ii) **Mechanical transmission:** The disease agent is transmitted mechanically by the arthropod as seen in the transmission of diarrhoea, dysentery, typhoid, food poisoning and trachoma by housefly.

(iii) **Biological transmission :** In this process the causative organism multiplies or undergoes some developmental change in the arthropod host. Malaria, filaria, plague and guinea worm disease are the examples of biological transmission. Arthropod-born diseases are symmarized in Table-4.2.

Table-4.2 Infections conveyed by arthropods

Name of arthropod	Genus	Disease (s) transmitted
Housefly	Musca	Dysenteries, enteric fevers, cholera, trachoma, salmonelloses, tropical ulcer.
Housefly	Tabanida	Tularemia, Anthrax
Oscinid fly	Hippelaes	Streptococcal dermatitis and nephritis, yaws
Tsetse fly	Glossina	African trypanosomiasis (sleeping sickness)
Mosquito	Anopheles	Malaria, Filaria
	Aedes	Yellow fever, dengue
	Culex	Filariasis, Japanese encephalitis, arboviruses.
Black fly	Simulium	Onchocerciasis
Soft ticks	Rhipicephalus	Typhus ever, KFD, Tularemia
Sand flies	Phlebotomus	Leishmaniasis, sandfly fever
Lice	Pediculus	Epidemic louse fever, french fever, louse- borne relapsing fever.
Mites	Leptotrombidium	Scrub Typhus fever
	Allodermanyssus	Rickettsial pox
Itch mite		Scabies
Winged bugs	Triatoma	Chagas disease
Fleas	Xenopsylla	Plague, Endemic typhus fever
Cyclops		Guineaworm disease.

Arthropod control:

There are a number of methods employed for the control of arthropods. They are based on the following principles:

(a) **Environmental Control** : Methods based on environmental control produce long lasting results. These include elimination of breeding places; filling and drainage operation, carefully planned water management; provision of piped water supply, proper disposal of refuse, cleanliness in and around houses and intensive health education of the community.

(b) **Chemical Control**: Chemical control is affected by a wide range of insecticides belonging to organochlorine, organophosphorus and carbamate compounds available for vector control. However, a number of arthropods have shown resistance to these insecticides. These compounds also possess inherent danger of environmental pollution and hence the highly persistent insecticides like DDT are now gradually replaced by readily biodegradable and less toxic compounds like methoxychlor.

(c) **Biological Control:** In order to minimize environmental pollution by toxic insecticides, more emphasis is now being given to biological control. The use of larvivorous fish gambusia is well known for mosquito control. Certain fungi are also known to be pathogenic to mosquitoes.

(d) **Genetic Control**: Significant progress has taken place in the genetic control of arthropod during the recent years. Genetic methods such as sterile male technique, cytoplasmic incompatibility, and chromosomal translocations have been found effective in the control of arthropods. However, these methods have not as yet exploited in the control of arthropods on a large scale.

(e) **Newer methods:** Amongst the newer methods which may be applied for the control of arthropods, the use of insect growth regulators, chemosterilants and sex attractants or pheromones may find some application in future.

Based upon these principles, a number of methods have been developed for the control of the spread of important arthropods. Some of the methods used for the control of mosquitoes, houseflies, lice, fleas, ticks and mites and cyclops are being described in some detail.

Measures of mosquito control:

The currently used methods for mosquito control are based on an integrated approach which produces maximum results without producing environmental pollution and insecticide resistance. These methods of mosquito control can be classified as under:

(1) Anti-larval measures:

(a) **Environmental Control** : It is achieved by eliminating the breeding places of mosquitoes which is known as "source reduction". It comprises of minor engineering methods such as filling, levelling and drainage of breeding places and water management. Source reduction also implies rendering the water unsuitable for mosquito breeding e.g., by changing the salinity of water. Adequate collection, removal and disposal of sewage and waste water helps in the control of mosquito breeding.

(b) **Chemical Control**: The commonly used chemical larvacides include mineral oils, Paris green and the synthetic insecticides. Mineral oils such as kerosene, diesel or special mosquito larvicidal oil, when applied on water, spread and form a thin film which cuts off the air supply to mosquito larvae and pupae and thus produce toxic effects on these insect stages. Oil is applied once in a week on all breeding places. Paris green or copper acetoarsenite is an emerald green, microcystalline powder containing 50 percent arsenious oxide. It is a stomach poison when ingested by larvae. It is applied as 2 percent dust with particles ranging from 20-50 microns by hand blowers or rotary blowers.

Synthetic insecticides used for larvae control are organophosphorus compounds like Abate, Chloropyrifos and Fenthion, as they quickly hydrolyse in water. abate at a concentration of 1.00 PPM is very effective larvacide and also the least toxic.

(c) **Biological Control** : Small fishes like Gambusia affinis and Lebistor reticulatus (Barbados millions) feed on mosquito larvae. They are used in burrow pits, sewage oxidation ponds, ornamental ponds, cisterns and farm ponds. However, biological control can be effective only when used in conjunction with other methods.

(2) Anti-adult measures :

(a) **Residual sprays** : DDT is the insecticide of choice for controlling adult mosquitoes by spraying it on the walls and other surfaces where mosquitoes rest. However, with continued use for many years DDT resistance is now frequently encountered. In such situations other insecticides like malathion, propoxur (OMS-33) and to a less extent lindane are used. It is now essential that periodical sensitivity tests should be made to determine the effectiveness of insecticides against different species of mosquitoes.

(b) **Space Sprays**: In this method an insecticidal formulation is sprayed into the atmosphere to form mist or fog which kills the insects. The common sprays are pyrethrum extract which contains nerve poison pyrethrin and the residual insecticides like malathion and fenitrothion are sprayed by a technique known as ultra-low-volume fogging.

(c) **Genetic Control**: Methods of genetic control are still under development and research phase. They include sterile male technique, cytoplasmic incompatibility, chromosomal translocation, sex distortion and gene replacement. Once developed they may prove cheaper, more effective and not subject to vector resistance.

(3) Protection against mosquito bites :

(a) **Mosquito net** : It is used for protection against mosquito bites during sleep. Ideally, the mosquito net should be white to allow easy detection of mosquitoes; all the sides of a net should be of netting; it should be of rectangular shape and the size of opening in the net should not exceed 0.0475 inch in any diameter.

(b) **Screening:** A complete screening of the house with copper or bronze gauge is highly effective in blocking the entry of mosquitoes. The aperture should not be larger than 0.0475 inch in any diameter.

(c) **Repellent**: Repellents are used for application on the skin. They provide a short duration of protection. Diethyltoluamide (Deet) has been employed as a very effective all purpose repellent. Other repellent compounds include indalone, dimethyl phthalate, dimethyl carbate and ethylhexanediol etc.

Fly Control Measures :

(a) **Environmental control**: Elimination of breeding places and improvement in environmental sanitation are the best methods for the control of flies. This would imply (i) proper storage of garbage and refuse in bins with tight lids (ii) efficient collection, removal and disposal of refuse by suitable and effective methods as described earlier (iii) provision of sanitary latrines (iv) stopping open air defecation (v) sanitary disposal of animal excreta and (vi) improvement of general sanitation inside the houses and of the surroundings are the most effective measures for controlling the fly problem.

(b) **Insecticidal control** : Residual sprays with organophosphorus and pesticides, use of cords and ribbons impregnated with insecticides, space sprays containing pyrethrin and other insecticides and application of larvicides at breeding places are the commonly used methods for the insecticides control of flies.

(c) **Fly papers:** Sticky flypapers are useful adjuncts to other methods of fly control. They are prepared by applying an adhesive mixture containing resin and castor oil on papers.

(d) **Protection against flies** : Screening of houses, hospitals, restaurants, food and meat shops and other such establishments can provide considerable protection against flies.

(e) **Health education** : In the absence of health education on the importance and benefits of fly control and other sanitary measures, no method of fly control can be effectively implemented. It is through constant health education that any community can be persuaded and motivated to adopt the desired measures for the control of flies and mosquitoes.

The methods of fly control described can be effectively employed with some modifications in the control of sand flies, tsetse fly and black flies, lice, fleas, bugs and ticks and mites.

Control of Cyclops:

Control of cyclops is particularly important as they are the intermediate hosts of Dracontiasis or guinea worm disease. Man acquires infestation by drinking water containing cyclops. Guineaworm disease is a public health problem in Rajasthan, Maharashtra, Madhya Pradesh, Andhra Pradesh and Tamil Nadu.

Cyclops are controlled by the following methods:

(a) **Physical**: Straining and boiling of water are physical methods useful for providing individual prophylaxis. Straining of water through a fine cloth removes cyclops and boiling of water kills cyclops readily as they cannot withstand a temperature beyond 600C.

(b) **Chemical** : Chlorine 5 ppm destroys cyclops and larvae of guineaworm. Lime at a concentration of 4 g per gallon of water is found very efficient for killing cyclops. Another insecticide, Abate at a concentration of 1 mg/l is effective in killing cyclops.

(c) **Biological:** Gambusia and barbel fishes feed on cyclops and they have been used for the eradication of cyclops in Karnataka state.

Apart from these measures which have to be employed in the endemic areas, the most satisfactory and permanent method for controlling cyclops in drinking water is to provide piped water supply or tube wells. Abolition of step wells must be accomplished in rural areas.

2. RODENTS

Rodents live in close association with man and they are part of our environment. In addition to their being hazard to our health, they can also cause damage to buildings, grains, food stuffs and other household commodities. Rodents are generally classified into two distinct groups, domestic and wild.

Domestic rodents: As they live close to man they are of greater public health concern. They include the common black rat (**Rattus rattus**) the Norway rat (**R.norvegicus**) and the houses mouse (**Mus musculus**). **Rattus rattus** is a domestic animal with a restricted area of movement. It is good climber and it generally infests the roofs of houses. It can also burrow and is capable of infesting even ships. Therefore it is of considerable public health importance. The Norway rat is a semidomestic animal and it frequents sewers, drains as well as houses.

R.rattus is generally called the house rat, whereas **R. norvegicus** is known as the sewer rat

Wild rodents: Wild rodents in our country include **Tatera indica** which is a natural reservoir of plague and **Bandicota bengalensis, B.indica, Millardia meltada, M.gleadowi** and **Mus booduga.**

Rats are instrumental in spreading a number of diseases. These are:

(i)	**Bacterial**	:	Plague, tularemia and salmonellosis
(ii)	**Viral**	:	Encephalitis, Lussa fever and hemorrhagic fever.
(iii)	**Rickettsial**	:	Scrub typhus, marine typhus and rickettsial pox.
(iv)	**Parasitic**	:	Leishmaniasis, amoebiasis, trichinosis, chagas disease and Hymenolepsis diminuata.
(v)	**Others**	:	Rat bite fever, leptospirosis, histoplasmosis and ring worm etc.

The mode of transmission may be direct through rat bite e.g. rat bite fever, through contamination of food and water e.g., salmonellosis, leptospirosis and through rat fleas e.g., plague and typhus.

Control of rodents:

(a) **Sanitary measures**: Environmental sanitation plays important role in the eradication of rats. If the basic requirements of food, water and shelter are denied to rats, their population will gradually decrease. The measures required for achieving this comprise of i) proper storage, collection and disposal of garbage, ii) proper storage of food stuffs and grains iii) construction of rat proof houses, godowns and ware houses, and iv) elimination of rat burrows permanently blocking them with concrete.

(b) **Trapping**: Trapping is a simple operation and can cause only temporary reduction of rat population. Haffkine Institute, Bombay has developed a trap which can trap 25 rats at a time. These rats are then killed by drowning them in water.

(c) **Rodenticides**: Single dose rodenticides are popularly used for controlling rats. These include barium carbonate and zinc phosphide. Barium carbonate is a weak rotenticide and is not fully reliable as it is easily detected by rats in the baits. Zinc phosphide is now extensively used in the ratio of 1 part to 10 parts of wheat or rice flour and mixed with a few drops of edible oil in order to make it more attractive for rats. Rats are killed within 3 hours after consuming the bait.

(d) **Fumigation**: It is a very effective method of destroying both rats and rat fleas. The fumigants used are calcium cyanide (Cyanogas), carbon disulphide, methyl bromide and sulphur dioxide etc. Cyanogas has been used very extensively in our country for the fumigation of rat burrows. It is pumped into rat burrows in powder form by a special pump called the cyanogas pump. About 2 ounces of poison is pumped into each burrow and thereafter the burrow is sealed promptly. On contact with moisture the cyanogas powder generates hydrogen cyanide gas which is lethal to both rats and their fleas.

3. OTHER ANIMALS

Like rodents some animals are also part of man's biologic environment and they serve as reservoir host of a number of diseases. The WHO lists more than 150 diseases and infections of these animals which are communicable to man. These diseases and infections are known as 'Zoonoses' or 'Zoonotic diseases'. Some of the important zoonoses are depicted in the Table-4.3.

Our country has the largest animal population in the world. India being basically a land of agriculture, the association between man and animals is also the closest. The available information shows that a large number of zoonotic infections (e.g. brucellosis, rabies, tuberculosis, leptospirosis and hydatid disease etc.) occur in different parts of the country.

Table 4.3 Important Zoonoses Prevalent in India

Diseases	Causative Agent	Animal(s) involved
Viral		
1. Rabies	Lyssavirus type 1	Dog, Fox, Jackal
2. Japanesè encephalitis	J.E. Virus	Birds, Pigs, Horses
3. KFD	KFD virus	Monkeys, rodents
Bacterial		
1. Anthrax	**B. anthracis**	Pigs, herbivores cattle,
2. Brucellosis	Brucella spp	Sheep, goats, pigs, dogs, horses.
3. Leptospirosis	**L. interrogans**	Rodents, cats, dogs.
4. Plague	**Y. pestis**	Rodents
5. Salmonellosis	Salmonella spp	Mammals, birds
6. Tuberculosis	**M. tuberculosis**	Cattle, sheep, goats, dogs, pigs.
Parastic		
1. Hydatidosis	**E. granulosis**	Dog, cow, sheep
2. Taeniasis	**T. saginata**	Cattle
3. Cysticercosis	**T. solium**	Swine
4. Leishmaniasis	**L. donovani**	Dogs, rodents
5. Toxoplasmosis	**T. gondil**	Cats, mammals, birds.

5

NUTRITION AND HEALTH

Nutrition and health — Classification of foods, requirements, diseases induced by deficiency of proteins, vitamins and minerals • their treatment and prevention.

Nutrition is defined as a function of living plants and animals, consisting of the taking in and assimilation of material through chemical changes (metabolism) whereby tissue is built up and energy liberated. The successive stages of metabolism are digestion, absorption, assimilation and excretion. Digestion is preceded by mastication and deglutition in man.

Excretion is effected by expiration, perspiration, urination and defecation. Not all the materials involved in human metabolism can be synthesized by the body. Therefore, these essential materials-nutrients must be provided by the diet.

The terms food and nutrition are often used synonymously though it is not abosolutely correct. Food is a composite mixture of substances including proteins, carbohydrates, fats, vitamins and minerals etc whereas nutrition signifies a dynamic process in which the food that is digested, absorbed and assimilated, is used for nourishing the body. The word nutrition comes from the Latin "nutrire" which means to breast feed or nurse. No clear distinction has yet been made between the food and the nutrients.

Classification of foods :

The dietary constituents of food include proteins, fats, carbohydrates, vitamins, minerals and water. A complete food should contain all these factors. Proteins, fats and carbohydrates are considered as proximate principles and alongwith water they form the main bulk of food.

Foods have been classified on the basis of their predominant function as :

(a) **Energy yielding foods:** These foods are rich in carbohydrates and fats, e.g., cereals, sugar, honey, jellies.

(b) **Body building (anabolic) foods :** e.g. meat, liver, fish, milk, pulses, eggs.

(c) **Protective foods :** These items are rich in proteins, vitamins and minerals e.g. milk, eggs, liver, green leafy vegetables and legumes.

The important functions of food are provision of energy, body building and repair, and the maintenance and regulation of tissue functions.

PROTEINS

Proteins are complex organic nitrogenous compounds. They are composed of carbon, hydrogen, oxygen, nitrogen and sulphur in varying amounts. Some of them also contain phosphorus, iron and other elements. Proteins provide about 24 amino acids of which eight are essential for normal synthesis of the different proteins in the body and for maintaining nitrogen balance in adults. As the human body cannot synthesize them in sufficient quantity they must be supplied from the dietary proteins. The essential amino acids include methionine, lysine, tryptophan, phenylalanine, leucine, isoleucine, threonine and valine. The quality of dietary protein is closely related to its pattern of amino acids. Proteins from milk and eggs have patterns of aminoacids which are considered most suitable for human consumption.

Proteins have an important role in the constitution of all tissues including body fluids such as blood. They are required for body building, repair and maintenance of body tissues and for the biosynthesis of plasma proteins, hemoglobin, antibodies, enzymes and hormones. They are also responsible for the cell-mediated immune response and the bactericidal activity of leucocytes. Proteins can also serve as a source of energy but under normal conditions human body does not utilize them for this purpose.

Proteins in our diet are generally obtained from two important sources.

(a) **Animal sources:** Milk, eggs, meat, fish, beef and poultry etc.

(b) **Vegetable sources:** Pulses, cereals, legumes, nuts and fruits etc.

On the basis of their nutritional value animal proteins are considered superior to vegetable proteins as they contain all the essential aminoacids and hence they are biologically complete whereas the vegetable proteins lack in one or two essential amino-acids. The "biological value" of different proteins depends on the relative proportions of essential aminoacids they contain. Thus the proteins obtained from eggs, milk and meat are generally of higher biological value than the proteins of vegetable origin. However, it is possible to have a diet of mixed vegetable proteins with high biological value if the principle of complementation is utilized. For example cereals, e.g., wheat contain about 10% protein and are relatively deficient in lysine. Legumes contain around 20% of protein which is relatively deficient in methionine. If two parts of wheat are mixed with one part of legume, a food results which contains 13% protein of biological value. This happens because cereals contain enough methionine and legumes enough lysine to supplement the other component of the mixture.

Requirements of proteins: According to the recommendations of the Indian Council of Medical Research the daily protein requirement for an adult is adequately met if the diet provides about 1 G of protein per kg of body weight. Growing children need more proteins in terms of body weight since new tissues are being laid during growth. Protein needs of women during pregnancy and lactation are also greater. Factors like burns, surgery, diabetes, worm infestation, emotional disturbances and stress situations also affect the protein requirements.

Deficiency of proteins: Protein-calorie malnutrition (PCM) is the most prominent form of protein deficiency state. It occurs frequently among infants and young children between 1-3 years of age. It is not only responsible for childhood morbidity and mortality but it may also lead to permanent impairment of physical and mental growth of surviving children. The most important etiological factors of PCM are : a) inadequate diet, both in quantity and quality due to poverty and ignorance and b) the infective and parasitic diseases. Two terms are used to describe PCM.

1. **Marasmus :** Its a chronic condition resulting from a deficiency of total energy intake. Consequently the individual's reserves of protein and energy are depleted (Fig. 5.1).
2. **Kwashiorkor:** It is common in patients who have adequate caloric intake but a relative protein deficiency and who are catabolic usually with trauma, infection or burns (Fig. 5.2).

Treatment of PCM : Treatment of PCM essentially comprises of adequate diet, treatment of infections and measures to prevent relapse. In most cases 3-5 g of good quality protein per Kg of body weight per day will suffice the child's needs. After deworming and treating other infections it may take about 3 months to obtain a complete cure of PCM. Health education of parents and taking adequate care of the child's nutritional requirement will prevent a relapse.

Prevention of PCM : A number of measures are essential for prevention of PCM in the developing countries like ours. These include (a) **Health education :** measures directed to pregnant and lactating

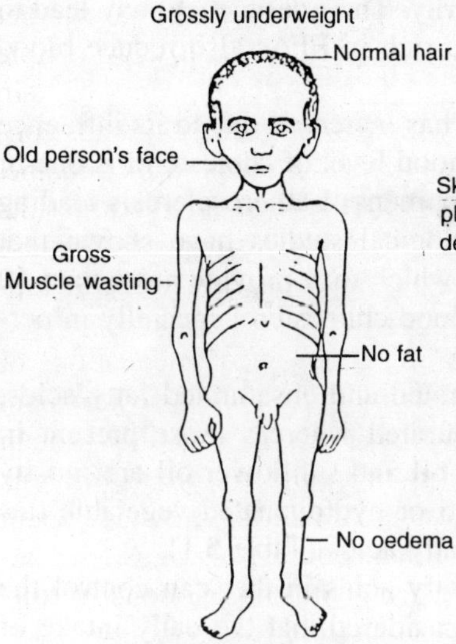

Fig 5.1 Marasmus

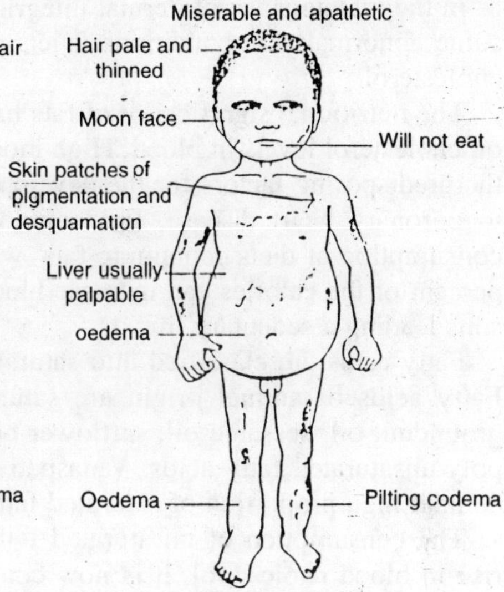

Fig. 5.2 Kwashiorkor

mothers, their education towards health consciousness, breast feeding, family planning, nutrition and food requirements of the family and growing children.

(b) **Specific protection of infants and children** :This can be achieved by timely immunization, and provision of protein and calorie rich foods like milk, eggs, and flesh foods wherever possible.

(c) **Early diagnosis, treatment and rehabilitation:** These can be achieved by periodic surveillance, proper treatment of diarrhoeas and worm infestations, development of supplementary feeding programmes and follow up care in case of hospitalized children.

FATS

Fats are concentrated sources of energy and thus form an essential part of our diet. They improve the palatability of food and are required for the absorption of Vitamins A, D, E and K. Dietary fats are derived from both animal sources like milk, ghee, butter, eggs, flesh foods and fish oil etc. and from vegetable sources like vegetable oils and nuts etc. Animal fats are in general poor sources of essential fatty acids but they are good sources of retinol and cholecalciferol, whereas the vegetable oils except cocount oil are rich sources of essential fatty acids.

Essential fatty acids (EFAs) include linoleic, linolenic and arachidonic acids. They are active in the promotion of growth as well as in the maintenance of dermal integrity. Their deficiency may lead to some abnormal skin conditions. Diets rich in EFAs also reduce blood cholesterol.

The nutritional significance of fats has increased due to its influence on cholesterol levels in blood. High blood level of cholesterol is one of the predisposing factors for the development of atherosclerosis leading to coronary heart disease. Epidemiological studies have shown that consumption of diets containing fats which may provide more than 50 percent of the calories can increase blood chlolesterol specially in persons leading a sedentary life.

Fatty acids are classified into saturated and unsaturated fatty acids. Fatty acids of animal origin are saturated whereas those present in groundnut oil, sessame oil, safflower oil and sunflower oil are mostly poly-unsaturated fatty acids. Vanaspati or hydrogenated vegetable fats contain high proportion of saturated fatty acids (Table 5.1).

The consumption of unsaturated fatty acids in diet can control the rise in blood cholesterol. It is now considered that the daily intake of fats should not account for more than 15-20 percent of the total calories in the diet and these should include some amount of vegetable fats which contain unsaturated fatty acids.

Table 5.1 : Percentage of Fatty Acids contents of commonly used Vegetable Oils

Vegetable oils	Saturated Fatty Acids	Monounsaturated Fatty Acids	Polyunsaturated Fatty Acids
Safflower oil	10	15	75
Sunflower-seed oil	08	27	65
Corn oil	08	27	65
Soyabeen oil	14	24	62
Cottonseed oil	25	25	50
Groundnut oil	19	50	31
Palm oil	46	44	10
Coconut oil	92	06	02
Butter	60	37	03

Blood fats are found in various forms but only two of these cholesterol and triglycerides are important from the point of view of health. In general plasma cholesterol level higher than 200 mg/100 ml plus the age of person in years and plasma triglyceride level exceeding

150 mg/100ml require medical attention. An excessively high quantity of fat in the blood vessels is likely to get deposited on the walls of the blood vessels and make them narrow. This narrowing of blood vessels is called atherosclerosis. The narrowing of coronary arteries may lead to decreased blood and oxygen supply to the myocardinm and cause diseases like angina and myocardial infarction which may be fatal unless treated immediately and cared for life time.

Hydrogenation: Hydrogenation converts the liquid oils into semi-solid and solid fats which are commonly known as "Vanaspati" and are popular cooking medium in our country. Hydrogen helps in maintaning the quality of vegetable oils even in hot and humid climates, but it drastically reduces the contents of EFAs. As vegetable oils do not contain fat soluble vitamins, these are added to the "Vanaspati" preparations by Government regulation to the extent of 2500 I.U. of Vitamin A and 175 I.U. of Vitamin D per 100 grams.

Refined oils: Refining of vegetable oils is done by treatment with steam and alkalies. It renders them free from unpleasant odour and colour and improves the taste. However, refining reduces the EFAs content of vegetable oils.

Invisible fats : Fats like butter, ghee, vegetable oils and Vanaspati are "Visible fats" as their daily intake can be estimated. On the other hand fats present in various food items like cereals, pulses, nuts, milk and milk products, meat, eggs and vegetables cannot be quantitated and hence they are called "invisible fats". In typical Indian diets the "invisible fats" provide for about 9 percent of the total calories.

OBESITY

Obesity represents an imbalance between energy intake and output resulting in a surplus of energy which is converted to fat and stored as adipose tissue. Individuals whose weight is 10-20% above the desirable weight for their age, sex and frame are defined as over-weight. When the weight exeeds 20% more than the desirable weight, a person is regarded as obese.

The association of obesity with increased morbidity and mortality rates is wellknown. Hypertension, diabetes mellitus, gall bladder disease, gout,oseto-arthritis, varicose veins, flat feet and coronary arteriosclerosis are frequently associated with obesity. There is an unexplained increase in the incidence of certain types of cancer (breast, endometrium, gall bladder, colon) in the obese individuals. Obesity also presents special hazards in pregnancy and surgical patients. An obesity-hypoventilation syndrome has been described in extremely obese individuals (Pickwickian Syndrome). (Fig. 5.3)

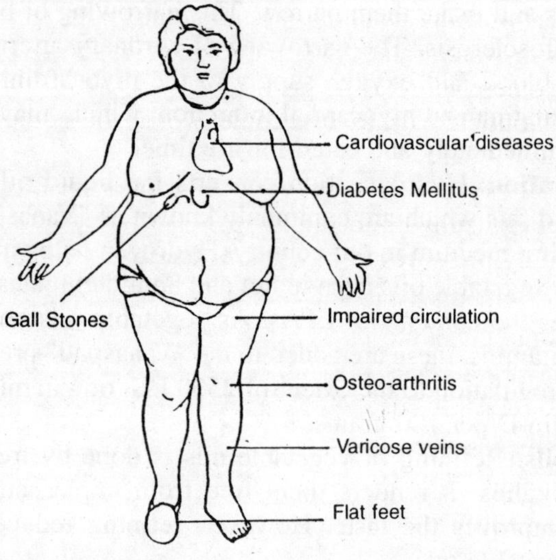

Fig. 5.3 Pickwickian Syndrome

Balancing One's Weight:

Gaining or losing weight is simply a question of balancing food calories with the body's need for calories. One kg of fat is equal to about 7500 Kcal. Thus, if you have 500 Kcal every day above what your body needs, you will gain about 0.5 kg in a week. On the other hand if your intake is 500 Kcal below your needs, you will lose about 0.5 kg in a week.

Fat deposition occurs when caloric intake exeeds caloric output. Modern living conditions contribute to the obesity problem because of several factors:

1. Family pattern of rich, high calorie foods, (mother often has reputation of being a good cook).
2. Good appetite, likes to eat, likes many rich foods, may dislike fruits and vegetables.
3. Ignorance of calorie value of foods.
4. Skips breakfast, is a frequent nibbler, coffee break with high calories snacks.
5. Pattern of living :
   (a) Sedentary occupation, idleness.
   (b) Riding to work or school.

(c) Little exercise during leisure.
(d) Less use of energy owing to mechanized instruments- lawn mower, washing machine, vacuum cleaner etc.
(e) Tends to watch rather than participates in sports.
(f) Often sleeps more as he grows older.

6. Emotional outlet: eats to overcome worry, boredom, loneliness, grief.
7. Many social events with rich foods, frequent eating in restaurants.
8. Lower metabolism with increasing age, but failure to reduce intake.
9. Influenced by pressures of advertising for many high calorie foods.

Treatment: Specific weight reducing agents and hormones (eg thyroid, chorionic gonadotropin) singly or in combination are either ineffective or hazardous and have no place in the treatment of obesity. Drugs like fenfluramine have limited value as anorexigenic agents. Juvenile onset obesity is often very difficult to treat, possibly because of unknown metabolic disorder and it is important to institute a therapeutic programme as early as possible.

Any programme of weight loss of more than a few pounds should be directed by a physician. If a weight-losing programme is to be successful, the individual must be convinced of the rewards that will come: better health, a slimmer figure, more energy, and perhaps a longer life. Although a low-calorie diet is used only so long as the weight needs to be lost, each obese person must be convinced that he needs to modify his lifetime eating habits. It he fails to do this, he will gain back all the pounds he has lost.

Diet: Diet is the most important factor in the management of obesity. Preventive education about diet should be started during the early years, at the time when eating habits are being established. The motivation to reduce caloric intake to normal levels is difficult to achieve in patients with long-standing overeating patterns. Diets that claim to offer easy weight reduction by reliance on certain special foods or unusual combinations of food not only are invalid but may actually be harmful. There are a number of basic points to be considered in planning a diet for an obese patient.

1. **Calories** — In order to lose weight, it is necessary to decrease the intake below the caloric requirements. An intake of 500 Kcal per day less than the required calories should lead to an average weight loss of approximately 0.5 kg a week. The number of calories per day to prescribe for a patient varies with age, occupation, temperament and urgency of the need for weight reduction. A daily caloric intake of 800-1200 Kcal is satisfactory for a modest

reducing diet. Complications of rapid weight reduction are largely associated with severe or prolonged caloric restriction and occur most commonly in patients who were obese as children. Weakness, postural hypotension, ketosis, metabolic acidosis, hyperuricemia, urolithiasis, ulcerative colitis, mental depression and sometimes even suicidal thoughts also occur.

2. **Protein —** A protein intake of about 1 g per kg should be maintained.
3. **Carbohydrate and fat —** To keep the calories and ketosis down, fats must be decreased. After the protein requirements have been met, the remaining calories may be supplied as half carbohydrate and half fat.
4. **Vitamins and minerals —** Vitamins and minerals be used to supply the average daily maintenance requirement during the time of weight reduction.

Table 5.2 outlines the contents of low calorie diets which should be distributed into regular meals during the day.

Table 5.2 : Low Calories Diets : Foods to be distributed into regular meals during the day

	800 kcal	1000 kcal	1200 kcal	1500 kcal
Bread, enriched white or whole-grain	1/2 slice	1 slice	2 slices	2 slices
Fruit, unsugared (1/2 cup)	3 servings	3 servings	3 servings	3 Servings
Eggs, any way but fried	One	One	One	One
Fats and oils, butter, margarine, mayonnaise, or oil	None	3 tsp	5 tsp	6 tsp
Milk (nonfat, skimmed or butter milk)	2 cups	2 cups	2 cups	2 cups
Meat, fish or poultry, any way but fried.	4 oz	5 oz	6 oz	6 oz
Vegetables, raw (salads) (1 servings = 1/2 cup)	2 servings	2 servings	2 servings	2 servings
Vegetables, cooked, green, yellow or soup (1 serving = 1/2 cup)	2 servings	2 servings	3 servings	3 servings
Starch, Potato, etc.	None	None	None	1 serving
Artificial sweetners	As desired	As desired	As desired	As desired

CARBOHYDRATES

Carbohydrates are the main sources of energy to the human body. They consist of starches, sugars and cellulose. Cereals, millets and roots and tubers used as vegetables are rich in starches and account for most of the dietary carbohydrate. Cane sugar and glucose are pure carbohydrates. Cellulose is the fibrous substance lining fruits, vegetables and cereals. Leafy vegetables, condiments and spices are also relatively rich in fibre . Dietary fibre has not been considered an important component of human diet probably because it has no nutritional value. Most of the fibre is removed from the cereals by milling, while peeling and boiling reduce the same in vegetables and fruits. Of late there has been a reawakening of interest about the useful role of dietary fibre. A wide range of diseases like constipation, colonic cancer, atherosclerosis, coronary heart disease, appendicitis and gall stones have been associated with the deficiency of dietary fibre.

Carbohydrates should provide 50-70 per cent of total caloric intake in the diet.

ENERGY METABOLISM

Energy is required for :

1. Basal metabolism (maintaining life)
2. Voluntary exercise and activity.
3. Additional needs such as growth.

Energy is derived from the oxidation of carbohydrates, fats and proteins in the diet. We measure the energy value of the foods or the energy needs of the body in units called calories or joules. The calorie or the joule is a measure of heat.

These units of energy are defined as under :

Calorie :One large calorie (kcal) is the amount of heat required to raise the temperature of 1000 g of water by 1° C. In nutrition the large calorie is always used. It is 1000 times as great as the small calorie unit used in Chemistry or Physics.

Joule :The International Unit for energy is the Joule. It is defined as the amount of heat needed to raise the temeperature of 240 g of water by 1° C. (kilojoule)

1 Kcal is equal to 4.184 Kilojoule

The energy value of food is measured in the laboratory by an instrument called a bomb calorimeter. e.g.

Carbohydrate : 4 kcal (17 kj)per gram

Fat : 9 kcal (38 kj) per gram
Protein : 4 kcal (17 kj) per gram

Thus if we know the carbohydrate, fat and protein contents of food or diet, we can calculate the caloric value.

Energy needs of the body: The body uses glycogen, sugars, fatty acids, glycerol and amino acids to supply energy. The breakdown of these substances requires numerous steps and is a very complex process. The rate of breakdown depends upon the total daily energy requirement: the basal metabolism, the amount of voluntary activity, the influence of food and the need for growth.

Basal Metabolism: Basal metabolism accounts for more than half the energy requirements of most people. It includes the involuntary activities of the body (activities over which we have no control e.g. respiration, cardiac function, circulation of blood, peristalsis, digestion, metabolic functions etc.) while at rest but awake.

The basal metabolism can be measured as Basal Metabolic Rate (BMR) . The following conditions are observed (Basal conditions).

1. The individual is awake but lying quietly in a comfortable room.
2. He is in the postabsorptive state i.e., he has had no food for 12-16 hours.
3. The body temperature is normal.
4. He is not tense or emotionally upset.

The BMR is then measured by indirect calorimetry, which is the measurement of oxygen consumption and carbon dioxide production arising from the combustion of specific nutritents. It is based on the fact that the amount of energy expended is always in direct relationship to the amount of oxygen utilised in the combustion of various food components.

In clinical practice BMR can be estimated accurately by measuring O_2 consumption of the patient for two 6 min periods under basal conditions. Thus :

O_2 Consumption per hour = Average O_2 Consumption x 10

1L of O_2 = 4.825 Kcal/hour.Convert O_2 Consumption/h into Kcal/h

$$BMR = \frac{\text{Kcal/hour}}{\text{Surface area}}$$

Surface area = Obtained from the Namogram for determining the body's surface area from height and weight.

$$= \text{K cal/m}^2\text{ /h}$$

Several factors affect the BMR: These include body size, muscle tissue, growth, age, thyroid status and climate.

Voluntary activity: Voluntary activity increases the energy requirements considerably. When calculating a person's energy needs the BMR may have to be doubled for a very active person. Under most conditions it is adequate to determine whether the individual is one whose normal life includes mainly light exercise (office workers, teachers), moderate exercise (those in light industry, nurses etc.) or heavy exercise (manual labourers).

Useful tables based on the type of activity, age and weight are available to help one determine quickly the needs of the individuals. One such table is being reproduced to determine caloric expenditure for various types of activities (Table 5.3)

VITAMINS

Vitamins are complex organic compounds required by the body in very small amounts. They are concerned with vital metabolic functions in the body, and hence essential for maintenance of health. Since vitamins cannot be manufactured in body, they have to be supplied through the diet. Vitamins are classified into two major groups:

1. **Fat Soluble Vitamins:** Vitamin A,D,E and K
2. **Water Soluble Vitamins:** Vitamin B complex and C (Ascorbic acid)

The chief functions, sources, deficiency diseases and daily requirements of vitamins are given in Table 5.4 and Table 5.5.

MINERALS

The human body consists of a number of minerals and trace elements which are required for various metabolic functions in the body. The important minerals involved are: Calcium, Phosphorus, Sodium, Potassium, Iron and Iodine.

Calcium : It is obtained from milk, cheese, eggs, green vegetables and some fish. A well-balanced diet provides adequate amount of calcium for the body's need.

Calcium in association with vitamin D and phosphorus is essential for the hardening of bone and teeth. There is no clear cut definition of signs and symptoms due to the deficiency of calcium. Children, expectant and nursing mothers require higher amount of calcium as it is needed for the growth of tissues and bones.

Phosphorus : Good sources of phosphorus are cheese, meat, liver, cereals, pulses, nuts and oil-seeds. If there is sufficient calcium in the diet, it is unlikely that there will be a deficiency of phosphorus.

Table 5.3 : Calorie Expenditure for various types of activities

Type of Activity*	Kcal per Hour
Sedentary activities, such as : Reading, writing eating, watching television or movies, listening to the radio, sewing, playing cards, and typing, miscellaneous office work ,and other activities done with sitting that require little or no arm movement.	80 to 100
Light activities, such as : Preparing and cooking food, doing dishes, dusting, handwashing small articles of clothing, ironing, walking slowly; personal care; miscellaneous office work and other activities done while standing that require some arm movement; and rapid typing and other activities done while sitting that are more strenuous.	110 to 160
Moderate activities, such as : Making beds, mopping and scrubbing, sweeping, light polishing and waxing, laundering by machine; light gardening and carpentry work; walking moderately fast; other activities done while standing that require moderate arm movement; and activities done while sitting that require more vigorous arm movement.	170 to 240
Vigorous activities, such as : Heavy scrubbing and waxing; hand-washing large articles of clothing, hanging out clothes; stripping beds; other heavy work, walking fast; bowling, golfing, and gardening	250 to 350
Strenuous activities, such as : Swimming; playing tennis, running, bicycling, dancing; ski-ing; and playing football.	350 or more

*During sleep the average caloric expenditure would range from 50 to 65 kcal per hour. These values include the basal metabolism. The lower level of calories is typical for women, the upper level is more appropriate for the average man.

L. Page, and L.J. Fincher, Food and Your Weight, Washington, D.C. Home and Garden Bulletin No. 74 U.S. Department of Agriculture, 1964 p. 4.

Table 5.4 :Summary of Fat Soluble Vitamins

Vitmin and its chemical name	Source	Functions	Deficiency Diseases	Daily Requirements (Adults)
Vitamin A Retinol	Milk,butter, cheese, egg yolk, fish liver oils, green leafy vegetables, ripe fruits, like mango, papaya, tomatoes	Maintenance of healthy epithelial tissues Proper functioning of retina and vision	Stunted growth Night blindness Xerophthalmia Keratinization	750 μ g.
Vitamin D Calciferol	Fish liver oils, milk, cheese egg yolk	Facilitates the absorption and utilization of calcium and phosphorus for healthy bones and teeth	Rickets Osteomalacia	2.5 μg.
Vitamin E Tocopherols	Egg yolk, milk, butter, green vegetables,nuts, oils of germs of cereals like wheat	Maintains healthy muscular system, anti-oxidant		8-10 mg
Vitamin K Phylloqu-inone	Cabbage, cauliflower, fish liver, fruits, leafy vegetables	Formation of Prothrombin and factors VII, IX and X in liver	Slow blood clotting, Hemorrhages in new born	70-140 g.

Bile is necessary for the absorption of fat soluble vitamins. Mineral oils reduce their absorption.

Phosphorus is associated with calcium and vitamin D in the hardening of bones and teeth and helps to maintain the constant composition of body fluids. Phosphates are essential part of systems of energy transport inside cells.

Sodium : Sodium is found in most foods specially in fish, meat,

Table 5 : Summary of Water Soluble Vitamins

Vitamin & its chemical name	Source	Function	Deficiency Diseases	Daily requirements (adults)
Vitamin B_1 Thiamine	Yeast, liver, germ of cereals, nuts, pulses, rice polishings, egg yolk, legumes	Proper utilization of carbohydrates in food, nutrition of nerve cells	General fatigue and loss of muscle tone, ultimately leads to Beri-beri	1-1.5 mg
Vitamin B_2 Riboflavin	Liver, yeast, milk, eggs, green vegetables	Necessary for tissue oxidation and growth	Angular stomatitis, cheilosis, dermatitis, eye lesions	1.5-2 mg
Vitamin B_6 Pyridoxine	Meat, liver, vegetables, bran of cereals egg yolk, beans, soyabeans	Protein metabolism, formation of RBCs and WBCs	Rarely observed	1-2 mg
Vitamin B_{12} Cyanacobalamin	Liver, milk, moulds, fermenting liquors, eggs	Maturation of RBCs	Pernicious Anemia, Degeneration of nerve fibre of spinal cord	2-3 g
Folic Acid	Dark green vegetables, liver, kidney, eggs	Formation of RBCs	Anemia	200 g
Nicotinic Acid (Niacin)	Yeast, offal, fish, pulses, wholemeal cereals, synthesized in body from tryptophan	Metabolic functions in cells necessary for tissue oxidation	Prolonged deficiency causes, pellagra i.e., dermatitis, diarrhoea, dementia	10-20mg
Pantothenic Acid	Liver, yeast, egg yolk, fresh vegetables	Formation of RBCs (Probable function)	Dermatitis, adrenal insufficiency	Unknown
Biotin	Yeast, liver, kidney, pulses, nuts	Carbohydrates, fat metabolism, growth of bacteria	dermatitis, conjunctivitis	Unknown
Vitamin C Ascorbic Acid	Citrus fruits, currants, berries, green vegetables, potatoes, liver and glandular tissues of animals	Formation and maintenance of healthy intercellular matrix, maturation of RBCs	Multiple hemorrhages, slow wound healing, anaemia, gross deficiency causes scurvy	30-45 mg

eggs, milk, artificially enriched bread and as cooking and table salt. The normal intake of sodium chloride per day varies from 5 to 20 g whereas the daily requirement is between 2 and 5 g. Excess amount is excreted in urine.

Sodium is the most commonly occurring extracellular cation and is associated with the contraction of muscle, transmission of nerve impulses in nerve fibres and the maintenance of electrolyte balance in the body.

Potassium : Potassium is to be found widely distributed in all foods. The normal intake of potassium chloride varies from 5 to 7g and this meets the body's potassium requirements.

Potassium is the most commonly occurring intracellular cation and it is involved in various chemical activities inside the cell. It also plays important role in the contraction of muscles, transmission of nerve impulses and maintenance of electrolyte balance in the body.

Iron : Iron as a soluble compound is found in green leafy vegetables, liver, kidney, egg yolk and wholemeal bread. Normal adults lose about 1 mg iron daily from the body. The normal daily diet may contain more but the amount absorbed is equal to the amount lost. Higher intake is necessary for women particularly during pregnancy.

Iron forms an important component of hemoglobin which functions as a carrier of oxygen in the blood. Iron is necessary for growing children and pregnant women and deficiency of this mineral leads to anemia. It is also necessary for tissue oxidation.

Iodine : Iodine is found in salt-water fish and in vegetables grown in soil containing iodine. In some parts of the world including India, where iodine is deficient in soil very small quantities (1 in 40,000) are added to table salt. The minimum daily requirement of iodine is 140µg. for an adult man and 100 µg for an adult woman.

Iodine is essential for the formation of thyroxine and triiodothyronine, the hormones secreted by thyroid gland. It's deficiency can lead to endemic goitre; hypothyroidism and impaired hearing and brain development.

Fluorine : Fluorine is never found free in the nature. About 96% of fluoride is found in bones and teeth. It is essential for the normal mineralization of bones and formation of dental enamel.

The main source of fluoride to man is drinking water. The fluoride content of drinking water in our country is 0.5-0.8 mg/l. The average adult man may ingest about 1 mg of fluoride from drinking water and his daily diet may provide another 0.25 to 0.35 mg of fluoride.

Fluorine is often considered a two edged sword. Ingestion of large amounts is associated with dental and skeletal fluorosis characterized by mottled enamel and osteosclerosis respectively.

On the other hand if the fluoride deficiency occurs due to less than optimum intake of fluoride, it may lead to development of dental caries. Dental caries may be prevented by fluoridation of community water suplies. The addition of fluoride to toothpastes has been a controversial issue as according to some reports it may lead to fluorosis in the long run. Fluoride levels below 0.5 mg/l in drinking water are usually associated with a high prevalence of dental caries.

Trace elements:

Apart from the above mentioned minerals, there are other elements which are required by body in very minute amount and hence they are known as trace elements.

Zinc : Zinc is present in small amounts in all the tissues and is a constituent of insulin and of many enzymes in the body. It is widely distributed in food stuffs both animal and vegetable. Daily intake in adults ranges from 5-10 mg. Low circulating zinc levels have been associated with liver disease, pernicious anemia and delayed wound healing.

Copper : Copper is widely distributed in nature. The deficiency or excess of this element is rarely observed. Copper requirement for adults is about 2 g per day. Hypocupremia is seen in patients with nephrosis, Wilson's disease and protein calorie malnutrition.

Cobalt : The only established function of cobalt in the human body is as a part of Vitamin B_{12} molecule. It may also be involved in the capture of iodine by the thyroid gland.

Other trace elements include **chromium,** which may play a role in relation to carbohydrate and insulin function, **selenium**, which is reduced in protein calorie malnutrition and **molybdenum** whose deficiency has been associated with mouth and oesophageal cancer.

6

DEMOGRAPHY AND FAMILY PLANNING

Demography and family planning—Demography cycle • fertility • family planning • contraceptive methods • behavioural methods • natural family planning methods • chemical methods • mechanical methods • hormonal contraceptives • population problem of India.

Demography is defined as the scientific study of human population. It is mainly concerned with a) changes in the population size, b) the composition of population and c) the distribution of population in space. It deals with five demographic processes namely fertility, mortality, marriage and social mobility. These processes are constantly at work within a population determining size, composition and distribution.

Demography cycle:

There are five stages of demographic cycle through which a nation passes:

1. **First Stage :** This stage is characterized by a high birth rate and a high death rate which act in aposition to each other and the population remains stationary. It is also known as high stationary stage.
2. **Second Stage :** In the "early expanding" stage death rate begins to decline while the birth rate remains unchanged.
3. **Third Stage :** This "late expanding" stage is characterized by further decline in death rate and the birth rate also falls. The population continues to grow because births exceed deaths. India appears to have entered this phase whereas in a number of countries like China and Singapore birth rates have declined rapidly.
4. **Fourth Stage :** This is the 'low stationary stage' which is characterized by low birth and low death rate with the result that

population remains stationary. Austria is one such country where zero population growth has been recorded.

5. **Fifth Stage :** This is the 'declining stage' in which the population begins to decline because the birth rate is lower than the death rate. Some East European countries like Germany and Hungary are undergoing this stage.

FERTILITY

Fertility denotes the actual bearing of children. Some demographers prefer to use the word 'natality' in place of fertility. Fertility depends on several factors. The high fertility in our country has been attributed to universality of marriage, lower age at marriage, low level of literacy, poverty, limited use of contraceptives and the traditional life styles. Some of these factors are discussed below:

1. **Age of marriage :** The age of a female at the time of marriage has a great impact on fertility. Demographic data show that females who marry before the age of 15 gave birth to a larger number of children than those who married later. Early marriage had been a long established custom in India. The child Marriage Restraint Act of 1978 raises the legal age of marriage to 18 years for girls and to 21 years for boys.
2. **Duration of married life :** It has been shown that 10-15% of all births occur within 1-5 years of married life and 50-55% of all births within 5-15 years of marriage. These data suggest that family planning efforts should be concentrated in first few years of married life.
3. **Spacing of children :** Spacing of children leads to significant reduction in fertility rates as well as it is good for the health of children already born and the mothers.
4. **Education status :** There is negative correlation between educational status of women and fertility rate. Based on a nation-wide study conducted by the Registrar General of India, the total fertility rate was 4.15 among the urban illiterate as compared 2.60 among the urban literate.
5. **Economic status :** Economic status also bears an inverse relationship with fertility. Economic development leading to increase in per capita expenditure of the household takes care of population growth and brings about reductions in fertility.
6. **Religion and Caste :** Muslims have higher fertility rate than Hindus and Hindus have higher fertility rate than the Christians.

Amongst Hindus the lower castes seem to have a higher fertility rates than the higher castes.

7. Nutritional status : Nutritional status has an indirect effect on the fertility rate. Well nourished societies have lower fertility than the poorly rourished societies who have high fertility.
8. Family planning : Family planning plays an important role in the reduction of fertility rate. In most of the developing countries family planning has been greatly responsible for declining fertility.

FAMILY PLANNING

An Expert Committee of World Health Organization (W.H.O.) in 1971 defined family planning as "a way of thinking and living that is adopted voluntarily, upon the basis of knowledge, attitudes and responsible decisions by individuals and couples, in order to promote the health and welfare of the family group and thus contribute effectively to the social development of a country.

Another Expert Committee of WHO in the same year came forward with a more precise and to the point definition of Family Planning as given below.

"Family planning refers to practices that help individuals or couples to attain certain objectives:

(a) to avoid unwanted births.
(b) to bring about wanted births
(c) to regulate the intervals between pregnancies.
(d) to control the time at which births occur in relation to the ages of the parent.
(e) to determine the number of children in the family.

Basic Human Right :

The United Nations Conference on Human Rights in 1968 recognized family planning as a basic human right. The World Conference of the International Women's Year in 1975 also declared the right of women to decide freely and responsibly on the number and spacing of their children and to have access to the information and means to enable them to exercise that right.

The Scope of Family Planning:

Family planning should not be taken as only synonymous with birth control. According to WHO family planning includes the following in its purview.

1. The proper spacing and limitation of births.
2. Advice on sterility.
3. Eduction for parenthood.
4. Sex education.
5. Screening for pathological conditions related to the reproductive system.
6. Genetic counselling.
7. Premarital consultation and examination.
8. Carrying out pregnancy test.
9. Marriage counselling.
10. The preparation of couples for the arrival of their first child.
11. Providing services to unmarried mothers.
12. Teaching home economics and nutrition.
13. Providing adoption services.

These activities may vary from country to country in accordance with the national objectives and policies with respect to family planning.

Family Planning and Health :

Family planning has direct effect on the health of the mother, foetus, infant and the children. These can be summarized as under:

Mothers health

Decrease in maternal mortality and morbidity.
Improves nutritional status.
Prevents complications of pregnancy and abortion.

Foetal health

Decrease in foetal mortality and abnormal development of foetus.

Infant and child health

Better health of the infant at birth
Decrease in vulnerability to diseases.
Decrease in preschool mortality.

CONTRACEPTIVE METHODS

A number of scientifically tested and reliable methods of contraception are available now. These make it possible for a couple to avoid having a baby unless they want to. In an intimate and personal matter like this, individual preferences vary and only they are the best judge of what is most suitable for them and perhaps most acceptable at a particular period of time. They may find different methods suitable at different stages of their life. The various birth control methods available to couples at present are summarized below. It must be remembered that it is necessary to consult a gynaecologist before adopting some to these methods of family planning. It is also necessary to understand the basic physiology of reproduction before the methods of contraception are discussed.

The sex glands of man (testes) produce sperms, while the sex glands of women (ovaries) produce ova, when the male sperm and woman's ova join together inside the woman's body, fertilization occurs and a new life begins to grow.

The woman produces ovum once every four weeks and this process is called ovulation. The ovum pass through the woman's fallopian tubes towards the uterus. At about this time an ova is met by a male sperm following the sexual inter-course; it can get fertilized and pregnancy can take place.

From the time a girl starts ovulating i.e. from the age of 12 or so until she is well past 45, her uterus grows a new lining with blood in about 28 days. If no ova is fertilized, this wall lining breaks up and slowly leaves the vagina. This shedding of lining and the blood is called menstruation. After the menstrual period is over, the uterus starts growing a new lining and the ovaries produce another lot of ovum. However, once an ova is fertilized, then no further ovum are released by the ovary and there is no menstruation until well after the childbirth. The period between the onset of menstruation (12-14 years) and it's stoppage (45-50 years) is called the reproductive span of a woman's life, i.e. the period during which she can bear a child.

The male sperms produced by testes pass through the spermatic duct and mix with the fluids produced by seminal vesicles and prostate glands. This is called semen. At the time of sexual climax, the semen which contains sperms, is ejaculated from the penis into the vagina. The sperms from the semen swim up to the uterus, where one of them can possibly meet an ova and fertilize it. The fertilized ova then grows into a baby inside the woman's womb i.e. uterus. (Fig. 6.1)

The family planning methods prevent this meeting of the sperm and

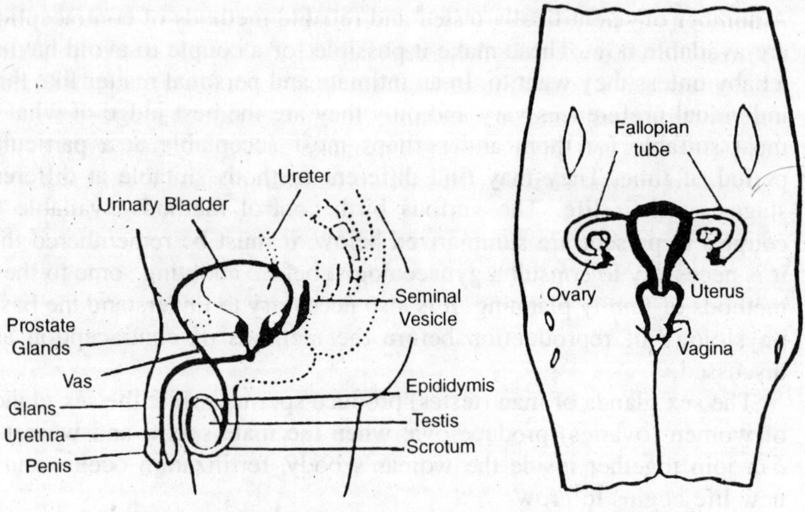

Fig. 6.1 Male and Female reproductive systems

ova to avoid pregnancy. These methods have been divided into following broad categories.

(a) Behavioural methods.
(b) Natural methods.
(c) Chemical methods.
(d) Mechanical methods.
(e) Hormonal contraceptives.
(f) Post-conceptional methods.

(A) BEHAVIOURAL METHODS

(i) **Abstinence :** This is the only fool proof method which is 100% effective. However, it amounts to repression of natural physiological instinct which may manifest in temperamental changes and nervous breakdown. Hence, this methods cannot be advocated to the masses.

(ii) **Coitus interruptus :** It is the oldest method of voluntary fertility control. In this method the male withdraws before ejaculation and thereby tries to prevent the deposition of semen into vagina. It has limited appeal and usefulness.

(iii) **Safe period :** This is also known as the calendar method. It is based on the fact that ovulation occurs from 12 to 16 days before the onset of menstruation. The couple is advised to avoid intercourse from 10th to 18th day of the menstrual cycle counting from the 1st day of the menstrual period. This is not a very reliable method as a woman's menstrual cycles are not always regular, and only educated and responsible couples with high degree of motivation and cooperation can make it work effectively. The following chart clarifies the safe and unsafe periods.

Safe and risky periods for family planning by calender method (For 28 days regular menstrual cycle)

		1	2	3	4	5
6	7	8	9	10	11	12
13	14	15	16	17	18	19
20	21	22	23	24	25	26
27	28					

Day 1 to day 5 denote the days of menstrulation
Day 6 to day 9 denote safe period, conception cannot occur.
Day 10 to day 18 denote unsafe period, conception can occur.
Day 19 to day 28 denote safe period, conception cannot occur.

(B) NATURAL FAMILY PLANNING METHODS

The principle underlying these methods is the same as that of calendar method. However, these methods are more objective as they depend on the self-recognition of certain physiological signs and symptoms by the women. These symptoms are correlated with the event of ovulation and thus ascertain the beginning of fertile period, during which sexual intercourse can be avoided by the couple. These include following 3 methods.

(i) **Basal body temperature method :** The basal body temperature shows a rise of 0.3 to 0.5^0C at the time of ovulation which is due to increased production of progesterone. The temperature is measured before getting out of bed in the morning. This method is reliable if intercourse is restricted to the postovulatory infertile period which starts 3 days after the ovulatory temperature rise and continues upto the beginning of menstrual cycle. Total abstinence is necessary for the entire preovulatory period.

(ii) **Cervical mucus method :** As ovulation starts cervical mucus becomes watery clear, resembling raw egg white, smooth, slippery and profuse. After ovulation it thickens and lessens in quantity. The woman uses a tissue paper to wipe the inside of the vagina and assesses the characteristic of mucus. This method can be used only by intelligent and motivated woman who can distinguish between different type of mucus.

(iii) **Symptothermic method :** In this method the physiological symptoms of rise in basal temperature, characteristics of mucus and the estimation of safe period can be combined and the woman can have a double check of her interpretation of the infertile period.

(C) CHEMICAL METHODS

Chemical contraceptives contain a base into which a spermicrde is incorporated. The commonly used spermicides are "surface active agents" which on contact inhibit oxygen uptake and kill the male sperms deposited in the woman's body during intercourse. The spermicides should be introduced in the vagina just 15 minutes before the intercourse.

Foam tablet:

The foam tablets are inserted by the woman into her birth canal before having sexual intercourse. Some foam is produced after the insertion which provides protective coating to the whole area and kills the sperm released during intercourse and thus prevents pregnancy. (Fig. 6.2).

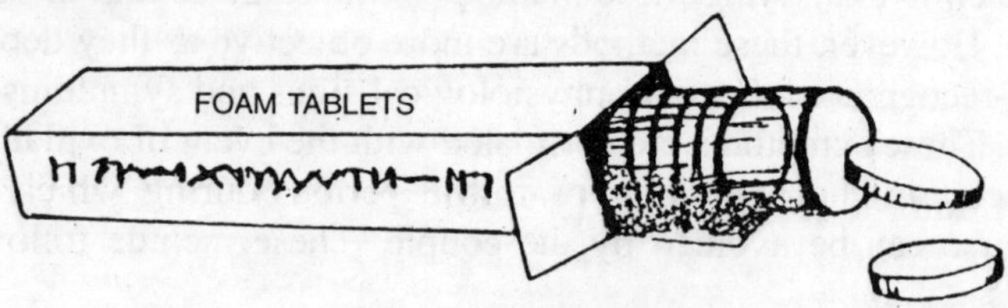

Fig. 6.2 Foam Tables

Jelly/cream/paste :

The spermicidal jelly, cream or paste is similary applied in the vagina with the help of an applicator. These preparations destroy the male sperms on contact in the vaginal canal itself (Fig. 6.3).

The spermicidal creams etc. are effective if used alongwith a diaphragm or Nirodh. Their main drawback are :

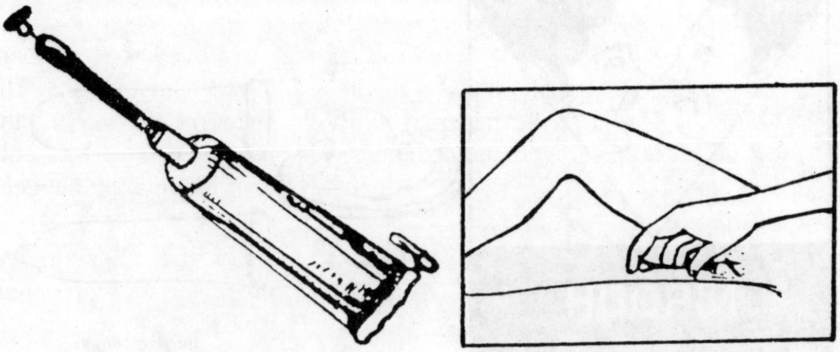

Jelly Cream tube with applicator

How to apply Jelly Cream

Fig. 6.3 Jelly cream and its application

(a) They have a high failure rate
(b) Being coitus-related procedures many couples find them cumbersome to use.
(c) They may cause mild burning or irritation.
(d) They are not fool-proof unless used in conjunction with a barrier method.

(D) MECHANICAL METHODS

A number of physical methods suitable for both men and women are now available. They function by preventing the live sperm from meeting the ovum. They have become quite popular because of the absence of any side effects and because they also afford protection from sexually transmitted diseases, cause reduction in the incidence of pelvic inflammatory disease and protection from the risk of cervical cancer. Thee methods include:

(a) **Condom or Nirodh:** The condom is an extremely thin rubber sheath used by the man. The Government of India have made available 3 brands of Nirodh;
  (i) Dry Nirodh
  (ii) Deluxe Nirodh which is a lubricated condom.
  (iii) Super-Delux Nirodh which is of thinner variety (0.03–0.04 mm), lubricated and coloured. (Fig. 6.4)

The condom is unrolled on the erect male sex organ before inter-

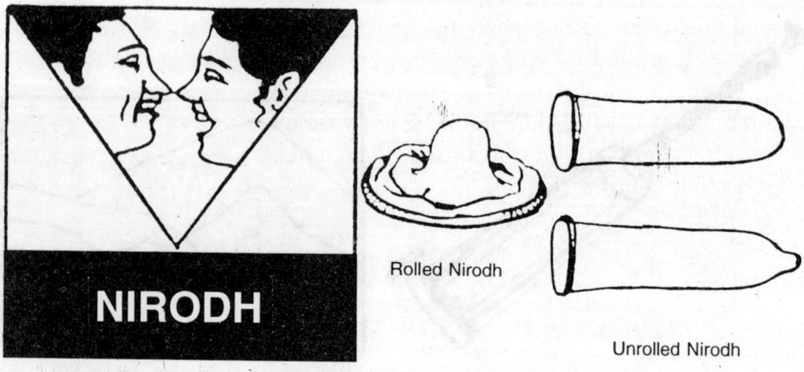

Fig. 6.4 Nirodh or Condom

course. As it covers the penis, the sperms cannot go inside the woman's body. While unrolling it on the male sex organ, a little space should be left at the end so that the fluid after discharge can spill into it. A new condom should be used for each sexual act. At the end of the intercourse the male must make sure to carefully withdraw his sex organ with the condom still in place to avoid spilling of semen into the vagina. The effectiveness of a condom can be increased by using it in conjunction with a spermicidal jelly or cream. The advantages of condom are that the are:

(a) Simplest, most effective and easily available.
(b) Easy to use, do not require medical supervision or consultation.
(c) Free of side effects.
(d) Protective against sexually transmitted diseases.
(e) Light, compact and disposable.
(f) Discontinued whenever a couple desires to have a child.

Their drawbacks are few as in rare cases an individual may be sensitive to rubber or they may tear off or slip during intercourse. a few couple complain that the rubber sheath interferes with the natural sexual sensation.

(b) **Diaphragm:** The diaphragm is a vaginal barrier. Also known as "Dutch cap" the diaphragm is a thin shallow rubber cap which is shaped like a dome with a spring in its ring. It ranges in diameter from 5 to 10 cm. The diaphragm is inserted before sexual intercourse and must remain in place for not less than 6 hour after sexual intercourse. It prevents pregnancy in a very simple way. The diaphragm blocks the opening of the womb with the result that the sperms cannot find their way towards the womb and no pregnancy can take place. To be most effective, a small amount of the jelly is smeared around the edge of the diaphragm and on both sides, and a teaspoon of the same is placed inside the cup. Because the diaphragm is to fit the vagina. Each woman has to take the proper size from a doctor who would also teach her how to fix and remove it so that later on she can do it herself. (Fig.6.5).

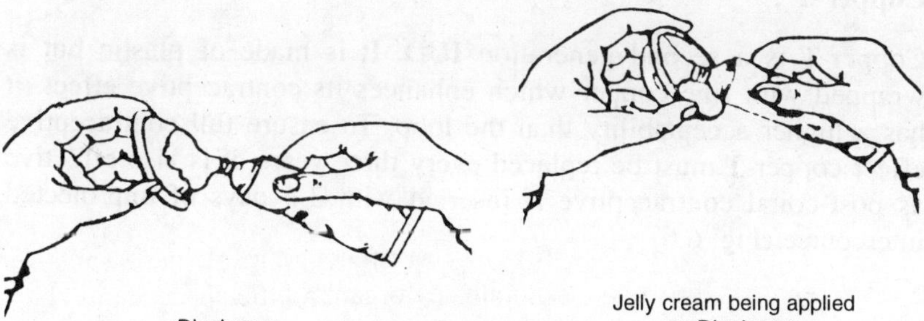

Diaphragm

Jelly cream being applied on Diaphragm

Fig. 6.5 Diaphragm

Diaphragm is a reversible non-invasive method and it does not interfere with sexual act. There is no risk associated with its use and there are no medical contraindications.

In rare cases an individual may be sensitive to rubber. If not used properly, the failure rate may be quite high. It also needs elaborate preparation before the sexual act, it has to be removed and washed each time after sexual act and a high standard of hygiene is necessary for its storage and use failing which it can be source of infection.

Intra-uterine devices (IUDs):

Intra-uterine devices are placed inside the uterus for the prevention of pregnancy. There are two basic types of IUDs: nonmedicated and medicated. both are usually made of polyethylene. The medicated IUDs release either metal ions (e.g., copper) or hormones (progestagens). The nonmedicated IUDs are often referred to as "first generation IUDs". "Second generation IUDs" comprise of copper IUDs and the "third generation IUDs" include the hormone releasing IUDs. The medicated IUDs have been developed to minimize the side effects and to enhance the contraceptive effectiveness.

Lippes Loop:

The loop is a small double 'S' shaped flexible device of fine polyethylene material that is nontoxic, nontissue reactive and extremely durable, and about one and a half inches in length. It has attached threads or 'tail' made of fine nylon, which project in to the vagina after insertion. The tail is easily felt by the user, reassures her that the loop is in place and makes it easy to remove the loop when desired.

Copper-T :

Copper-T is a second generation IUD. It is made of plastic but is wrapped with fine copper which enhances its contraceptive effect. it has a higher acceptability than the loop. To ensure full contraceptive effect copper-T must be replaced every three years. it is also effective as post-coital contraceptive if inserted with 3-5 days of unprotected intercourse (Fig. 6.6).

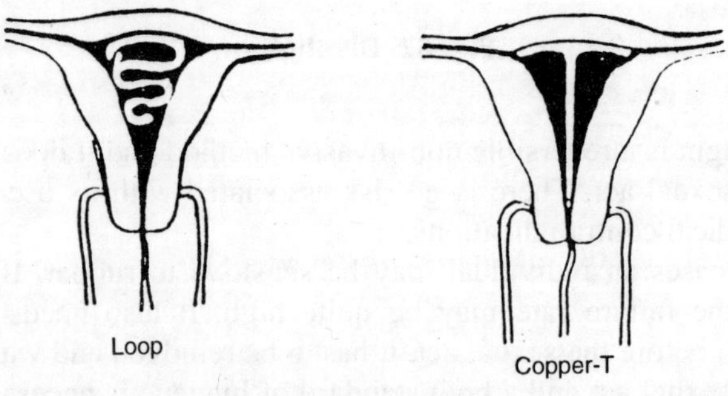

Fig. 6.6 Copper T and loop

Progestasert:

This is the most widely used third generation hormonal contraceptive. It is a T-shaped device filled with progesterone, the natural hormone. The hormone is released slowly in the uterus at a rate of 65 μg daily. It has direct local effect on the uterine lining and cervical mucus. As the hormone supply is gradually depleted, regular replacement of the device is necessary. Another long active hormonal IUD has recently been introduced. It releases 20 μg of levonorgestral daily, shows a low pregnancy rate 0.3 per 100 women, less menstrual blood loss and an effective life of 5 years.

Mechanism of action of IUDs:

Nonmedicated IUDs cause a foreign body reaction in the uterus causing cellular and biochemical changes in the endometrium and uterine fluids and these changes impair the viability of the gamete and thus reduce its chances of fertilization.

Copper seems to enhance the cellular response in the endometrium and affects the enzymes in the uterus, thus by altering the biochemical composition of cervical mucus, copper ions may affect sperm motility and its survival.

The hormone releasing devices increase the viscosity of cervical mucus and thereby prevent sperm from entering the cervix. They also maintain high levels of progesterone in the endometrium and render it unfavourable for implantation.

Advantages :

The IUDs have many advantages:

(i) Simple devices, insertion does not require hospitalization.
(ii) Do not interfere with the sexual act and their presence is not felt.
(iii) It is a reversible method, can be easily removed when a couple desire their next child.
(iv) Its failure rate is almost nil.
(v) Virtually free from systemic side effects.
(vi) Highest acceptability and continuation rate.
(vii) There is no need for continuous motivation.

Drawback:

(i) Side effects such as heavier bleeding, backache and abdominal cramps have been reported in some cases. These complaints however, invariably disappear after a few days or weeks.
(ii) This method is not advised for delaying the first pregnancy.
(iii) Sometimes the device is automatically expelled.

(E) HORMONAL CONTRACEPTIVES

Hormonal contraceptives are the most effective spacing methods of contraception. Combined oral contraceptive pills are almost 100% effective in preventing pregnancy. They are the best means of ensuring a desired gap between one childbirth to another. Apart from the combined pill the other hormonal contraceptive preparations include, progester one only pill, post-coital pill, once-a-month pill and injectables and subdermal implants. However, none of them have received wide acceptance and they have number of drawbacks.

The Combined Pill:

The combined pill is the most successful spacing method of contraception. At present most formulations of the combined pill contain 30-35 μg of a synthetic estrogen and 0.5 to 1.0 mg of a progestagen.

The pill is taken orally for 21 consecutive days beginning on the 5th day of the menstrual cycle, followed by a break of 7 days during which period the menstruation occurs. Even if the bleeding (menstrual) does not occur, the woman is advised to start the next course of pills one week after the preceding one.

The regularity is the most important aspect which ensures the high efficacy of this method. However, if a pill is missed on a particular day, the missed tablet should be taken as soon as possible and the next day's pill should be taken at the usual time. The pill must be taken every day at fixed time, preferably before going to bed.

The pill is prescribed by a doctor after proper medical examination of a woman and following a well defined guide line. The pill should not be prescribed if the woman is:

(i) already pregnant
(ii) over 35 years of age
(iii) has either diabetes or a family history of diabetes
(iv) has had jaundice during the last six months
(v) has cancer of the breast or genital organs or
(vi) is breast feeding a child

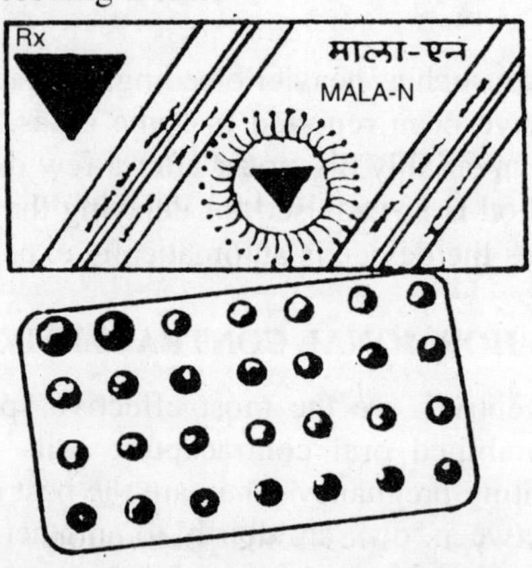

Fig. 6.7 Hormonal combined pill

Advantages of combined pill :

(i) It is a reversible method of family planning, ii) If taken regularly, it is 100% effective, iii) It is not coitus-related and hence does not interfere with the normal sexual life of the couple, iv) It corrects pre-existing menstrual problems, or irregular cycles, v) Because of regular medical check-ups, early detection of breast and cervical cancers become possible.

Drawbacks :

As the combined pill acts by inhibiting the ovulation, it can simulate in some women the signs and symptoms of early pregnancy. This is more so in the initial starting period. The complaints of dizziness, weight gain, vomiting, sickness and usually tenderness of breasts are generally noted which disappear within 3-4 months. Sometimes there may be irregular vaginal bleeding. The pill is not to be used by women over 35 years particularly so if they are smokers.

Terminal methods :

The methods, discussed so far, are useful for delaying the first pregnancy or for ensuring a reasonable gap between two children. The terminal methods are used after the family is complete and they put an end to the need for contraceptives or other methods.

Operation for sterilisation of either the husband or the wife provides permanent protection against pregnancy and the couple can then enjoy married life without fear of pregnancy. Following four methods are considered for this purpose.

(i) **Vasectomy :** Vasectomy of the male is very simple outpatient surgical procedure which takes about 20 minutes. Small cut equal to the size of a grain of wheat is made above the man's scrotum on both the sides. On each side a small portion of the vas deferens is removed, and the cut ends are tied up. The male's sex glands are not touched. This operation does not affect the strength or virility of the person and he continues with his normal sex life. He ejaculates but now his semen does not contain sperms.

Advantages :

Vasectomy is a very simple surgical procedure, it is hundred percent effective and provides life long protection against unwanted

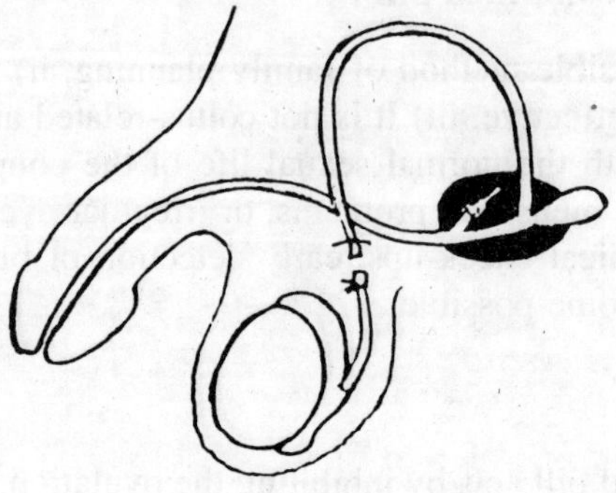

Fig. 6.8 Vasectomy

pregnancies. There are no side effects and complications associated with this procedure when performed under aseptic conditions and adequate care is taken to see that the wound doesn't get infected till it completely heals.

Drawbacks :

Though in some cases surgical recanalization has been successfully done, for all practical purposes this method should be accepted as irreversible.

Tubectomy:

In this sterilization procedure of the female, the surgeon removes a small piece of each fallopian tube and the cut ends are tied-up to block the passage of ovum. Following this procedure the ova will not be able to meet the sperm during the sexual intercourse and no pregnancy will take place. For tubectomy the female has to remain in the hospital for 2-3 days and will need a few days rest after the operation (Fig.6.9)

Laparascopy :

Now the female sterilization has become very simple by the use of a modern instrument called laparascope. It resembles a telescope and is introduced in the abdomen through a very small opening of hardly an inch. This procedure requires hospitalization for only a few hours. This operation is undertaken only in those centres where specialist obstetrician-gynaecologists are available. The abdomen is inflated with

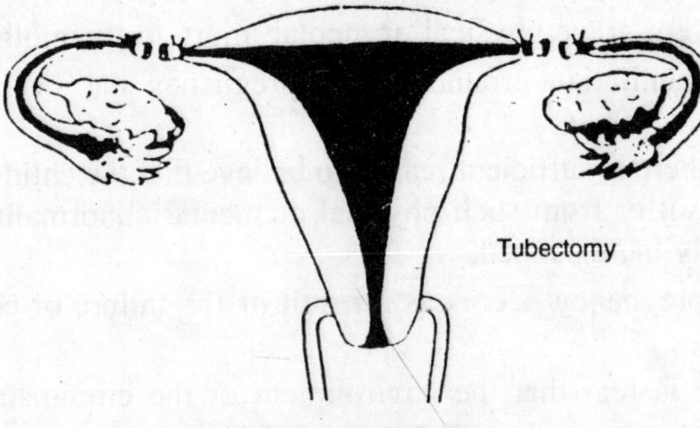

Fig. 6.9 Tubectomy

a gas or air, and as the fallopian tubes become visible and accessible, the falope rings or clips are applied to occlude them.

Laparoscopy and tubectomy provide permanent safeguard against unwanted pregnancies and there are no side effect or complications when performed by a competent surgeon (Fig. 6.10).

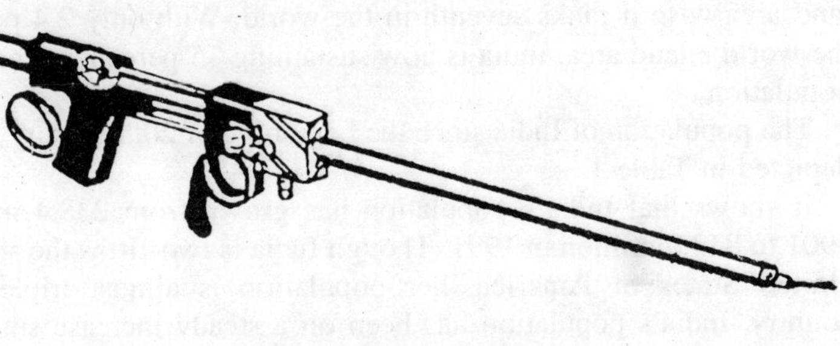

Fig. 6.10 Laparoscope

MEDICAL TERMINATION OF PREGNANCY (MTP)

MTP should never be used as a method of family planning as repeated termination of pregnancy is harmful to the woman. However, when pregnancy occurs as a result of a failure of contraceptive measures taken by the couple, and a woman does not want to continue with it, she has full right to seek its termination before 12 weeks under the Medical Termination of Pregnancy Act, 1971.

MTP is comparatively easy and safe when performed within 12 weeks of pregnancy by a qualified medical practitioner. Under the Medical Termination of Pregnancy Act, 1971, MTP is done free of charge in all public hospitals under the following conditions:

(i) To save the life of a pregnant woman.

(ii) To prevent grave physical or mental injury to the mother.

(iii) On humanitarian grounds when pregnancy has been caused by rape.

(iv) When there is sufficient reason to believe that the child to be borne, would suffer from such physical or mental abnormalities as to be seriously handicapped.

(v) When pregnancy occurs as a result of the failure of contraceptive measures.

(vi) If there is fear that the environment or the circumstances of the pregnant woman may cause injury to her health.

MTP should be done as early as possible and only in an officially recognized hospital and by well qualified and trained doctors. There are usually no complications after MTP and normal routine work can be assumed from the third day onwards.

POPULATION PROBLEM OF INDIA

India is the second most populous country of the world whereas total land area wise it ranks seventh in the world. With only 2.4 percent of the world's land area, India is now sustaining 15 percent of the world's population.

The population of India since the beginning of 20th century has been depicted in Table-1.

It shows that India's population has grown from 238.4 million in 1901 to 843.9 million in 1991. Though India is two-fifths the size of the United States of America, her population is almost triple of that country. India's population has been on a steady increase since 1921. The year 1921 is called the 'big divide' because the absolute number of people during each decade has been on the increase since 1921.

At the time of our independence in 1947 we were 344 million people living in India. within a period of 34 years after independence we added a second India to our population and we were 685 million in 1981. According to the population projection prepared by the Registrar General, Government of India, our country's population would be between 959 and 1053 million at the turn of the century.

The other parameters related to population are being discussed briefly.

(a) **Birth rate :** The world's birth rate fell below 30 per thousand for the first time around 1975 and had declined to 27.3 during 1980-85. This decline reflects a global trend toward smaller families. The outstanding examples are Singapore and China. In Singapore in 25 years the birth rate fell from 38 in 1960 to 17 in 1985 an in China from 36 to 18 during the same period. In India the birth rate fell from 43 in 1960 to 32.7 in 1985.

Table 6.1 Population of India 1901-1994

Census Year	Total Population in millions
1901	238.4
1911	252.1
1921	251.3
1931	279.4
1941	318.7
1951	361.1
1961	439.2
1961	439.2
1971	548.2
1981	685.2
1988	792.0
1991	843.9
1994	906.5

(b) **Density of Population :** Population density has increased by 23.6 percent over the last decade from 216 to 267 per sq.km. This density of population is considered high relating to the present state of our economic development.

(c) **Family size :** The completed family size indicates the total number of children borne by a woman upto the age of her child bearing. The total fertility rate (TFR) gives the approximate magnitude of completed family size. The total fertility rate recorded in 1985 shows TFR of 4.5 for India which is much higher as compared to 1.8 in U.K., U.S.A and Japan and 1.5 in Switzerland.

(d) **Life Expectancy :** Life expectancy is one of the best indicators of a country's level of development and overall health status of its population. The life expectancy at birth range from 40 years in some of the least developed countries to 75-80 years in most developed countries. The world's average is estimated at 61 years. One of the goals of the "Health For All by 2000 AD" is the attainment of life expectancy of 64 years at birth for both males and females. The 1985 figures show a life expectancy of 57 for males and 51 for females in India which is only higher than the life expectancy rates of countries like Nepal, Bhutan and Bangladesh.

National Demographic Goals:

India has adopted a long term demographic goal for reducing the Net Reproduction Rate to one by the year 2000. The implications of this goal have been spelt out as under :

(a) The average size of the family would be reduced from 4.2 children in 1985 to 2-3 children.

(b) The birth rate per thousand population would be reduced to 21 from 32.7 in 1985

(c) The death rate per thousand population would be reduced to 9 from 11.7 prevailing in 1985.

(d) The infant mortality rate would be reduced to 60 or less.

If these goals are achieved, the population of India would be around 950 million by the turn of the century. It may be noted here that we have already crossed the 906 million mark before September, 1994.

7

FUNDAMENTAL PRINCIPLES OF MICROBIOLOGY

Characteristics and classification of microbes • isolation and staining techniques • organisms producing common diseases

Microbiology can be defined as the study of living organisms of microscopic size which include bacteria, fungi, algae, protozoa and viruses. It is concerned with their morphology, physiology, metabolism, reproduction and classification. Microbes are closely associated with the health and welfare of human beings. Some of them are beneficial and others are harmful to man. On one hand they are involved in the making of yoghart, cheese and wine, in the production of penicillins, interferon and alcohol and in the processing and recycling of domestic and industrial wastes, while on the other hand they can cause serious and at times life threatening diseases, and deterioration of food and other useful materials. Microbiology has therefore become increasingly important to our society and has emerged as one of the most important branches of the life sciences. In order to fully understand and appreciate the science of microbiology, it is worthwhile reviewing the important historical aspects relating to the development of this subject.

Recognition of organisms as cause of disease :

The idea that diseases may be caused and transmitted by living organisms was first put forward by Fracastoro of Verona in the early 16th century but no experimental evidence was recorded to substantiate it. The first report of a direct observation is credited to a monk Athanasius Kircher (1659) who reported the presence of minute worm like structures in the blood of patients suffering from plague.

The microscope:

Microbiology began when people learned to grind lenses from pieces of glass and combine them to produce magnifications great enough for the study of microbes. Antony van Leeuwenhoek was the first to develop a microscope and report his observations with accurate descriptions and drawings in 1677. It was he who first saw microbes and called them "animalcules".

Louis Pasteur (1822-1895)

It was in the latter years of 19th century that special organisms were recognised as the causative agents of contagious diseases by Louis Pasteur. He suggested that infection was due to micro-organisms that multiplied in the host producing disease and that each disease was caused by a particular organism. He also established the role of micro-organisms in the process of fermentation and showed that by proper selection of the microbes the manufacturer can be assured of consistently good and uniform products.

Variation in susceptibility to disease and variation in virulence were two important discoveries made by Pasteur. He isolated the bacterium responsible for chicken cholera and grew it in culture. He found that when he injected several weeks old culture to chicken, they failed to get sick and die. He reported that bacteria could lose their ability to produce disease i.e., their virulence after standing and growing old. But these attenuated (having decreased virulence) bacteria still retained their capacity for stimulating the host to produce substances i.e., antibodies, that protect against subsequent exposure to virulent organisms. He called the attenuated cultures as vaccines.

He applied this principle to the prevention of anthrax and developed a vaccine against it. Later on Pasteur also developed a vaccine for another deadly disease known as hydrophobia or rabies, which is transmitted by bites of dogs, cats and other animals.

Robert Koch (1843-1910)

Koch found small rod like structures in the blood of animals that had died of anthrax. These were not present in the blood of healthy animals and were the actual cause of anthrax. He discovered that under certain conditions small oval bodies appeared inside the anthrax organisms and these structures, known as spores were not affected by drying or storage. When transferred to suitable medium these spores developed into ordinary cells which then multiplied rapidly. He also found that spores were never present in the body of an infected animal during life but developed shortly after its death while the body was still warm. Spores from dead carcasses remained viable in the soil for months, ready to germinate when they gained access to healthy animals. He introduced a new method of fighting epidemics when it was not possible to burn the carcasses immediately after death; namely immediate burial deep in the soil where temperature would be low enough to kill the ordinary form of bacterium before the formation of resistant spores could take place.

Koch further refined the methods for the study of bacteria in order to obtain isolated growths of organisms known as colonies, each of which contained millions of individual bacterial cells packed tightly together. From these colonies pure cultures could be transferred to other media using the improvised techniques. Koch studied with painstaking care the material taken from patients with pulmonary tuberculosis. After performing a number of rigid tests, he announced the discovery of the organism that causes tuberculosis, which is also called as Koch's bacillus.

Koch, Pasteur and their other associates attempted to find curative or preventive measures against various infective diseases. Koch showed how infection spreads (e.g., anthrax by the formation of resistant spores soon after the death of the animal and cholera through water polluted by fecal matter) and indicated the modes of checking these diseases. Pasteur showed that immunity could be produced against certain diseases by injecting the causative organism in an attenuated form. Further researches led to the discovery of safer and effective measures of acquiring immunity and combating the infection already present in a host. The different vaccines, antitoxins and toxoids used for the prevention of a number of infective diseases have been discussed elsewhere in this book.

Joseph Lister (1872-1912)

Prior to the discoveries of Pasteur and Koch that diseases were caused by microbes, surgery was performed without any precautions to prevent infection. Collins in Dublin and Semmelweis in Vienna had shown that puerperal fever could be transferred by midwives and obstetricians and controlled by cleaning the hand with bleach between examinations of patients. Conditions that proved fatal to patients after surgery were septicemia, gas-gangrene and tetanus. Pasteur established that gas-gangrene was a fermentation caused by airborne microbes gaining access to wounds. Lister lost more than 40% of his post-operative patients before he used a dilute solution of phenol (carbolic acid) to soak surgical dressings. Wounds protected in this way did not become infected and healing took placc rapidly. Lister's success was so remarkable that the technique was quickly accepted and the system he developed became known as Listerian system of antiseptic surgery and later established the principles of present-day antiseptic techniques. Nowadays all the equipment that can be subjected to heat safely is sterilized by wet heat in an autoclave or dry heat in an oven and only the skin of the patient, surgeons and nurses is sterilized by chemical means.

Paul Ehrlich (1854-1915)

In spite of the above-mentioned advances made in the new science of bacteriology, some infections could not be treated by the methods that had proved so successful with diphtheria, anthrax and tetanus. Satisfactory antisera against malaria, tuberculosis and syphilis could not be produced. Hence other methods of treating these diseases were sought. Paul Ehrlich who is now known as the Father of Modern Chemotherapy, was first to make progress in this direction. While studying aspects of diphtheria, Ehrlich was surprised by the body's ability to generate antibodies which were specific to particular infective organisms. He was determined to find synthetic chemical substances which like antibodies, would destroy organisms and yet be comparatively nontoxic to hosts.

In 1891, Ehrlich and an associate successfully treated malaria with methylene blue and then they turned their attention to the treponemas responsible for syphilis. Arsenical compounds were known to be effective against trypanosomes responsible for sleeping sickness but the preparation used, called Atoxyl was liable to damage optic nerve. Ehrlich applied arsenical compounds to treponemas and introduced arsphenamine (Salvarsan) in 1910 for the treatment of syphilis. Later on other arsenicals like neoarsphenamine, carbarsone and acetarsol etc. were also added to the list of antisyphilitic arsenic compounds. Ehrlich's work led to intensive efforts to find chemotherapeutic agents for other diseases, like stibophen, an organic antimony compound for the treatment of kalazar, cloquinol for amoebic dysentry and crystal violet, brilliant green and other derivatives for the prevention of pyogenic cocci in wounds and burns, and for treating fungal diseases like tinea pedis.

Subsequent progress in chemotherapy was very slow. Close co-operation between chemists and biologists was difficult to arrange. Pharmaceutical companies were still immature and the drug development occurred either as a byproduct of scientific investigations or as a part of the development of industrial chemistry. Till 1935 only a few compounds were available for chemotherapeutic use which included quinine for malaria, emetine for amoebiasis, arsenical and antimony compounds for syphilis, amoebiasis and kalazar etc.

The situation changed in the mid 1930s when Gerhard Domagk announced the discovery of Prontosil a diazo dye which was capable of destroying hemolytic streptococci in mice. This was followed by the introduction of a number of sulpha drugs like sulphapyridine (M&B 693) sulphathiazole, sulphadiazine, sulphacetamide, sulphathiazole and a host of other sulphonamides which have specific chemotherapeutic uses. The discovery of penicillin and subsequent families of antibiotics further enlarged the scope of chemotherapeutic attack. Penicillin was first identified by Sir Alexander Fleming in 1928 and proved to be one of the most effective chemotherapeutic agents of all, with demonstrated effectiveness against most pus forming cocci as well as pneumococcus, gonococcus, meningococcus, anthrax, diphtheria bacterium, tetanus and syphilis. However, it became available for widespread clinical use only in the mid 1940s. A further weapon was added in 1944 by Selman A. Waksman when he isolated streptomycin from a fungus **Streptomyces griseus.** This substance proved effective against the tubercle bacillus and with other compounds, it opened the way to an ultimately successful chemotherapy leading to complete cure of tuberculosis in most of the patients. Eighteen years later Selman A. Waksman was present alongside Pandit Jawaharlal Nehru when the first streptomycin plant in India was inaugurated at the Hindustan Antibiotics Ltd. Pimpri in 1962. Paul Ehrlich, Gerhard Domagk, Sir Alexander Fleming and Selman A Waksman were awarded Nobel Prizes for their contributions to Chemotherapy.

At present, chemotherapy is one of the most active fields of medicine. Research aims not only at developing new drugs and discovering new therapeutic substances but also at learning more about the action of established drugs. Apart from toxic effects, the sulphonamides, the antibiotics and penicillin have all been reduced in effectiveness by the development of bacterial strains which are immune (resistant) to the drugs' actions. Combinations of drugs can counter some immunity problems while the search for acceptable alternative continues.

IMPORTANT CHARACTERISTICS OF MIRO-ORGANISMS

In order to classify and identify the micro-organisms, it is essential to learn about their characteristics. It is usually not possible to study the characteristics of single micro-organism because of its small size;

therefore we study the characteristics of a culture containing many micro-organisms of only one kind. Micro-organisms play many important and essential roles in nature. It is, therefore desirable to determine the characteristics of species that enable these activities to occur. The important characteristics of micro-organisms can be described as under:

1. Morphological characteristics :

These include cell shape, size and structure; cell arrangement, occurrence of special structures and developmental forms; staining; and motility and flagellar arrangement. Determination of morphological features usually requires studying individual cells of a pure culture. Routine examination of microbial cells requires the use of a high power microscope usually at a magnification of about 1000 times.

2. Chemical Composition:

Microbial cells consist of a wide variety of chemical constituents. When the cell components are chemically analysed, each kind of micro-organism is found to have a characteristic chemical composition. For example cell walls of gram negative bacteria contain lipopolysaccharide which is not present in the cell wall of gram positive bacteria. On the other hand cell wall of gram positive bacteria contain teichoic acid which is not found in gram negative bacteria. Fungi and algae have also different chemical constituents than those of bacteria. A very important distinction is made amongst the viruses on the basis of their nucleic acid constitution namely ribonucleic acid (RNA) or deoxyribonucleic acid (DNA).

3. Cultural Characteristics:

Different micro-organisms require different nutrients and physical conditions for growth and also differ in the manner in which the growth occurs. Some microbes can grow in a medium containing only inorganic compounds whereas other require a medium containing organic compounds (amino acids, sugars, vitamins etc.). Some require still complex medium containing natural substances (peptone, yeast, blood cells or serum) and some cannot be grown in artificial laboratory medium and can be cultured only in a living host or living cells. In addition to specific nutrients different micro-organisms also vary in their requirements of physical conditions like temperature, light and oxygen. Each kind of micro-organism grows in a specific manner. Growth in a liquid medium can be abundant or sparse. It may be evenly distributed throughout the medium or it may occur as a sediment in the bottom or may appear only as a thin film or pellicle at the top. On solid media microbes grow in colonies which may differ in size, shape, texture, consistency and color etc.

4. Metabolic characteristics:

The life processes of different microbial cells vary in the way they obtain and use their energy, carry out chemical reactions and regulate these reactions. The various chemical reactions of any organism are catalysed by proteins called enzymes and the complement of enzymes possessed by one kind of organism and the way in which these enzymes are regulated may differ significantly from that of other organisms.

5. Antigenic characteristics:

Antigens are special large chemical components of the bacterial cell and they are distinctive of certain kinds of micro-organisms. They induce the production of specific antibodies in the host following the invasion of bacteria. A single bacterium may carry several antigens which are classified according to the position occupied by them. Flagellar (H) antigens are present on the flagella. Surface antigens are associated with structures of the surface of the cell, e.g., the capsule or cell wall. Somatic antigens are present in the body of the bacterium and may occur in several layers within the cell.

When microbial cells enter the animal body, the animal responds to their antigens by forming specific blood serum proteins called antibodies, which bind to antigens. Antibodies are highly specific for the antigens that induce their formation. As different kinds of micro-organisms have different antigens, antibodies are widely used as tools for the rapid identification of particular kinds of organisms.

6. Pathogenicity :

The phenomenon of invasion and destruction of tissues is known as pathogenicity. This includes the complete sequence of events by which invading organisms enter the host, establish growth within its tissues and eventually give rise to the symptoms of disease. Some micro-organisms may cause disease in other organisms such as viruses called bacteriophages can infect and destroy bacterial cells.

7. Genetic Characteristics:

The double-stranded chromosomal DNA of each kind of micro-organism has certain features. These are constant and characteristic of that organism. DNA base composition and the sequence of nucleotide bases in the DNA are the examples of such features.

In addition to the chromosomal DNA, plasmid DNA may also be present in microbial cells. Plasmid DNAs confer the ability to make toxins, to develop resistance to various antibiotics and to use some unusual chemical compounds as nutrients.

8. Ecological Characteristics :

The habitat of a micro-organism is an important characteristic of certain microbial species. The microbial population of oral cavity differs from that of intestinal tract. Similarly micro-organisms normally found in marine environment differ from those in freshwater environment.

Groups of Micro-organisms:

The major groups of micro-organisms are briefly described below. They include

1. Bacteria (0.1-15 μm)
2. Fungi & yeasts (2 μm-20 cm)
3. Viruses and Bacteriophages (0.01-02 μm)
4. Algae (1 μm-meters)
5. Protozoa (5-250 μm)

Bacteria:

Bacteria are widely spread in the nature in large numbers. They are present in animals, plants, solid, water and the atmosphere. Majority of them are nonpathogenic and serve as useful scavengers in the breakdown of organic matter and its resynthesis into living organisms, they are essential in the cycle of life.

Morphology:

The individual cell (Fig. 7.1)

Slime layer : This is outer layer of bacterium. It consists of polysaccharide or polypeptide. Its physiological function appears to be the protection of organism against changes in environment.

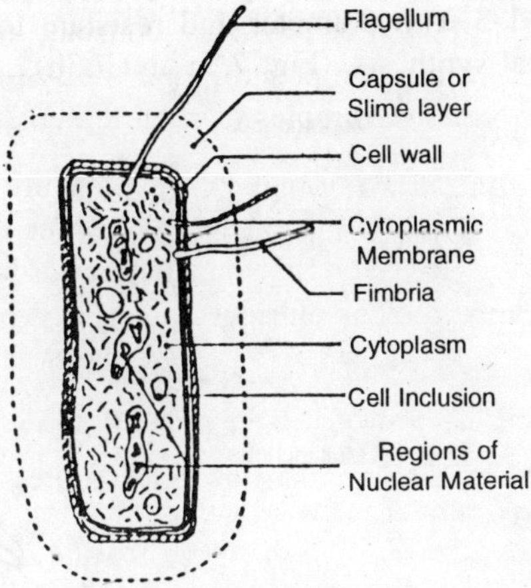

Fig. 7.1 An Individual bacterial cell

Cell wall : It is a rigid structure that renders the cell capable of survival even when there are great differences of osmotic pressure between cell and environment. In majority of bacteria which are of importance in pharmacy, the cell wall consists of protein and polypeptide with mucin, polysaccharide or phospholipid components.

Flagella and Fimbria :

These are outgrowths of the protoplasm protruding through the cell wall. They are responsible for movement in most types of motile bacteria and are useful in identification and important in immunology. (Fig.7.2)

Cytoplasmic membrane :

It is a limiting semipermeable membrane within the cell wall, a closely packed lipoprotein sheet, two to four molecules thick, having low affinity for water.

Cytoplasmic constituents :

Nuclear material : Bacterial cell does not have a well defined nucleus. However, it does contain genetic material.

Endospores : Under unfavourable conditions for their continued growth certain bacteria can produce a resting body (spore) within the cell wall. They are 1-3 μ in diameter and resistant to wide range of chemical and physical synthesis. (Fig. 7.3a and 7.3b).

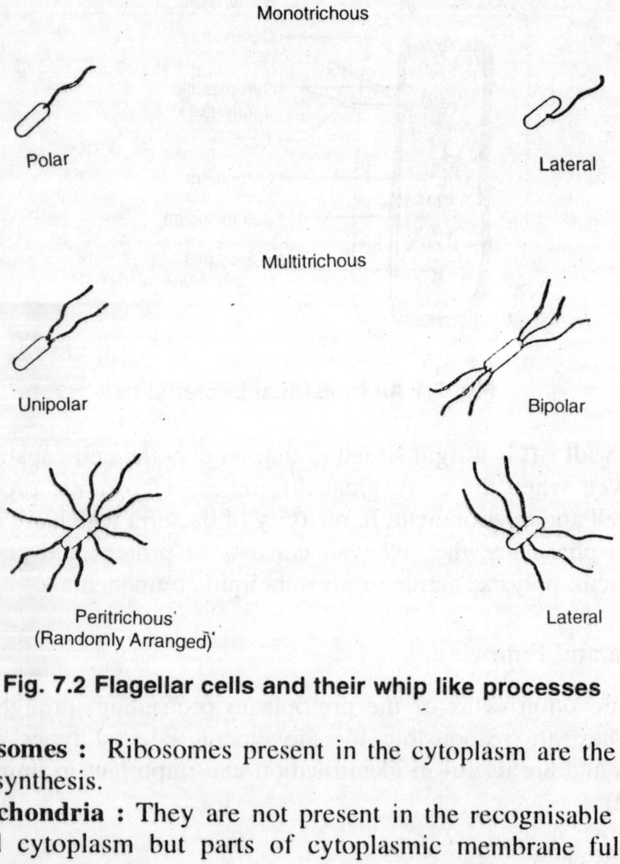

Fig. 7.2 Flagellar cells and their whip like processes

Ribosomes : Ribosomes present in the cytoplasm are the sites of protein synthesis.

Mitochondria : They are not present in the recognisable form in bacterial cytoplasm but parts of cytoplasmic membrane fulfil their function.

Vacuoles : Vacuoles appear in cytoplasm of bacteria only under special cultural conditions.

Similarly oil and fats droplets and other crystalline material also appear in the cytoplasm depending on the constitution of the media.

Shape and size :

Bacterial cells exhibit many shapes and sizes which may differ for the same species depending on the age of culture and type of culture

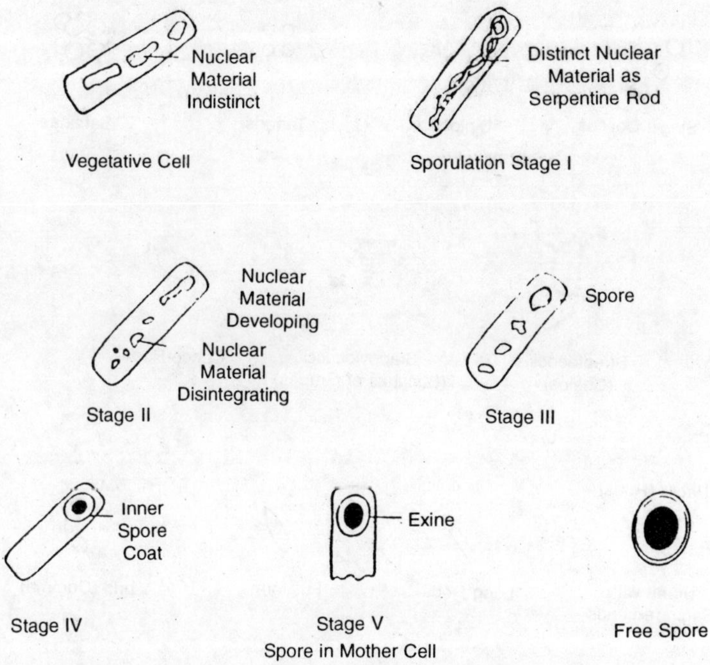

Fig. 7.3a Stages of formation of a bacterial spore

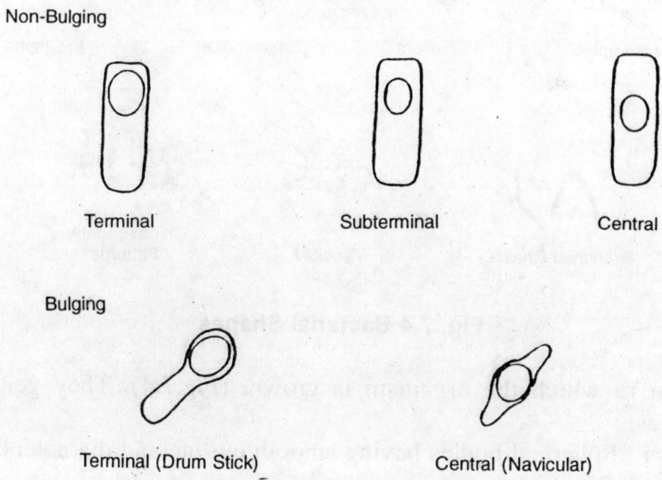

Fig. 7.3b Position of spores in cells

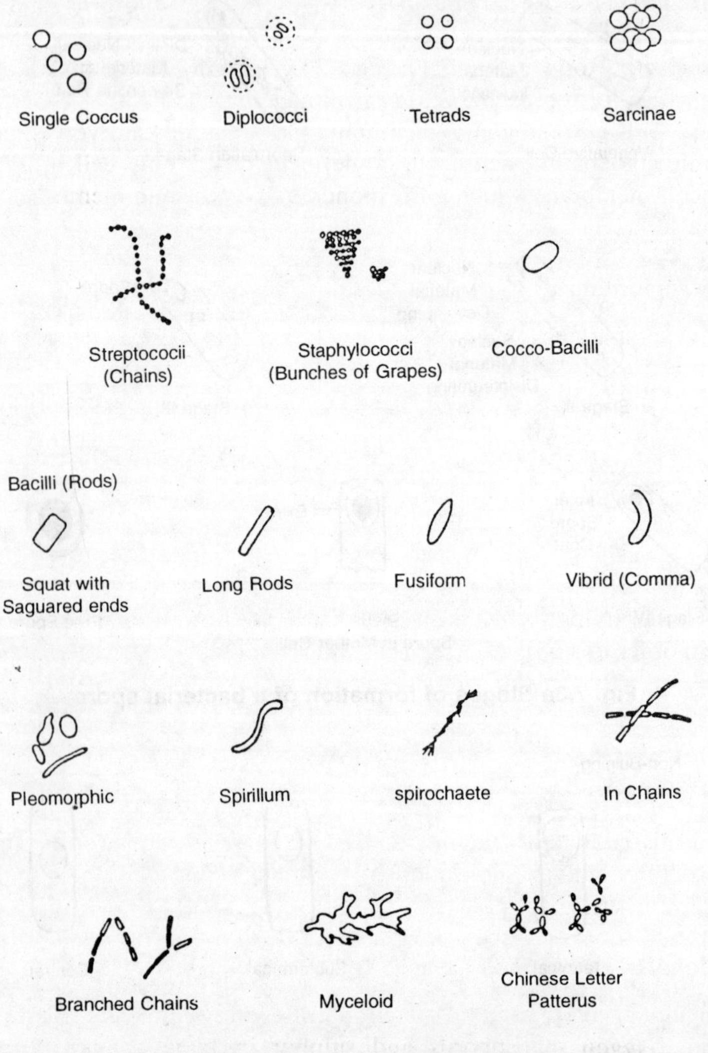

Fig. 7.4 Bacterial Shapes

medium in which the organism is grown. (Fig.7.4). They generally appear as:

Cocci : Spherical bodies having smooth outline and diameters ranging from 0.75 to 3.0 μ.

Rods : Rods are cylindrical in shape and vary greatly in length and diameter.

Spirochaetes : An organism having a number of turns and is flexuous, is known as spirochaete.

Branching Rods : Some bacteria like genera Actinomyces and Streptomyces form branches and remain adherent in chains.

Amoeboids : Some pleuropneumonia like organims are very small, nonmotile amoeba like cells with no defined shape or no cell wall but only a cell membrane which corresponds to cytoplasmic membrane of other bacteria.

Colony formation :

When bacteria are grown on the surface of a solid medium, they divide according to their normal habit and after a few generations a small colony is produced. It gradually adopts a characteristic shape and form determined by growth characteristics and adhesiveness of the cells. Bacilli like Anthrax form long chains and produce thin threads that make the colony look like a head of unruly hair (Medusa head).

Physiology :

Like all other living forms, bacteria perform the fundamental processes of life in order to survive but in bacteria all the functions are performed in one cell. Two major groups of enzymes are involved in these processes:

Exo-enzymes : They are released from the cell and they convert the food materials into assimilable forms.

Endo-enzymes : They are confined to protoplasmic membrane and transport material across the membrane and are responsible for the synthesis of the complex molecular components of the cell and for the production of energy.

Nutritional requirements :

For their survival bacteria require following elements: Carbon, nitrogen, oxygen, phosphorus and sulphur in large amounts; iron, calcium, magnesium, potassium and sodium in smaller quantities and manganese, zinc, copper, silica, bromine and iodine in traces, depending upon the species.

They can be classified into two major groups depending on their nutritional requirements.

Autotrophic bacteria : They can synthesize carbohydrates and obtain energy from simple inorganic sources of carbon like carbon dioxide and carbonates. A few can also utilize nitrates and ammonia as sole sources of nitrogen. Autotrophs are of interest to pharmaceutical industries because they cause deterioration of products and packaging materials.

Heterotrophic bacteria : This group of higher bacteria is unable to grow without elaborate sources of carbohydrates and aminoacids. They are subdivided into two classes:

(i) **Parasites :** These require the environment of living cells. They can be grown using highly specialized media.

(ii) **Saprophytes :** These organisms can grow on organic matter from dead plants or animals. They cause the decay of the dead material and hence are of supreme importance in nature. Generally they are nonpathogenic but if they get access to diseased tissues, they may produce harmful toxins and certain diseases which are difficult to cure.

Heat relationships :

Bacteria are also classified according to their thermal characteristics, which are of two kinds.

(a) Growth characteristics :

Psychrotrophs : Organisms that will grow at a temperature below 25°C are known as psychrotrophs. As some of them can grow slightly at 0-4°C, they are capable of spoiling blood and unsterilized pharmaceutical preparations stored in refrigerators.

Mesophiles : The favourable temperature for the growth of these bacteria lies between 25-45°C. Most of the pathogenic microorganisms are found in this group.

Thermophiles : These bacteria will not grow properly below 45°C and their optimal temperature lie between 55 and 65°C. In tropical climates they cause spoilage of food in sealed containers.

(b) Tolerance characteristics :

Microbes which are highly, resistant to heat treatments are known as thermoduric. This resistance is of two types.

(i) Many soil organisms form spores, which because of their low water content, can resist heat treatment and survive a temperature of 121°C for 20 minutes or more in an autoclave and upto 160°C for three hours in a hot air oven.

(ii) Some vegetative bacteria can survive abnormally long periods at above 60°C, whereas majority of pathogens in vegetative form will not survive 55°C for more than 15 minutes.

Oxygen requirements :

Bacteria can be classified in four categories according to their oxygen requirements:

(i) **Aerobes :** They must receive atmcspheric oxygen for their growth.

(ii) **Anaerobes :** They do not need molecular oxygen as a hydrogen acceptor. Further, if an organism is an obligate anaerobe, oxygen can have a lethal effect on it and such organism can survive only if they can form spores.

(iii) **Microaerophiles :** These can grow satisfactorily at very low oxygen levels but not in its complete absence.

(iv) **Facultative anaerobes :** These microorganisms are capable of growth under aerobic or anaerobic conditions.

Reproduction

(a) **Binary fission :**

Bacteria belong to Schizomycetes, i.e. the organism which multiply by binary fission. The protoplasm enlarges to a limiting size, the genetic materials forms into two units, cross walls are laid down and the cells separate. Some bacteria divide very rapidly, e.g. **E. Coli** divides about every 20 minutes under ideal conditions while **M. tuberculosis** takes upto a day to make its first division after transfer to a synthetic medium, subsequently dividing every five hours or so. Once the culture has settled down to a steady state, the interval between successive divisions remains almost constant. This interval is known as mean generation time.

(b) **Sexual reproduction :**

As bacteria are so small, it has been difficult to establish that sexual reproduction is feasible in these organisms. Marked variation in their characteristics and in the genetic patterns have indicated that sexual behaviour may be present in bacteria and this has been confirmed by recent improvements in genetic techniques.

Protozoa :

Protozoa (singular protozoan) is a greek word which splits into protos and zoo meaning the first animal. They occur generally as single cells, have ability to move at some stage of their life cycle and are distinguished by the lack of cell walls. They are predominantly microscopic in size. The majority are between 5 and 250 μ in diameter. They occur in colonies where individual cells are joined by cytoplasmic threads or, are embedded in a common matrix. Thus, the colonies of protozoa are essentially aggregates of independent cells.

Protozoa are found in all moist habitats. They are common in the sea, in soil and in fresh water. Many protozoa survive dry conditions by the formation of a resistant cyst, or dormant stage. Parasitic protozoa can modify their morphology and physiology to cope with a change in host.

Some protozoa can cause diseases in human beings and animals. They cause serious infections and make life miserable. Such parasitic protozoa multiply within the host much as bacteria do. Some live only as obligate parasites and may produce chronic or acute disease in humans. Some wellknown protozoan diseases in humans are intestinal amoebiasis, African sleeping sickness and malaria.

Fungi and Yeasts :

The fungi (singular fungus) are a group of organisms that are of great practical and scientific interest. The gross appearance of many multicellular fungi is familiar to us as we see the velvety blue and green growth on rotting oranges and lemons as well as on stale cheese, the whitish gray furry outgrowths on bread and jam. These are the bodies of various fungi. Fungi comprise the molds and yeasts. Molds are filamentous and multicellular and yeasts are usually unicellular.

The fungi are heterotrophic organisms as they require organic compounds for nutrition. When they feed on dead organic matter, they are known as saprophytes. Saprophytes decompose complex plant and animal remains, breaking them into simpler chemical substances that are returned to the soil, thereby increasing its fertility. They are also important in industrial fermentations e.g., brewing of beer, making of wine and production of antibiotics such as penicillin. As parasites fungi cause disease in plants, humans and animals.

Viruses and bacteriophages :

Viruses differ from bacteria as they are much smaller obligate intracellular parasites which contain only one type of nucleic acid, do not reproduce by binary fission and most of them are not sensitive to antibiotics. Animal viruses range in size from about 10 nm to 250 nm. All except the very large ones are invisible under the light microscope and will pass through conventional bacteria proof filters.

Since viruses will grow only within living cells, they cannot be cultivated in ordinary bacteriological culture media. A living system is necessary for their growth.

Viruses consist of a central core containing a single nucleic acid, surrounded by protein shell. The nucleic acid may be either DNA, as in vaccinia virus or RNA as in poliomyelitis virus. The shell known as the capsid, is built up of large number of small units (capsomeres) arranged symmetrically around the core.

The life cycle of virus involves the following important sequence of events:

(a) **Adsorption on to the host cell membrane :** The virus attaches itself to a chemically complementary receptor on the host cell by means of structures like the hemagglutin-containing spikes of influenza virus.

(b) **Penetration of the host cell :** The host cell may behave like an amoeba and engulf the complete virus.

(c) **The eclipse phase :** After penetration the infective virus cannot be detected within the cell during the first few hours and this period is known as the eclipse phase. In the meantime the capsid of the virus disintegrates freeing the nucleic acid core which inhibits the functioning of the host nucleic acid and then takes over the cell's metabolic activity and directs it to synthesize virus protein and nucleic acid.

(d) **Virus replication :** The virus nucleic acid replicates itself and synthesizes protein. As the new molecules become available, the protein components are gradually built up around the nucleic acid in the geometric arrangement characteristic of the virus type. The cell membrane of the host contributes to the formation of an envelope and the virus buds out by a process which is the reversal of penetration mechanism.

(e) **Liberation from the cell :** Generally the release of enveloped viruses does not damage the host cell immediately although deleterious changes may occur later. On the other hand some viruses like small pox and poliomyelitis cause the cell to disintegrate completely.

Bacteriophages : Bacteriophages (often called phages) are viruses that are parasitic on bacteria. They are widely distributed in the nature. Phages exist for most, if not all bacteria. Phages like all viruses are composed of a nucleic acid core surrounded by a protein coat. They occur in different shapes and many have a tail through which they inoculate the host cell with viral nucleic acid.

There are two main types of bacterial viruses: Lytic or virulent and temperate or avirulent. When lytic phages infect cells, the cells respond by producing large number of new viruses. In temperate type of infection, the result is not so readily apparent. The viral nucleic acid is carried and replicated in the host bacterial cells from one generation to another without any cell lysis.

Since virulent or lytic phages can destroy their host bacterial cells, it was logically considered that inoculation of such phages into bacteria-infected individuals would result in elimination of the pathogens. However, after numerous studies, there is no evidence to show that phages can be used therapeutically to destroy bacterial pathogens in the human body, principally because phages do not persist in the body. The primary uses of bacteriophages are thus confined to the identification of bacterial strains and as genetic models in molecular biology.

The lytic phages have been used in the detection and identification of pathogenic bacteria. Strains of bacteria are characterized by their resistance or susceptibility to lysis by specific virulent phages. The resulting pattern of lysis of a bacterial strain by different phages types gives an indication of the identity of the bacterium. This laboratory procedure is termed bacteriophage-typing and is used routinely for the identification of certain strains of bacterial pathogen such as staphylococci and for medical diagnosis and for tracing of the source of disease spreading in a community.

Rickettsiae :

Most of these tiny, nonmotile, Gram-negative bacteria are obligate parasites, able to grow only within host cells. Although their size in some instances approaches that of some large viruses, they are classified as bacteria on the basis of their much closer relationship to bacteria, for example :

- (i) They are retained by bacteria proof filters.
- (ii) They are visible under light microscope.
- (iii) They can be stained e.g., they are gram-negative.
- (iv) They reproduce by binary fission.
- (v) They have a cell wall similar to that of bacteria.
- (vi) They contain both DNA and RNA and produce metabolic enzymes.
- (vii) They are sensitive to a number of antibiotics.

The features of this genus are:

- (a) Transmission to human occurs via an arthropod vector (lice, fleas, ticks or mites)
- (b) The organisms multiply within the cytoplasm and sometimes within the nucleus of host cells.

Diseases caused by Rickettsia species and the arthropod vector which transmit them include Rocky Mountain spotted fever (ticks), classical typhus fever (lice), murine typhus fever (fleas), rickettsial pox (mites) and scrub typhus (mites).

Algae :

These organisms are ubiquitous; many live in aquatic environment but many also thrive as terrestrial and subterranean algae. Many of them are unicellular micro-organisms. Algae contain chlorophyll and are photosynthetic. They differ from other green plants in having simple reproductive structures for sexual reproduction.

Algae are of great interest to biologists because single algal cells are complete organisms capable of photosynthesis and the synthesis of many other compounds which constitute the cell. In size, habitat and reproductive processes algae are a heterogeneous group. They range from microscopic unicellular forms comparable in size to bacteria, to seaweeds that may grow to many feet in length.

Many products of economic value useful in pharmaceutical and food industries are derived from algae. Agar and carrageenans are polymers of galactose with sulphate groups. Alginic acid consists of uronic acid residues. All three compounds are used either to make gels or to make solutions more viscous. Carrageenan is also used as a thickeing agent in shaving creams and lotions. Agar is wellknown as solidifying agent in the preparation of microbiological media. It is also used as a carrier for drugs and lotions and ointments can also contain some agar. An alginate material is used by dentists for making impressions of the teeth for crown etc. The stipe of the brown algae Luminary Japonica has been used by physicians for producing cervical dilatation and/or softening of cervix in performing an abortion or placing a radium implant.

Algae are rarely pathogenic. One Prototheca has been found to be a probable pathogen of humans. It has been involved in systemic and subcutaneous infections as well as in bursitis, an inflammation of the joints.

MICROBIOLOGICAL METHODS

Culture techniques : Microorganisms can be grown in fluid or semisolid media or on a solid media. Semisolid media are less widely used.

Fluid media for aerobic organisms are placed in tubes closed with cotton plugs or loose-fitting metal caps.

Solid media are used in flat dishes (petri dishes) or in small wide-mouthed bottles. In dishes the organisms are mixed with medium before it solidifies or are spread or dropped on to the surface after solidification. In bottles the medium may be allowed to set with the container placed in vertical position or at an angle to produce a slope or slant. Organism can be inoculated with a straight wire in the vertically placed bottle or can be spread on the slanted medium. Carrel flasks and Roux bottles are used for culturing large quantities of bacteria (Fig.7.5).

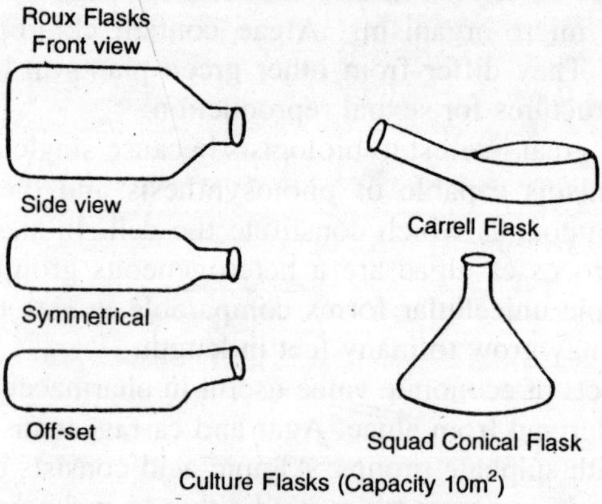

Fig. 7.5 Culture flasks

Transfer of culture :

The transfer of micro-organisms from one container to another is done under aseptic conditions, i.e., without introducing extraneous organisms. Suitable equipments are necessary for this purpose which include different types of calibrated capillary dropping pipettes, wires, loops and spreaders (Fig.7.6a, b, c & d).

However, if the concentration of an organism in a suspension is low, e.g., drinking water, transfer is not adequate by above mentioned methods.

The organism is concentrated by filtering a large volume of liquid through a bacteria proof membrane. Then the membrane is placed on a pad impregnated with a nutrient medium and incubated in a closed container.

Isolation of pure cultures :

In order to correctly identify a bacterial species, it must be obtained in pure culture. The following methods are commonly used to isolate bacteria from a mixture.

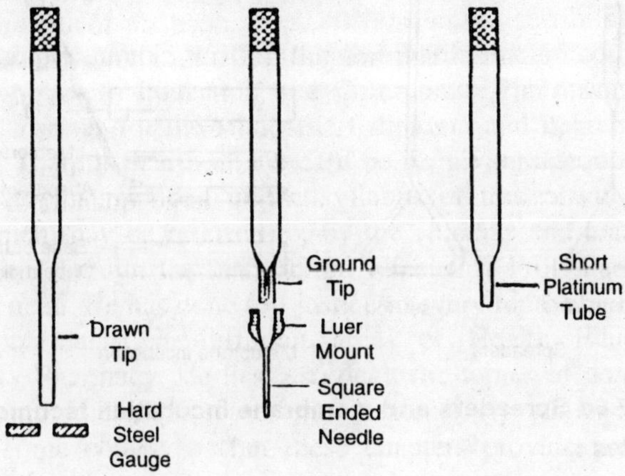

Fig. 7.6a Capillary dropping pipettes

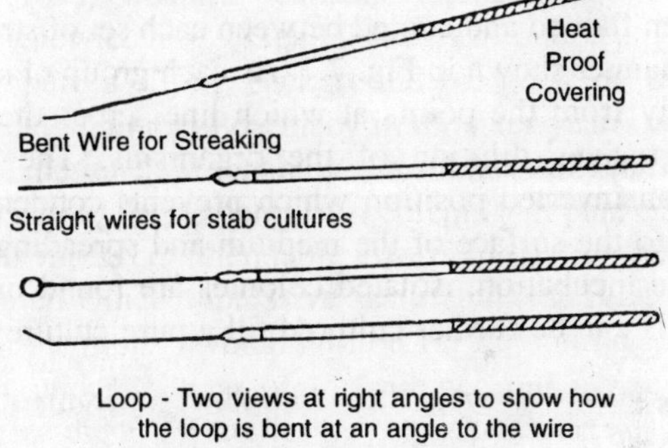

Fig. 7.6b Loops and wires

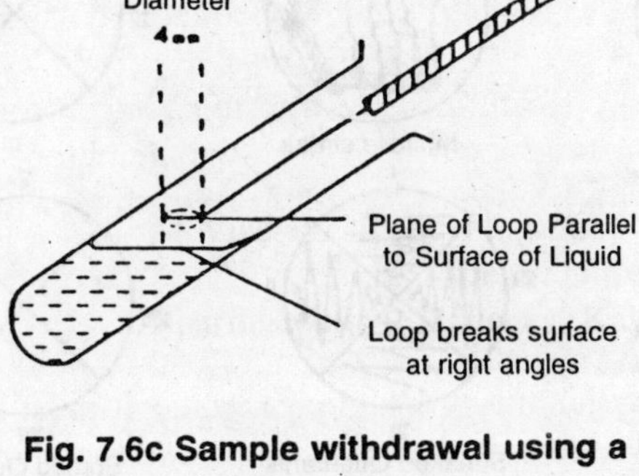

Fig. 7.6c Sample withdrawal using a loop

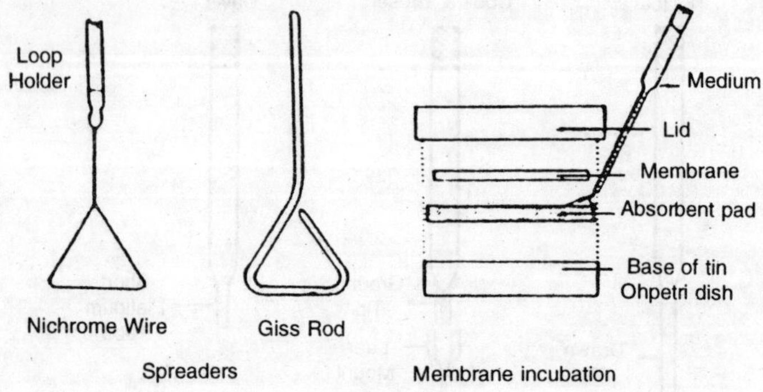

Fig. 7.6d Spreaders and membrane incubation technique

Streak plates :

A plate of solid medium (e.g., nutrient agar) is opened and inverted in an incubator for about 30 min to dry the surface. Then using a bent wire which has been flamed and cooled between each set of streaks, lines are made in the manner shown in Fig. 7.7. As each group of streaks obtains organisms only from the points at which lines cross the previous set, there is progresives dilution of the organisms. The plate is then incubated in an inverted position which prevents condensate from the lid falling on to the surface of the medium and spreading the colonies. After adequate incubation, isolated colonies are found in the later sets of streaks. This can be further cultured till a pure culture is obtained.

Spread plates :

In this method the base of a poured plate is marked into quadrants with

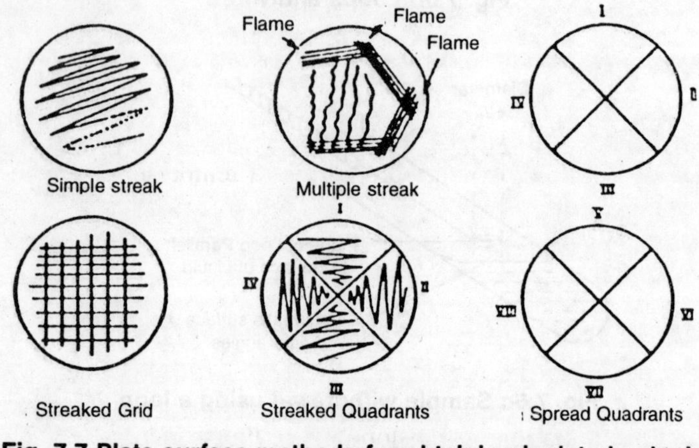

Fig. 7.7 Plate surface methods for obtaining isolated colonies

a waxed pencil and a drop of very dilute culture is placed on the medium within one quadrant and spread over that area with a flamed spreader. Then the spreader is moved to second, third and fourth quadrants in succession and the organisms carried on it are thus spread in all the four quadrants. After a few minutes of absorption of the liquid by the medium, the plates are incubated in inverted position.

Pour plates :

In this method initial suspension is diluted to a concentation of about 100 organisms/cm^3. Then volumes of 1 cm^3 are pipetted into empty petri dishes and mixed with nutrient agar by moving them gently five times in the directions shown (Fig. 7.8).

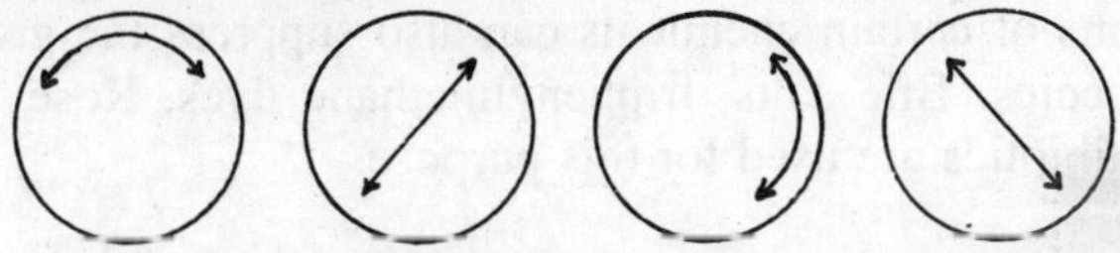

Fig. 7.8 The Milk Marketing Board method of mixing in plates

The temperature of agar is not allowed to exceed 47°C to avoid damage to the micro-organisms. The amount of agar also should not exceed 15 cm^3 in a 75 mm petri dish. This technique is also known as the Milk Marketing Board method of mixing in plates.

Micromanipulation :

An instrument called, micromanipulator is used in this method to remove single organisms from a suspension on a microscope slide. A high degree of skill is required for using this technique and it is used only when the species to be isolated differ morphologically.

Heat differentiation :

When a mixed culture is subjected to stepwise increase in temperature in a thermoregulated water bath, the number of heat sensitive species in samples will decrease as time progresses. If temperatures above 70°C are used only spores will be isolated after about 10 minutes and further heating will separate the sporing species according to their heat tolerance.

Motility :

In this method, a mixed culture is inoculated at the bottom of a moist slope and it is then incubated upright. The motile organisms are recovered from the top of the slope where they reach by swimming in the film of liquid on the surface. This method is helpful for the isolation of motile micro-organisms.

Enrichment media :

In this method a medium is chosen that favours the growth of a particular species and suppresses the growth of other organisms. Such methods are very useful in tracing the source of an epidemic by Public Health Departments. For example sewage contains most of the normal bacteria of the human gut and to isolate a few typhoid organisms is virtually impossible by normal culture methods. In such situations the use of enrichment media is made which would favour the growth of typhoid organisms.

Additions of certain chemicals can also suppress the growth of unwanted species. Bile salts, triphenylmethane dyes, Rose Bengal and certain antibiotics are used for this purpose.

IDENTIFICATION OF MICROORGANISMS

Light Microscope examinations :

Two methods are used to prepare specimens for light microscope examination.. One is to suspend organisms in a liquid (the wet-mount or hanging-drop technique) and the other is to dry, fix and stain films or smears of the specimen.

The wet-mount and hanging drop techniques :

Organisms can be examined in normal living conditions using wet preparations. A wet mount is made by placing a drop of fluid containing the organisms on to a glass slide and covering the drop with a coverslip. In order to reduce the rate of evaporation and exclude the effect of air currents, the drop is ringed by petroleum jelly to provide a seal between the slide and coverslip.

In hanging drop method, a special slide with a circular concave depression is used for examination of wet preparations. A suspension of microbial specimen is placed on a coverslip, then inverted over the concave depression to produce hanging drop of the specimen.

These wet methods are used to a) study the morphology of spiral bacteria as they are significantly distorted on drying and staining, b) determine whether the organisms are motile and c) observe cytological changes occurring during cell division. These characteristics can only be observed and studied when the organism is in the living state.

Fixed and stained smears :

Fixed and stained preparations are used for studying the morphological characteristics of microorganisms. In this method the cells are made more clearly visible after they are colored and the differences between the cells of different species and within the same species can be demonstrated by use of appropriate staining reagents. The essential steps in the preparation of a fixed, stained smear are a) preparation of the film or smear, b) fixation and c) application of one or more staining reagents.

Microbiological stains :

A large number of organic dyes are used for staining the micro-organisms. They are classified on the basis of their chemical behaviour, namely acid, basic or neutral. An acid dye is one in which the charge on the dye ion is negative, a basic dye is one in which the charge carried by dye ion is positive. A neutral dye is complex salt of a dye acid with a dye base, e.g. eosinate of methylene blue. Acid dyes generally stain basic cell components and the basic dyes generally stain acidic cell components.

Simple staining

The coloration of an organism by applying a single solution of stain to a fixed smear is called simple staining. The fixed smear is flooded with dye solution for a specified period of time after which this solution is washed off with water and the slide blotted dry. The cells usually stain uniformly.

Simple staining of microorganisms may be positive, where the stain is attracted to the microbial cells so that cells appear dark or coloured on a light or clear background, or may be negative, in which case the background is stained and the microorganisms appear bright on a dark background. Nigrosin and India ink are frequently used for negative staining of microbial cells. These staining procedures depend on the fact that bacteria and other cellular microorganisms have a negative charge associated with the outer surface of cell, largely because of the phosphate group of cell membrane.

Differential staining

Differential staining techniques make visible the differences between the bacterial cells or parts of a bacterial cell. These techniques are more elaborate as the cells are exposed to more than one staining reagent.

Gram staining

This is one of the most important and widely used differential staining techniques in microbiology. In this process the fixed bacterial smear is subjected to the following staining reagents in the order listed. Crystal violet, iodine solution, alcohol (decolorizing agent) and safranin or some other suitable counter stains. Bacteria stained by the Gram method fall into two groups: **Gram positive** bacteria, which retain the crystal violet and hence appear deep violet in color; and **Gram negative** bacteria, which lose the crystal violet, are counterstained by the safranin and hence appear red in color.

Examples of **Gram positive** bacteria are:

Micrococcus	Corynebacterium	Bacillus
Diplococcus	Mycobacterium	Clostridium
Streptococcus	Staphylococcus	Actinomycetes

Examples of **Gram negative** bacteria are

Vibrio	Escherichia	Pseudomonas
Proteus	Salmonella	Pasteurella
Neisseria	Shigella	Bordetella

Acid Fastness :

Certain organisms are not easily stained by the usual dyes probably due to the presence of a water repellant outer layer or a high lipid content, but when stained with acid fast stain they may retain the color even when washed with acid. Such organisms are called acid fast. The mycobacteria that cause leprosy and tuberculosis are both acid and alcohol fast. Most bacteria are neither acid nor alcohol fast.

Other Differential Stains :

There are several other staining techniques which have been designed to identify some particular features of cell structure or composition. They also identify the presence of capsules, spores and flagella.

These techniques are summarized as under :

Endospore stain : Demonstrates spore structure in bacteria as well as free spores

Capsule stain : Demonstrates presence of capsules surrounding cells

Flagella stain : Demonstrates the presence and arrangement of flagella

Cytoplasmic Inclusion Stain : Identifies intracellular deposits of starch, glycogen, polyphosphates, hydroxybutyrate and other substances.

Giemsa Stain : Particularly applicable for staining rickettsias and some protozoa.

CLASSIFICATION OF COMMON DISEASE PRODUCING BACTERIA

Bacteria can be classified either on the basis of staining reactions or on the basis of their zoological order, family, genera, species and variety. In this text they have been classified according to their staining reaction which is simple and more practical classification for the students of pharmacy and community medicine. Attempt has also been made to outline important diseases produced by the pathogenic organisms.

Name of the order, family, genus and species etc.	Characteristics	Disease(s) produced by them
Gram positive cocci		
Staphylococcus	Grow in grape like aggregates, Nonmotile, non sporing	
Staphylococcus aureus		Boils, abscesses, sties, osteomyelitis, food poisoning impetigo, conjunctivitis
Streptococcus	Ovoid rods, Grow in Chains like a string of beads, extremely dangerous pathogens	
Streptococcus pyogens		Scarlet fever, acute tonsilitis, Puerperal sepsis, Rheumatic fever, Inflammation of Kidney
Diplococcus	Similar to steptococcus, grow in pairs	
Diplococcus pneumonia		Causes acute lobar pneumonia, meningitis, peritonitis and conjunctivitis

(*Contd.*)

Gram-Negative Cocci		
Neisseriae	Seen typically in pairs, likened to kidney bean in shape, found embedded in pus cells	
Neisseria gonorrhoee		Causes venereal disease gonorrhoea
Neisseria meningitidis		Causes cerebrospinal fever or meningococcal meningitis
Gram positive rods		
Bacilli	Large rod, aerobic spore forming, widespread in air, soil, water, hair, wool, carcasses; some are pathogenic	
Bacillus anthracis	Most dangerous	Causes anthrax
Bacillus cereus		Implicated in food poisoning
Bacillus subtilis and B. pumilis		They are used in antibiotics assays.
B. megaterium	They are sources of	Used to produce penicillinase
B. Polymyxa, B. brevis & B. licheniformis	polymyxin,	tyrothricin and bacitracin respectively
Clostridia	Aerobic, spore forming rods, many species are dangerous pathogens	
Clostridium tetani		Causes tetanus
Clostridium botulinum		Nerve poison, causes fatal food poisoning
Cl. septicum, Cl. welchii and C.oedematiens		Causal organisms of gas gangrene, all produce powerful toxins
Corynebacterium	Slightly curved rods, clubbed ends	
Corynebacterium diphtheriae		Causes diphtheria, produces a dangerous exotoxin
Gram-Negative rods		
Pseudomonas	Straight rods, produce water soluble pigment	
Pseudomonas aeruginosa	Dangerous pathogen	Infects wounds, burns, can cause serous eye infections

(*Contd.*)

Vibrio	Comma shaped rods, water borne	
Vibrio cholerae		Causes cholera which is still endemic in India.
Yersinia	Nonmotile, shows bipolar staining	
Pasteurella pestis	Causes bubonic plague	
Bordetella	Ovoid rods	
Bordetella pertussis		Causes Whooping cough
Escherichia	Motile or non-motile rods, ferments carbohydrates, commensal in gut	
Escherichia coli		Causes gastroenteritis, in infants, common pathogen of urinary tract in adults, causes pyelitis, pyelonephritis and cystitis.
Salmonella	Usually motile rods,	
Salmonella typhi		Cause of typhoid fever
Shigella	Nonmotile rods	
Shigella shiga and other species		Cause bacillary dysentery
Proteus	Highly motile rods, produce characteristic seminal odour, commensal in bowel	
Proteus vulgaris		Causes severe wound infection and urinary tract infection, difficult to eradicate
Serratia	Very small pigmented rods (0.5 1.0 μ long)	
Serratia marcesens		Used to test the efficiency of bacterial filters
Chlamydia	Possess cell wall containing muramic acid	
Chlamydia trachomatis		Causes trachoma, conjunctivitis and non-gonococcal urethritis

(*Contd..*)

Acid Fast Organisms		
Mycobacteria	Straight or slightly curved rods, grow slowly, highly pathogenic	
Mycobacterium tuberculosis		Causes tuberculosis
Mycobacterium leprae		Causes leprosy
Spirochaetes	Slender, non-rigid spiral forms, motile	
Treponema pallidum		Causes syphilis
Leptospira ictero-haemorrhagiae		Cause of jaundice in man called Weils' disease encountered in sewage workers

8

COMMUNICABLE DISEASES

(Causative agents • mode of transmission and prevention)

A. RESPIRATORY INFECTIONS

Chicken Pox, Measles, Influenza, Diphtheria, Whooping cough and Tuberculosis.

• • •

B. INTESTINAL INFECTIONS

Poliomyelitis, Hepatitis, Cholera, Typhoid and Paratyphoid Fevers, Food poisoning, Hookworm infection and Amoebiasis.

• • •

C. ARTHROPOD BORNE INFECTIONS

Plague, Malaria and Filariasis.

• • •

D. SURFACE INFECTIONS

Rabies, Trachoma, Tetanus, Leprosy, Scabies and Pediculosis

• • •

E. SEXUALLY TRANSMITTED DISEASES

Syphilis, Gonorrhoea and AIDS

A. RESPIRATORY INFECTIONS

CHICKEN POX (VARICELLA)

Etiology and Incidence:

Chickenpox is caused by the varicella-zoster virus. Its spread is mostly by the droplets from the upper respiratory tract of the infected person or through the discharge from ruptured lesions on the skin or through contact with herpes zoster. Herpes zoster is due to the reactivation of the varicella-zoster virus and it is often accompanied by a varicelliform rash.Chickenpox is highly infectious and it mainly affects children under 10 years of age. Most children tolerate this disease well but as it generally happens with viral infections, adults may develop a more severe illness. In patients with leukemia who are otherwise immunocompromised, chickenpox may be severe or even fatal. The incubation period is 14 to 21 days.

Clinical presentation:

Chickenpox produces usually brief and mild constitutional symptoms. The first sign of the disease is often the rash. Sometimes the lesions are present on the palate before the characteristic rash appears on the trunk on the second day of the illness. Thereafter the face and finally the limbs are affected. The spots reach their maximum density upon the trunk and are more sparse on the periphery of the limbs. Macules are first to appear and within a few hours the lesions become papular and then vesicular, and within 24 hours pustular. Damage from scratching is frequent since itching is often troublesome and irresistable. The pustules may or may not rupture but they dry up in a few days to form scabs. The spots appear in crops, so that the lesions at all stages of development are seen in any area at the same time.

Complications:

The course of chickenpox is usually uneventful but complications do occur occasionally. These are listed in the Table 8.1 below.

Table 8.1 Complications of Chickenpox

Complications
Direct Viral effects
Pneumonia (in adults or immunocompromized individuals)
Myocarditis (in adults or immunocompromized individuals)
Post Viral effects
Encephalitis (cerebellar)
Glomerulonephritis
Secondary bacterial infections
Skin
Septicemia
Osteomyelitis/septic arthritis
Intra-uterine infection
Congenital hypoplasia of limbs (rare)

Management:

For majority of patients no treatment is necessary, however, acyclovir may be used in the immunocompromized patients. In case of a secondary infection on the skin, a local antiseptic should be applied to the affected area, e.g., chlorhexidine. In the presence of a systemic bacterial infection flucloxacillin may be prescribed. Immunocompromized children who have been in contact with chickenpox patients, should be given an injection of human antivaricella gammaglobulin.

MEASLES

Etiology and Incidence:

The causative organism is a paramyxovirus which spreads by droplet infection. One attack infers a high degree of immunity. Most people suffer from measles in childhood and a mother who has had measles confers passive immunity on her infant for the first six months of life. Measles is very severe with a high mortality in many tropical countries. The incubation period is about 10 days to the commencement of catarrhal stage.

Clinical presentation:

Catarrhal stage: Measles commences almost like common cold. There is a febrile onset with nasal catarrh, sneezing, redness of the conjunctivae and watering of the eyes. In addition to these symptoms, cough, hoarseness of voice due to laryngitis and photophobia generally appear by the second day. At this stage, a diagnosis of measles can be made from the presence of Koplik's spots on the mucous membrane of the mouth. These spots are white, small and surrounded by a narrow zone of inflammation. Chicken pox is highly infectious during the catarrhal stage and the child is irritable and suffers miserably.

Exanthematous stage: After 3-4 days the diagnostic Koplik's spots disappear and the dark red macular or maculopapular rash develops initially at the back of ears and at the junction of the forehead and hair. Then within a few hours there is invasion of whole skin and as the spots rapidly become more numerous, they fuse to form the characteristic blotchy appearance of measles. In 2-3 days as the rash is fully erupted, it tends to deepen in colour and then fades into a faint brown staining followed by a fine desquamation. The malaise and fever subside as the rash fades.

Complications:

A number of complications may occur during the course of an attack of measles. They have been summarized in the Table 8.2 given below :

Table 8.2 Important Complications of measles

Due to the effect of measles virus
Stomatitis
Enteritis
Pneumonia
Secondary bacterial infections
Otitis media
Bronchopneumonia
Conjunctivitis
Neurological Complications
Post-viral encephalitis
Sub-acute sclerosing panencephalitis
Nutritional Complications
Severe weight loss
Kwashiorkor
Corneal ulceration

Prevention:

Acute immunization: One injection of live attenuated measles virus (in association with mumps and rubella vaccines: MMR Vaccine) should be given to children of 15 months or older who have not had the disease.

Passive immunization: For passive immunization Immune Serum Globulin Human (Gamma Globulin) is used. Given intramuscularly it is recommended for the prevention or attenuation of measles, for contacts under 18 months of age and for debilitated children especially those with malignant disease. The dose is 250 mg. for children under one year and 500 mg for those older than one year.

INFLUENZA

Etiology:

Influenza is a specific acute illness involving the respiratory tract, which is caused by a group of myxoviruses. It occurs in endemics and occasionally in pandemics striking many continents simultaneously or in sequence. It is often explosive in nature. There are two common types of virus, influenza A and B. At least four serologically distinct strains of influenza A, which is responsible for pandemics have been identified. Influenza B is usually associated with smaller and less virulent outbreaks. The immunity which follows infection is type specific and is of relatively short duration. This has caused problems in the development of an effective influenza vaccine.

Clinical presentation:

The disease may spread rapidly throughout a household or institution. During the epidemics, the diagnosis is very easy. Most sporadic cases are identifiable only as respiratory or viral infections. Diagnosis can be confirmed only after the virus is isolated or demonstrated by fluorescent antibody techniques or if serological tests for specific antibodies are positive. The clinical features are listed in the Table 8.3 below:

Table 8.3 Important Clinical Features of Influenza

Incubation period	:	24-28 hours
Onset	:	Sudden pyrexia associated with chills, headache, severe generalized myalgia, anorexia, nausea, vomiting, inflammation of nasal mucosa; pharynx and conjunctiva
Chest symptoms	:	Harsh and unproductive cough
Clinical signs	:	Fauces hyperaemic, usually no abnormalities on examination of chest in the initial stage.
W.B.C. Count	:	Leucopenia
Course	:	Acute symptoms subside within 3-5 days if there are no complications. Post-influenzal asthenia may persist for a few weeks.

Complications:

Complications of influenza include tracheitis, bronchitis, bronchiolitis and bronchopneumonia. A necrotizing bronchitis and interstitial pneumonia are prominent features of severe influenza and account for the susceptibility of patients to secondary bacterial pneumonia due to **Streptococcus pneumoniae, Haemophilus influenzae** and **Streptococcus aureus.** Toxic cardiomyopathy in the presence of pre-existing cardiac disease may cause sudden death. Post-influenzal asthenia and depression are common and may persist for several weeks.

Management :

There is no specific treatment for influenza. Bed rest is advised until the fever subsides. A mild analgesic-antipyretic like paracetamol 0.5-1 g every 4-6 hours reduces fever and relieves the headache and generalized pains. Pholcodine 5-10 mg, 3-4 times daily or any other antitussive may be used to suppress unproductive cough. Specific treatment of complications such as bronchitis and pneumonia may be necessary.

Prevention :

Immunity to influenza virus is type specific and if the antigenic constitution of a new strain can be established early, a specific vaccine may give about 70% protection. The currently available Influenza Virus Vaccine, Trivalent, types A and B is indicated only for immunization against those strains of viruses from which the vaccine is prepared or against closely related strains. Annual routine immunization is recommended only for persons, children and adults who are at increased risk of adverse consequences from influenza infection. Groups at greatest risk include: (a)adults and children with chronic disorders of pulmonary or cardiovascular systems requiring regular medical follow up or hospitalization during the preceding year, including children with asthma and (b) resident of nursing homes and other chronic-care facilities housing patients of any age with chronic medical conditions.

DIPHTHERIA

Etiology:

Diphtheria is an acute infectious disease caused by the toxigenic gram-positive bacillus **Corynebacterium diphtheriae.** In many parts of the world diphtheria is still an important cause of illness.

Pathology :

Infections with **Corynebacterium diphtheriae** occur most commonly in the upper respiratory tract and sore throat is the most common presenting feature. The disease is usually spread by droplet infection from cases or carriers. The organisms remain localized at the site of infection and serious consequences result from the absorption of soluble exotoxin which may damage the heart muscle or the nervous system. The average incubation period is 2-4 days. Cases are isolated until cultures from 6 daily nose and throat swabs are negative.

Clinical presentation :

The disease begins insidiously. The temperature is seldom raised although the tachycardia is usually marked. The diagnostic feature is the "wash leather" elevated greyish-green membrane of variable extent on the tonsils with a well-defined edge and surrounded by a zone of inflammation. The membrane is firm and adherent. There may be swelling of the neck (bull-neck) and tender enlargement of the lymph nodes.

With anterior nasal infection there is also nasal discharge which is tinged with blood. In laryngeal diphtheria there is husky voice, a high pitched cough and a danger of respiratory obstruction which can be fatal if tracheostomy is not carried out. As the infection spreads towards the uvula, to the fauces and then to nasopharynx, the patient is often gravely ill. The pulse is weak but rapid and blood pressure is low. Death from circulatory failure may occur within the first 10 days. Those who survive the earlier toxemia may later develop arrhythmias or cardiac failure. There is no permanent damage to heart in those who survive.

Involvement of the nervous system occurs sometimes and it commences with palatal palsy after about 10 days of the illness in cases of tonsilar or pharyngeal diphtheria. Paralysis of accommodation often follows. A week or two later weakness and parasthesia in limbs may occur which may be due to the development of polyneuritis. Recovery from such neuritis is always complete.

Management :

Upon making a clinical diagnosis of diphtheria, Diphtheria Antitoxin should be injected intramuscularly without awaiting the report on a throat swab. Delay increases the danger to the patient because toxin once fixed to the tissues can no longer be neutralized by antitoxin. Penicillin should be administered for one week to eliminate **C.diphtheriae.** Patients allergic to penicillin can be given erythromycin. Diphtheria antitoxin being a foreign protein can lead to undesirable reactions including anaphylaxis and serum sickness with urticaria. Care should be taken to control such reactions and treatment be continued for the infection.

Prevention :

Acute immunization should be given to all children as discussed under the use of DTP to prevent tetanus. In case of diphtheria occurring in a close community, all close contacts should be treated with erythromycin which is more effective than penicillin in eradicating the organism in carriers. Further, all contacts should be advised to have active immunization or a booster of toxoid.

WHOOPING COUGH
(Pertussis)

Etiology :

Whooping cough is a highly infectious disease caused by **Bordetella pertussis**. It is spread by droplet infection. Clinical diagnosis in the early stage which is most contagious is virtually impossible and that results in epidemics. Whooping cough can occur at all ages but about 90% cases occur in children under 5 years of age. The incubation periods is 7 to 14 days.

Clinical presentation :

The first stage of whooping cough which consists of highly infectious upper respiratory catarrh, is characterized by slight fever, sneezing, running of the nose and dry cough. In a week or two the distinctive paroxysmal stage begins with the characteristic paroxysmal cough. This consists of deep inspiration, followed by a series of quick, short coughs continuing until the air is expelled from the lungs. During the paroxysm, the face becomes cyanosed, the eyes injected and the veins distended. The cough frequently induces vomiting and in severe cases epistaxis may also take place. The close of paroxysm is marked by a long-drawn shrill, whooping inspiration due to spasmodic closure of the glottis. The number of such paroxysm in 24 hours varies from 10 or 12 to 40 or 50 and they are more severe at night. This stage lasts from 3 to 4 weeks and is followed by the stage of convalescence during which the paroxysms grow less frequent and less violent and finally cease. The disease is much more prevalent in cold weather.

Complications :

The complications of whooping cough occur more commonly in the respiratory tract and they include bronchopneumonia, atelectasis and bronchiectasis. Other complications consist of convulsions, conjunctival hemorrhage, ulceration of frenum and prolapse of the rectum.

Management :

Erythromycin is effective in reducing the severity of infection if given during the catarrhal stage. Cough suppressants like pholcodine and methadone are helpful in controlling the severity of paroxysms. When the illness is of long duration accompanied by frequent vomiting, skilled nursing will be required to maintain nutrition especially in infants and young children. Feeds are generally accepted and retained if they are given immediately after the vomiting which follows a paroxysm of coughing.

Prevention :

Pertussis vaccine is available in the multiple immunogen form of Diphtheria and Tetanus Toxoid and Pertussis Vaccine Adsorbed (DTP) which is recommended for active immunization of infants and children, 6 weeks through 6 years against diphtheria, tetanus and pertussis simultaneously. The schedule of vaccination has been described under tetanus.

TUBERCULOSIS

Throughout history, tuberculosis has assumed a prominent role as a frightening disease that has affected society as well as the practice of medicine. It has also been referred to as the white plague and as phthisis, which indicates its wasting character.

Human tuberculosis is almost invariably caused by **Mycobacterium tuberculosis,** a nonmotile, slow-growing, nonspore-forming aerobic bacillus that resides primarily in humans. In man, the lung is the most common site of infection, although other areas like bones, meninges, joints, peritoneum, genitourinary tract and skin may also get infected. **Mycobacterium tuberculosis** is an aerobic bacillus and because of its ability to resist decolorization with acid-alcohol after staining with carbolfuchsin (Ziehl-Neelsen method or fluorescence technique), it is also referred to as 'acid-fast' bacillus. It can thrive in organs of relatively high oxygen tension such as apices of the lung, the renal parenchyma, the growing ends of the bones and the cerebral cortex. It is also tolerant to the acid environment of the stomach and it has been isolated from the gastric contents of the patients suffering from tuberculosis.

Epidemiology: Tubercle bacilli are transmitted by aerosolized droplets, expectorated from a person with pulmonary tuberculosis which remain airborne for a considerable time. Transmission of these particles can be prevented by adequate room ventilation, ultraviolet light and chemotherapy of the source case. Tubercle bacilli are not transmitted on objects such as dishes, clothing or bedding.

The presence or absence of certain factors will influence an individual's likelihood of acquiring tuberculosis. Persons exposed to individuals with active pulmonary tuberculosis constitute the group at highest risk for acquiring the disease. Conversion rates may be as high as 27% depending on the infectivity of the patients sputum. Upto 15% of these converters may go on to develop the active form of the disease. Family household contacts and those in institutions e.g. hospitals, nursing homes, prisons sharing an enclosed environment with an open case are at a major risk for infection.

Geographic location also influences the propensity for developing tuberculosis. Individuals from underdeveloped countries are at extremely high risk.

Age has not generally been considered a risk for acquisition of tuberculosis. Recent studies, however, have documented an increased incidence of newly acquired skin test positivity in elderly patients, particularly those residing in nursing homes. Elderly patients may therefore be at risk for contacting tuberculosis as a nosocomial disease. It has also been suggested that children may also constitute a high-risk group for acquiring the disease particularly due to household contacts of infected individuals. Other patient factors associated with an increased risk for contacting tuberculosis include low socio-economic status, non-caucasian race and male sex.

Certain risk factors such as diabetes mellitus, silicosis, gastrectomy, crowded living conditions, alcohol abuse, chronic renal failure, hematological disease, reticuloendothelial disease and corticosteroid use enhance the chances of developing clinical tuberculosis.

Lastly, it appears that patients with AIDs or AIDs-related complex are at increased risk for acquiring tuberculosis. The diagnosis of tuberculosis should not be excluded in AIDs patients with respiratory tract infections who do not possess other risk factors.

There has been a dramatic decline in the incidence of tuberculosis after 1950s largely due to effective chemotherapy, early recognition of source cases and use of BCG vaccination in the underdeveloped countries. Some of the factors contributing to the decreasing incidence of tuberculosis are given in Table 8.4.

Table 8.4 Factors responsible for decreasing the incidence of tuberculosis.

1. Effective chemotherapy
2. Early detection of disease.
3. BCG vaccination.
4. Isolation of infectious open cases.
5. Less crowded living conditions.
6. Adequate nutrition.
7. Declining rate of infection in adults.
8. Medicosocial awareness.

With the recognition that tuberculosis can be effectively treated with outpatient drug therapy, the responsibility of treatment has now shifted from the sanatorium to the community hospital, private physician and general practitioners. The need for early detection and treatment necessitates that all the practioners and paramedical workers become familiar with the disease process and the principles of treatment of this one time dreaded disease.

Pathophysiology: The host-Mycobacterium relationship in man is incredibly diverse. The extent of infection may range from a solitary granuloma that is undetectable on chest X ray to a widely disseminated disease involving virtually every organ system in the body.

Tuberculosis is invariably transmitted from person to person via microsize droplet nuclei which are dispersed by either coughing or sneezing. The primary infection is initiated by the alveolar implantation of organisms in droplet nuclei that are small enough to escape the ciliary epithelial cells of the upper respiratory tract. This initial infection usually occurs in the lower segment(s) of the lung. Persons that have been previously infected with tuberculosis are protected from re-infection by a specific immunity mediated by T lymphocytes. In the susceptable (non-immune) host the bacteria multiply initially unopposed by normal host defense mechanisms. The tubercle bacilli that enter into the macrophage during phagocytosis may remain viable for long time. They may enter the lymphatic system and disseminate to other organs of the body.After a period of 3-10 weeks, a specific T-lymphocyte-mediated immune response develops and prevents further multiplication of these bacilli. The T-lymphocytes cause release of lysosomal enzymes from macrophages which destroy some bacilli but at the same time damage host tissues.

This immune response leads to tissue healing and granuloma formation. The bacilli present in the granuloma may survive and remain dormant for many years. These granulomas may break down in later years and lead to either pulmonary or extrapulmonary disease. Most of the cases of tuberculosis result from a reactivation (breakdown of a granuloma) of an earlier infection rather than a new infection.

In order to understand the pathophysiology of tuberculosis it is necessary to make a clear distinction between infection and clinical disease. Infection with tuberculosis refers to harboring the bacilli within the body with no X-ray changes, negative bacteriological profile and no clinical symptoms. Clinical disease results when a lack of host defense mechanisms allow infection to progress to one or more organs and produce clinical symptoms, X-ray changes, or positive bacteriological profile. A confirmed diagnosis of tuberculosis is dependent on the isolation of M. tuberculosis from the sputum, spinal fluid, urine or tissue biopsy. It takes 6-8 weeks for this culture to become positive. The risk of developing clinical disease within 5 years after infection is 5-15% if left untreated and the highest risk occurs in first one to two years after infection.

Diagnosis:

PPD Skin Test : The PPD skin test (Mantoux test) is used for the detection of infection with M.tuberculosis. It refers to the purified protein derivative of M.tuberculosis which is prepared from a culture of tubercle bacilli. The skin test (intermediate strength PPD, is performed by injecting 0.1 ml of solution containing 5 tuberculin units (TU) intracutaneously into the volar or dorsal portion of the forearm. The solution stabilized with tween 80, should be administered immediately after its withdrawal from the vial.

In the presence of mycobacterial infection, a delayed hypersensitivity reaction to the tubercle bacillus or to its components develops in the host. Upon re-exposure to the tuberculin antigen (PPD skin Test) the host's immune system responds with a characteristic inflammatory reaction at the site of exposure. This reaction generally develops within 2 to 10 weeks after infection.

A palpable induration of greater than 10 mm diameter, 48-72 hours after administration is considered to be a positive reaction; a reading of 5-9 mm is considered doubtful and 0-4 mm is interpreted as negative reaction. This measurement is not based on the erythematous zone, but rather on the palpable induration which represents localized thickening of the skin due to oedema and accumulation of sensitized leucocytes. The greatest value of PPD skin testing can be attributed to a negative test. With very few exceptions, a negative test rules out active tuberculosis.

Bacterial culture: Isolation of M.tuberculosis from an infected site provides confirmatory proof of tuberculosis in the patient. The most frequent source of the bacillus is sputum and tracheal or gastric washings. Material from washings or biopsy should be cultured for identification of the bacillus. Examination of sputum is important in providing microbiologic evidence of tuberculosis. Acid fast bacilli may be detected in the sputa of virtually all patients with active pulmonary tuberculosis.

X-Rays Chest X-rays are very valuable in the identification of pulmonary tuberculosis. Repeated films are usually necessary to establish the presence of the disease. X-rays are also essential in evaluating the progress and effectiveness of chemotherapy.,

Clinical Presentation: The clinical presentation of pulmonary tuberculosis is nonspecific, indicative of a slowly evolving infectious process. A patient with subclinical or early disease may be completely asymptomatic. When the severity of infection rises to a certain point, the patient begins to complain of generalized malaise, anorexia, weight loss and fatigue as well as intermittent fevers with alternating chills and night sweats. Subsequently, a cough with increasing sputum formation develops. Pleuritic chest pain may or may not be a concurrent complaint. Hemoptysis, when occurs, indicates advanced disease.

Expectoration and swallowing of sputum containing large number of organisms may result in extension of disease involving upper respiratory or gastrointestinal tract. Ulceration of pharynx, larynx, tongue and oral mucosa as well as otitis media, gastric ulceration and perirectal abscess may occur.

Physical examination suggests only slowly progressive pulmonary disease. Dullness to chest percussion suggests consolidation in involved areas of lungs. Rales and increased vocal fremitus are frequently observed upon ausculation. In patients in whom impaired oxygenation has developed, cyanosis and clubbing of digits may be seen.

Abnormal laboratory data are limited to moderate elevation of white blood cells count with a lymphocyte predominence.

Clinical features associated with extrapulmonary tuberculosis vary depending on the organ system(s) involved but typically consist of slowly progressive compromise of organ function with low grade fever and other constitutional symptoms. Concurrent pulmonary tuberculosis may or may not be present.

Complications : The complications associated with tuberculosis are dependent on the organs involved. In acute pulmonary tuberculosis, necrosis with liquefaction develops. As this fluid empties, cavities remain. Arteries leading to the resulting cavities may burst causing frank pulmonary hemorrhage. Atelactasis is a further complication associated with respiratory lesions. A similar process occurs with renal involvement. When lesions are in the kidney, cavitation may also occur. Ruptured blood vessels in this area lead to hematuria. In females tuberculosis of the fallopian tubes and uterus may result in abdominal pain, vaginal discharge, sterility or ectopic pregnancy. Tuberculosis of the adrenal glands may cause total destruction of the glands and results in Addison's disease. When tuberculosis strikes the linings of organs in the body such as peritoneum, pleura and pericardium several types of complaints may occur including tuberculous peritonitis, adhesions between peritoneal surfaces or fibrous membranes leading to constriction and impairment of intestinal motility etc.

Two very serious complications are miliary tuberculosis and tubercular meningitis. Miliary tuberculosis is a hematogenous disease allowing widespread infection throughout the body due to massive dissemination of tubercle bacilli. Lesions are also found in the liver, spleen, bone marrow and other organs which do not have a high oxygen tension. The signs and symptoms are nonspecific and include dyspnea, weight loss, weakness, fever, night sweats and gastrointestinal disturbances. Death is certain unless appropriate treatment is instituted promptly. Diagnosis is based on a biopsy of the liver or bone marrow showing caseating granulomas. In tubercular meningitis fluid collects around the base of the brain causing adhesion. Since these lesions are in the area of hypothalamus, fatal brain damage may be encountered. Signs and symptoms include headache, restlessness, irritability, nausea vomiting and stiffness of the neck.

Prophylaxis:

BCG Vaccine: BCG (Bacillus of Calmette and Guerin) is a human vaccine derived from a strain of bovine mycobacterium. It is the most common prophylactic measure used in the under-developed countries where there is a high rate of primary infection as well as inadequate facilities for diagnostic screening of patients with tuberculosis. It is used to prevent the disease in persons who are tuberculin negative (no immunity to tuberculous infection) There are many different BCG vaccines available worldwide and all of them differ with respect to immunogenicity, efficacy and reactogenicity. These factors may account for the varied degrees of protection afforded by the vaccine. Vaccination with BCG, at best, can provide 80% protection against tuberculosis. Prior vaccination with BCG usually results in a positive tuberculin skin test. It is impossible to differentiate between a positive skin test due to BCG and that due to infection with M. tuberculosis. Adverse reactions to BCG vaccine vary according to the type, dosage and age of the vaccine. Osteomyelitis, prolonged ulceration at the vaccination site, lupoid reactions, lymphadenitis, disseminated BCG infection and death have all been reported. Hence its routine use is not advocated.

However, it is administered to high risk patients who are in an environment where contact with tuberculosis is unavoidable. Such circumstances include children of parents with tuberculosis, family and friends of a tuberculous patient and hospital and rest home employees where contact is most likely to occur.

Prophylactic INH Therapy: Preventive therapy of tuberculosis with isoniazid decreases the bacterial population in those taking the drug. Therefore INH preventive therapy is not really prophylactic therapy but in actuality reflects treatment of an infection.Such therapy reduces future morbidity from tuberculosis in the groups at high risk of developing active disease. Persons treated with INH who have not received prior chemotherapy for tuberculosis had a 60% reduction in bacteriologically proven disease over a seven year period when compared to persons receiving a placebo. The American Thoracic Society and the Centre for Disease Control have balanced the risks of developing active tuberculosis against the risks of INH toxicity and have jointly established guidelines and priorities for determining the type of patients who should receive preventive INH therapy.

Prognosis: Tuberculosis was a major cause of death in the first half of the 20th century and earlier. Though a bane to mankind, tuberculosis was paradoxically the impetus for many of the early discoveries in medicine, including the monumental findings of Robert Koch and discovery of streptomycin leading to the award of Noble Prize in Medicine and Physiology to Dr. S.A. Waksman. Prior to the advent of chemotherapy for tuberculosis mortality figures were very high. Eminent personalities who fell victims to this disease included Smt. Kamla Nehru, Mohamed Ali Zinna and famous English poets John Keats and P.B. Shelley. Today few people die of this disease. Early detection and prompt treatment with correct drug regimen are usually sufficient to render patients free of active infection. An infected person is considered no longer contagious after about two weeks of appropriate chemotherapy. Patients should be able to return to work as soon as sputum cultures are negative. Patients should be instructed to report for an examination if symptoms of reactivation are noted. The most serious danger exists in miliary tuberculosis but even in this instance therapy usually results in remarkable clinical improvement within two months. In conclusion, chemotherapy of tuberculosis is the cornerstone of effective treatment. Three goals of chemotherapy exist i) to eliminate as many organisms from the body as possible, therapy limiting the incidence of relapse to less than 5%; (ii) to prevent the development of resistance which could result in treatment failure and (iii) to minimize toxicity and cost of treatment while maximizing patient compliance.

Management :

For an effective treatment of tuberculosis continuous and intensive drug therapy with at least two bactericidal drugs is necessary for a definite period of time. A combination of isoniazid (INH) 300 mg and rifampicin 600 mg daily for 2-3 months is prescribed for the treatment of uncomplicated cases of pulmonary tuberculosis. This INH-rifampicin combination sterilizes the lesions and sputum faster than the standard three drug regimen of INH, streptomycin and ethambutol used earlier. The dosage of rifampicin is extremely important when using this two drug regimen. Doses of rifampicin less than 600 mg a day in combination with INH are associated with decreased effectiveness.

Multiple drug therapy is required for preventing the development of resistance strains of bacilli and to sterilize the sputum and lesions as quickly as possible. The drugs available for the treatment of tuberculosis vary in their effectiveness to accomplish these tasks as described below in Table 8.5.

Table 8.5 Effectiveness of antibacterial drugs in tuberculosis

Activity	Prevention of Drug of Resistance	Sterilization Potential
High	Isoniazid	Rifampicin
	Rifampicin	Pyrazinamide
	Streptomycin	Isoniazid
	Ethambutol	Streptomycin
	Thiacetazone	Ethambutol
Low	Pyrazinamide	Thiacetazone

D.A. Mitchison, Basic mechanisms of chemotherapy. Chest, 76 (Suppl.): 771, 1979.

The antitubercular drugs can be divided in two groups on the basis of their use in clinical practice. The primary drugs INH and rifampicin are used initially as first line drugs. Both of them are bactericidal against the fast growing extracellular bacilli in the lung cavity. Rifampicin also has activity against intracellular organisms that are usually dormant but undergo periods of active growth. This ability to penetrate and destroy the slow growing persistent intracellular organisms makes rifampicin extremely valuable in short course chemotherapy regimens.

The secondary drugs streptomycin, ethambutol and pyrazinamide are generally less effective and more toxic than primary agents. They are mostly used in combination with INH and rifampicin when drug resistant organisms are suspected or to treat extrapulmonary tuberculosis infections. Streptomycin is active against the fast multiplying extracellular organisms and is very effective when given daily for two months followed by two or three times a week administration. Streptomycin must be given intramuscularly which is painful and hence there is poor patient compliance. Ethambutol is bacteriostatic and is moderately effective against the fast growing bacilli. It has poor sterilizing activity and is used primarily for the prevention of drug resistant organisms. Pyrazinamide is effective against intracellular bacilli and is very effective in sterilizing the lesions and appears to be most active in the first two months of the treatment.

The other drugs used in the treatment of tuberculosis, capreomycin, kanamycin, cycloserine, ethionamide and aminosalicylic acid are usually reserved for cases involving drug resistant organisms, drug toxicity or patient intolerance to other drugs.

B. INTESTINAL INFECTIONS

POLIOMYELITIS

Etiology: Poliomyelitis is caused by one of the three related polio viruses which comprise a subdivision of the group of enteroviruses. Its incidence has significantly declined following the widespread use of oral vaccine but it is still a major problem in developing countries. Infection usually occurs through the nasopharynx.

The virus is liable to affect the grey matter of the spinal cord, brain stem and cortex and has a particular propensity to damage anterior horn cells especially those within the lumbar segments. The incubation period is 7-14 days.

Clinical presentation: Its an acute viral disease, occurring sporadically and in epidemics and characterized clinically by fever, sore throat, headache and vomiting, often with stiffness of the neck and back. In the minor illness these may be the only symptoms. In other instances after a period of well-being lasting for about a week, there is recurrence of pyrexia and headache. The major illness, that follows, is characterized by the involvement of central nervous system, stiff neck, pleocytosis in the spinal fluid and meningeal irritation. Paralysis may occur and is of variable extent. Weakness of one muscle group may progress to widespread paresis. There may be subsequent atrophy of group of muscles, ending in contraction and permanent deformity. Respiratory failure may supervene if intercostal muscles are paralysed or the medullary motor nuclei are affected. The major illness is also called acute anterior poliomyelitis or infantile paralysis.

Management: In the early stages bed rest is absolutely necessary. At the onset of respiratory difficulties, a tracheostomy and intermittent positive pressure ventilation are required. Subsequent treatment is done by physiotherapy and orthopaedic measures.

Prognosis : Epidemics show wide variation in the incidence of abortive and non-paralytic cases and also in the mortality rate. Death occurs due to respiratory paralysis. Muscle weakness is maximal at the end of the first week and gradual recovery may then take place for several months. Any muscle not showing signs of recovery by the end of a month, will not regain useful function. It is difficult to make a more definitive prediction about the extent of permanent disability until 3-6 months after the onset. Subsequent attacks are very rare but occasional patients show late deterioration in muscle bulk and power, many years after the initial infection.

Prevention : Poliovirus Vaccine Live Oral (Trivalent Oral Polio Vaccine, Sabin Vaccine) is considered the vaccine of choice for primary immunization of children. It is indicated for active immunization against infections of poliovirus caused by poliovirus Types 1,2 and 3 in infants starting at 6-12 week and all unimmunized children and adolescents upto 18 years of age.

Dose: Oral two doses 6 to 8 week apart followed by a third dose 8 to 12 months after the second dose and a booster upon entering elementary school. Recently , the W.H.O. has strongly recommended reduction of the age of initial immunization with TOPV to birth. The recommended WHO schedule has been described elsewhere in this book.

HEPTATITIS

Heptatitis or inflammation of liver which may lead to hepatic cell necrosis is caused by various factors such as viruses, bacteria or chemicals. Acute viral hepatitis is a systemic infection affecting predominantly but not exclusively the liver. The pharmacist should be aware of the causes and treatment of viral hepatitis because of its comparatively high prevalence and also understand drug induced causes to help identify and eliminate their occurrence.

Etiology: Viral hepatitis can be caused by at least three distinct etiologic agents- hepatitis A virus (HAV), hepatitis B virus (HBV) and hepatitis non-A non-B viruses (HNANB). Although hepatitis A and B viruses produce clinically similar disease in man, the two forms generally differ in their incubation period, mode of transmission and sequelae. Precise differentiation can be made by their antigenic properties. The third type, non-A non-B hepatitis resembles hepatitis B, but is serologically distinct. Because it is not detected by the routine antigenic screening employed by blood banks HNANB causes about 90% of post transfusion hepatitis. HAV is a RNA virus while HBV is a DNA virus. Not much is known about the nucleic acid composition of NANB virus.

Epidemiology: Direct personal contact is the main route of transmission of HAV and the fecal-oral route is most often involved. Children and young adults are most commonly infected with HA which often occurs in epidemic form especially in the areas where sanitation is poor. Contaminated water, uncooked shellfish, other foods and poor hygienic conditions play a role in the spread of HA.

Transmission of HBV is most often by parenteral inoculation of the virus containing material. It can also be transmitted transcutaneously, orally and sexually. It is also spread by intimate physical contact and transmitted from mothers to their fetuses or neonates. Others shown to be at high risk of contacting HBV are surgeons, dentists, oncologists and renal dialysis unit personnel in the hospitals and drug abusers.

HNANB virus is transmitted mainly by transfusion of blood products containing the agent. Specific blood products can be classified as high risk, average risk or safe (Table 8.6). The actual risk of infection following transfusion depends on the donor population, the number of units transfused and the susceptibility of the recipient to viral hepatitis. Generally the risk of hepatitis following transfusion of pooled blood or of blood obtained from commercial/professional donors is greater than the risk following transfusion of blood from volunteer donors.

Table 8.6 Risk of Transmission of Hepatitis from Blood Products:

A.	**High risk:** Pooled, cannot be sterilized 1. UV light exposed pooled plasma. 2. Platelets 3. Fibrinogen and clotting factor concentrates. 4. Antihemophiliac concentrate. 5. Factor IX complex.
B.	**Average risk:** Single donor,cannot be sterilized. 1. Whole blood. 2. Single donor plasma. 3. Packed RBCs (2-6° C) 4. Frozen RBCs 5. Platelets. 6. Antihemophiliac concentrate.
C.	**Safe:** Sterilized products(prepared by heating for 10 h at 60°C or by ethanol fractionation) 1. Human serum albumin. 2. Immune and hyperimmune gamma-globulin 3. Plasma protein fraction. 4. Thrombin. 5. Fibrinolysin.

Pathophysiology: The pathological changes induced by three viruses include panlobular infiltrations with small lymphocytes or monocytes, hepatic cell degenerative swelling, ballooning and necrosis, hyperplasia of Kupffer cells and cholestasis without fatty infiltration. In uncomplicated cases the reticulum framework remains intact and orderly regeneration of liver cells occurs. In severe cases extensive necrosis, destruction of reticulum framework and fibrosis between liver lobules occurs. In massive hepatic necrosis a small shrunken liver is found at autopsy.

In HB the liver cells replicate the virus and the virus or its fragments are incorporated into liver cell membranes. Humoral antibodies, IgG and IgM are formed against the virus. These antibodies attack the foreign plasma membranes. Cellular immunity is thus involved in the liver damage. Circulating immune complexes and complement activation are responsible for the systemic manifestations seen in hepatitis. The consequences of HB are thus largely due to immune response to infection rather than to the cytotoxicity of the virus.

Clinical presentation: Symptoms of infection with HA are usually acute in onset and infections occur primarily in children and young adults. The incubation period is short ranging between 15 to 50 days (mean 25-28 days) . On the other hand symptoms of infection due to hepatitis B can be either acute or insidious in onset, infections occur in all age groups and the virus has a longer incubation period of 45 to 180 days. HA is a comparatively mild disease with complete recovery and does not appear to produce a chronic carrier state, chronic liver disease or cirrhosis. It tends to be benign and self limited. With the exception of some elderly patients HA virus rarely produces fulminant hepatitis.

HB may be a severe disease with a poor prognosis, the clinical course is frequently longer for HB than for HA, it can progress to chronic hepatitis and a carrier state may develop. HNANB resembles HB.

The prodromal symptoms vary and may include anorexia, nausea, vomiting, changes in the sense of smell and taste, fatigue, malaise, arthralgias, myalgias, headache, photophobia, pharyngitis, cough, coryza and fever. The symptoms usually appear 1-2 weeks before the onset of jaundice. Dark urine and clay-colored stools may occur 1 to 5 days before the jaundice. During the icteric phase the liver is enlarged and tender and there may be right upper quadrant pain. Splenomegaly and cervical lymphadenopathy may also be present. The symptoms subside during the recovery phase but the abnormal laboratory findings may still persist. The recovery phase may last 2 to 12 weeks and is longer in HB. Laboratory indices may take 3 to 4 months to normalize.

Several liver cell enzymes including serum aminotransferases and lactic dehydrogenases increase during the prodromal phase of acute viral hepatitis. The degree of rise does not correlate well with the severity of disease. The liver-cell enzymes peak with the onset of jaundice. Jaundice is usually visible in the skin and sclera when the serum bilirubin levels exceed 2.5 mg/100 ml.

Almost all the patients with HA and the majority of patients with HB and HNANB recover without sequelae. Poor prognostic signs include the presence of subacute hepatic necrosis, a serum bilirubin level of greater than 20mg/100ml, that persists and an elevated prothombin time which indicates extensive hepatocellular damage. Elderly patients or patients with underlying disease generally suffer from a more severe form of hepatitis. The mortality rate is 0.1% for HA and 1-2% for HB. Chronic hepatitis occurs as a complication of HB in 5-10% of patients and in 30% patients with HNANB. About 0.1 to 1.0% patients of HB develop a carrier state. The virus DNA becomes integrated into the hepatocyte genome in some patients. They are usually asymptomatic and noninfectious but carry an increased risk of developing hepatocel-

Prophylaxis:

Prophylactic use of γ-globulin has been advised for persons with suspected exposure to hepatitis or who live in the endemic areas. It is administered intramuscularly 0.01ml/lb, early in the incubation period after exposure to hepatitis A. It is possible that the individual may still develop a subclinical infection but will not be symptomatic. A dose of 0.05 to 0.06 ml/lb is given for protection upto 4 months in endemic areas. It has however not proved effective in the prophylaxis of HB even when used in much higher doses. A HB Immune Globulin containing high titres of anti-HB has been developed which can be given either preceding or concomitant with Hepatitis B vaccine to provide a more rapid achievement of protective levels of hepatitis B antibody. Given alone it remains effective for about four weeks. These measures are recommended for immunization against infections caused by all known subtypes of HB virus especially for persons who are or will be at higher risk of infection with HB. These higher risk groups include health care personnel, morticians, embalmers, homosexually active males and users of illicit injectable drugs etc. However, the high cost of immune globulins and Hepatitis B vaccine precludes their wide spread use for routine prophylaxis.

CHOLERA

Cholera is severe acute gastrointestinal infection caused by **Vibrio cholerae**. It is generally confined to the valleys of the Ganges and other great rivers of the far east where high humidity and population density have maintained the disease. In these valleys devastating epidemics have occurred often following large religious festivals and pandemics have spread throughout Asia and Europe even to North America. The biotype of **V.cholerae, El Tor** that is responsible for the pandemic is more resistant than the classic vibrio and amenable to more prolonged carriage following infection.

The organism is spread through the stools, vomitus, patients with cholera and a large number of subclinical cases who excrete it for a few days. It survives upto two weeks in fresh water and 8 weeks in salt water. Transmission is normally through infected drinking water, contaminated food, flies and infected hands.

Pathology : Vibrio cholerae multiplies in the lumen of the small intestine and is noninvasive. It secretes a powerful exotoxin (enterotoxin) which stimulates the adenyl-cyclase-adenosine monophosphate pathway of the mucosa and this results in an outpouring of normal alkaline, small bowel fluid. Severe dehydration follows rapidly in spite of the fact that absorption of fluid by the bowel is hardly impaired. There may be acidosis and depletion of sodium and potassium ions. This may lead to further complications of which renal failure is the most important. The incubation period of **V.cholerae** is few hours to 5 days.

Clinical presentation : There is sudden onset of severe diarrhoea without pain or colic which is followed by vomiting. After the normal fecal contents of the gut are evacuated the typical "rice-water" matcrial is passed which consists of clear fluid with flecks of mucus.This enormous loss of fluids and electrolytes leads to severe dehydration and muscular cramps. The skin becomes cold, clammy and wrinkled and the eyes get sunken. The blood pressure falls, the pulse becomes extremely weak and the urine output diminishes. The patient usually remains mentally clear and the perception is not affected. Death occurs within a few hours due to circulatory failure unless the fluid and electrolytes are adequatcly replaced.With proper treatment improvement is rapid. In rare circumstances anuria may persist and lead to death.

Complications: The complications of cholera are mainly due to electrolyte imbalance. They include hypocalcemia, tetany, hypernatremia, acidosis and hypoglycemia. Some patients develop febrile convulsions. In rare instances overtreatment may lead to pulmonary oedema.

Management: The most important measure in the treatment of cholera is to maintain circulation by the replacement of water and electrolytes. The earlier this is started the better will be the prognosis. Fluids are given intravenously in severe cases or when there is vomiting. Fluid is run as fast as possible until pulse and blood pressure return to normal levels.

Vomiting usually stops once the patient is adequately rehydrated and fluids are then given orally every hour. Patients are made to drink upto 500 ml hourly. The quantity of fluid to be administered is calculated every 8 hours from the output of urine, stool, vomitus and estimated insensible loss which may be as much as 5 litres in 24 hours in a hot and humid climate.

Total fluid requirement can be in excess of 50 litres in a period of 2-5 days.

The ideal solutions for replacement of fluids and electrolytes are given in the Table 8.7.

Table 8.7 Recommended solution for treatment of cholera

Intravenous	g/l	Oral	g/l
Sodium chloride	5.0	Common salt	3.5
Potassium chloride	1.0	Potassium chloride 1.5	
		or citrate	2.7
Sodium bicrbonate	4.0	Sodium bicarbonate	2.5
or acetate	8.0	Glucose	20.0

Other satisfactory fluids, which can be used, include Ringer lactate or Hartman's solution or Darrow's solution in which event supplements of potassium are required or given separately. The presence of glucose in oral fluid has been shown to promote electrolyte absorption. Chlorpromazine, 50 mg, 6-hourly reduces intestinal secretion and fluid loss. Three days treatment with tetracycline 250 mg, 6-hourly or co-trimoxazole one tablet daily reduces the duration of excretion of vibrios and the total volume of fluid needed for replacement.

Prevention: Strict personal hygiene is the best method of personal prophylaxis. Drinking water should come from a clean supply or it should be boiled. Access of flies to food must be totally restricted. Vaccination with a killed suspension of **V.cholera** may provide limited protection. Control of water sources and of population movement and public education are the most important measures during an epidemic. Mass vaccination with a single dose vaccine and mass treatment with tetracycline are valuable. Proper disinfection of infective discharges and soiled clothing and scrupulous washing of hands by medical attendants reduces the danger of spread from the treatment centres.

TYPHOID AND PARATYPHOID (ENTERIC) FEVERS

Typhoid and paratyphoid fevers, which are usually transmitted by faecal-oral route, are important causes of illness in many countries where sanitation is primitive.

Etiology : The enteric fevers are caused by infections with **Salmonella typhi** and **Salmonella paratyphi A** and **B**. They are usually spread by carriers, food handlers and contaminated food, milk or water supplies. The bacilli may survive in the gall bladders of carriers for months or years after clinical recovery and pass intermittently in the stool. The incubation period for typhoid fever is about 10-14 days and that of paratyphoid is somewhat shorter.

Pathology : After a few days of bacteremia, the bacilli localise mainly in the lymphoid tissue of small intestine. They produce typical lesions in the Peyer patches and follicles which swell at first, then ulcerate and ultimately heal, and during this process they may perforate or bleed.

Clinical presentation:

Typhoid fever : The onset may be insidious. The temperature rises in a step-ladder fashion for 4-5 days and is accompanied by malaise, headache, drowsiness and aching in the limbs. Cough and epistaxis occur. The pulse is often lower than would be expected from the rise in temperature. Constipation may be present although in children diarrhoea and vomiting may be prominent early in the illness.

At the end of the first week typical rash appears on the abdomen. About the 7th to 10th day the spleen becomes palpable. At this time constipation is succeeded by diarrhoea. Bronchitis and delirium may develop. By the end of second week the patient may be profoundly ill unless the disease is modified by antibiotic treatment. In the third week toxaemia increases and the patient may pass into coma and die.

Paratyphoid fever: The course of paratyphoid fever tends to be shorter and milder than that of typhoid fever but onset is generally more abrupt with acute enteritis. The rash may be more abundant and the intestinal complications less frequent.

Complications: Hemorrhage from Peyer's patches or their perforation may occur at the end of the second week or during third week of the illness. Additional complications, due to septicemia present during the second week include cholecystitis, pneumonia, myocarditis, arthritis, osteomyelitis and meningitis.

Management : The patient is preferably isolated and treated in bed. Proper attention must be paid to adequate nutrition and fluid intake, care of the mouth and prevention of pressure sores. Several antibiotics are effective in enteric fever. These include amoxycillin, ciprofloxacin, chloramphenicol and co-trimoxazole. Treatment should be continued for 14 days. Pyrexia may persist for upto 5 days after the start of specific therapy. Even with effective chemotherapy, there is still a danger of complications of recrudescence of the disease and the development of a carrier state. The chronic carrier should be treated for 4 weeks with ciprofloxacin.

Prevention: Monovalent typhoid vaccine is used for prevention of the disease in countries where enteric infections are endemic.

FOOD POISONING

Food poisoning (gastroenteritis) can be due to a number of causes which have been summarized in the Table 8.8.

Table 8.8 Causes of Food Poisoning

INFECTIVE		
	Non-toxin mediated	
		Salmonella species
		Campylobacter jejuni
		Bacillus cereus
		Viruses (e.g. Norwalk viruses)
		Listeria monocytogens (causes meningitis)
		Bacillus anthracis (Anthrax)
		Protozoa (Giardia; Cryptosporidium)
	Toxin-mediated	
		Staphylococcus aureus
		Clostridium perfringens
		Clostridium botulinum (Botulism)
		E.Coli 0157 (Verocytotoxin producing)
NON-INFECTIVE:		
	Allergic	
		Shell fish, strawberries
	Non-allergic	
		Scrombotoxin (fish)
		Ciguatoxin (tropical fish)
		Fungi (Amanita phalloides-mushroom)

Food poisoning presents with vomiting, diarrhoea or both, usually within 48 hours of the consumption of contaminated food or drink. Outbreaks are common especially in institutions and restaurants and following community lunches or dinners. Non-infective causes and bacterial toxins which are pre-formed in the infected food produce symptoms within minutes or hours of a meal whereas the other infections may not produce symptoms upto 48 hours. Infective gastroenteritis can be classified as nontoxin type and toxin type.

Non-toxin type: Salmonella species other than S.typhi are very commonly involved in the production of food poisoning. The domestic fowl is the most common source of infection which may be contacted from inadequately defrosted and undercooked chicken or from undercooked or raw eggs. Symptomless faecal carriers of salmonella who are food handlers are also source of infection. Campylobacter jejuni is another common bacterial cause of food poisoning. Sources of infection include poultry, dogs, water and unpasteurized milk.

Bacillus cereus infection. This is a hazard of eating rice which has been cooked and then consumed at a later date.

Listeria monocytogens: It contaminates food items including poultry and cheese. It rarely causes gastroenteritis but it can produce septicemia and meningitis especially in pregnancy, neonate, immunocompromized patients, diabetics and alcoholics.

Viruses: Viruses like Norwalk viruses which contaminate shell fish can cause food poisoning.

Protozoal Organisms: Amongst the protozoa **Giardia lamblia** and Cryptosporidium species can cause food poisoning or waterborne outbreaks of diarrhoeal disease.

Toxin type: Food poisoning of toxin type is generally caused by the enterotoxin of **Staphylococcus aureus.** It often orginates from a food handler with a septic lesion on the hand. Incubation at a favourable temperature leads to growth of the organism which is heat resistant and may not be destroyed by cooking. Strains of heat resistant clostridia can contaminate certain foods like meat. Precooking of stews and pies does not destroy all the spores and storing of such items will lead to formation of heat stable toxins which may give rise to severe gastroenteritis. A particular strain of **Escherichia coli** (enterohemorhagic **E.Coli** type 0157) which produces verocytotoxin, has been found to produce food poisoning originating in meat, which may present as haemorrhagic colitis.

Clinical presentation: The incubation period points towards the etiology of food poisoning to a great extent. If vomiting occurs within 30 minutes of the ingestion of suspected food, it is likely to be due to a chemical poison, if it occurs after 12-48 hours, the most likely cause may be a **salmonella** or **compylobacter** infection. The incubation periods of **staphylococcal** and **clostridial** food poisoning are intermediate between these. The **E.Coli** infection produces bloody diarrhoea after 12-48 hours which is generally not preceded by vomiting.

Management: With mild cases symptoms subside in a few days. Solids should be withheld and the patient is advised to take fluids only. Patients who are sick and dehydrated require intravenous fluid therapy. Codeine phosphate, loperamide, a combination of diphenoxylate and atropine (Lomotil) may be useful in controlling non-infective diarrhoea in adults.

Antibiotics should be given only when they are indicated for the treatment of an infective organism. If **salmonella** infection is confirmed or suspected with severe and prolonged diarrhoea, ciprofloxacin or trimethoprim should be given. **Campylobacter** enteritis is treated with ciprofloxacin or erythromycin. **Listeria monocytogenes** is sensitive to ampicillin or erythromycin. Gentamicin is combined with ampicillin for the treatment of **L.monocytogenes** induced meningitis. If the poisoning is due to a chemical or poisonous food, the patients stomach should be washed out with tepid water.

Botulism: Botulism is an ususual type of food poisoning caused by the ingestion of toxin produced by **C.botulinum** in imperfectly treated tinned food or preserved fish contaminated with this organism. The clinical features are quite different from other types of food poisoning and consist mainly of vomiting and slight paralysis of skeletal, ocular, pharyngeal and respiratory muscles. The mortality rate can be high in botulism.

Prevention of Food Poisoning : Prevention of the high incidence of food poisoning can best be achieved by improving the standard of personal hygiene especially in those handling food and by stressing the importance of washing of hands after using the lavatory and before taking the meals. Frozen food particularly poultry has to be properly thawed at room temperature for at least 12 hours before cooking otherwise pathogens may survive unharmed at the centre.

HOOKWORM INFECTION
(ANCYLOSTOMIASIS)

Hookworm infection is one of the main causes of anemia in the tropics. It is caused by the parasitisation of the small intestine with **Ancylostoma duodenale** or **Necator americanus.**

The adult hookworm is a greyish-white nematode, about 1 cm in length and lives in large numbers in the duodenum and upper jejunum. Hookworm eggs are passed in the faeces. In the warm, moist and shady soil the larvae develop and reach the filariform infective stage which penetrate human skin and from there carried to the lungs through the blood stream. After entering the alveoli, they ascend the bronchi, are swallowed and grow in the small intestine reaching maturity in 4-7 weeks after infection. Hookworm infection is widespread under insanitary conditions in the tropics and subtropics.

Pathology: The larvae of hookworm may cause allergic inflammation at the site of entry through the skin. If the infection is heavy, the passage of larvae through the lungs may cause pulmonary eosinophilia. The worms attach themselves to the mucosa of the small intestine by their buccal capsule and suck the blood. The mean daily loss of blood from one **A. duodenale** is 0.15 ml and for **N.americanus**

0.03 ml. The degree of iron and protein deficiency which develops is dependent not only on the load of worms but also on the general nutrional status of the patient and especially on the iron stores. Thus, if the infection is light it may not lead to anemia. However, in the early stage of infection eosinophilia is common (Fig. 8.1).

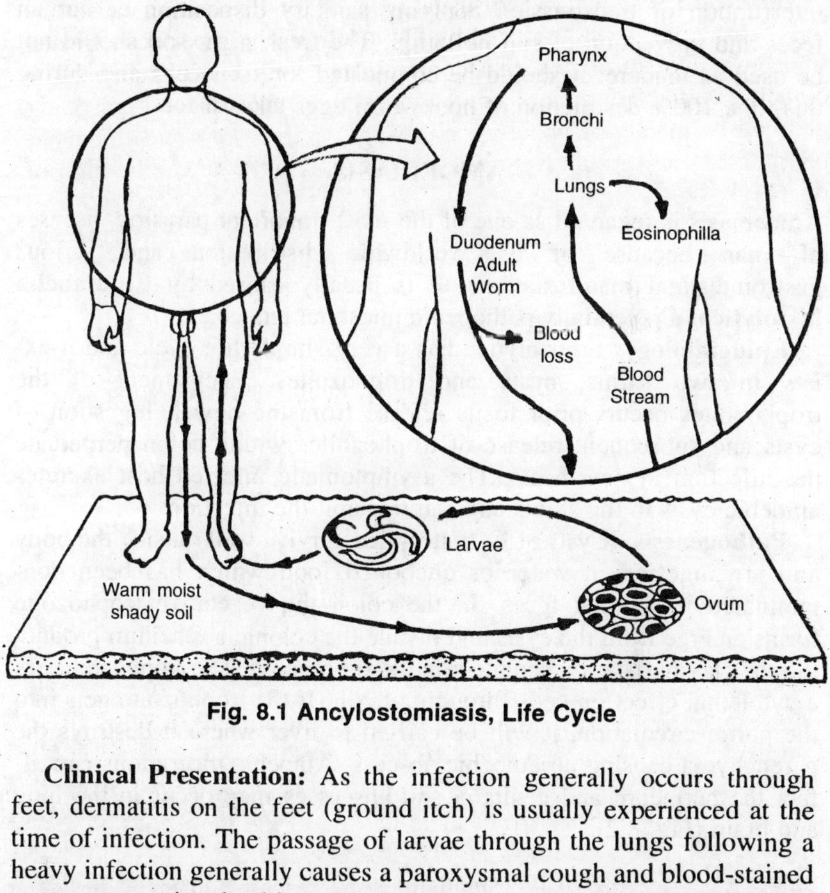

Fig. 8.1 Ancylostomiasis, Life Cycle

Clinical Presentation: As the infection generally occurs through feet, dermatitis on the feet (ground itch) is usually experienced at the time of infection. The passage of larvae through the lungs following a heavy infection generally causes a paroxysmal cough and blood-stained sputum, associated with patchy pulmonary consolidation. When the worms have reached the small intestine, vomiting and epigastric pain resembling peptic ulcer disease may ensue. Sometimes the conditions may resemble early sprue or giardiasis and frequent loose stools are passed. In the undernourished patients anaemia and hypoproteinemia may soon develop. In children the mental and physical development may be retarded. Following a light infection, a well nourished and healthy person may not show any symptom.

Management: Effective anthelmintic drugs are now available for the eradication of hookworm infection. Mebendazole 100 mg twice daily for 3 days is preferred. However, for single dose treatment pyrantel pamoate 10 mg/kg is the drug of choice. Anemia, associated with hookworm infection, can be best treated with oral iron preparations.

Control : Control of hookworm infestation is best achieved by the interruption of transmission applying sanitary disposition of human feces and prevention of soil pollution. The fresh night soil should not be used as manure. It should be composted for six weeks and during this time 100% destruction of hookworm eggs takes place.

AMOEBIASIS

Amoebiasis is regarded as one of the most important parasitic diseases of man because of its worldwide distribution and serious gastrointestinal manifestations. It is usually caused by **Entamoeba histolytica,** a potentially pathogenic intestinal amoeba.

Epidemiology: E.histolytica has a very simple life cycle and it exists in two forms, cysts and trophozoites. Encystment of the trophozoites occurs prior to its release from the bowel. Ingestion of cysts and subsequent release of trophozoites within colon perpetuate the infection in new hosts. The asymptomatic infected host excretes amoebic cysts in the stools and can transmit the infection.

Pathogenesis : Cysts of **E. histolytica** survive well outside the body and are ingested in water or uncooked food which has been contaminated by human feces. In the colon the vegetative trophozoite forms emerge from the cysts and invade the colonic epithelium producing the classic flask shaped ulcer in the submucosa. The trophozoite has a cytolethal effect on cells through a toxin. If the trophozoite gets into the portal circulation, it will be carried to liver where it destroys the parenchyma causing an amoebic abscess. Amoebic ulcerations can affect the perineum and genitalia and abscesses may occur in the lung and brain (Fig. 8.2).

Clinical presentation :

Intestinal amoebiasis : The most frequent clinical manifestation of the disease are gastro-intestinal, with vague complaints of abdominal discomfort and malaise to severe abdominal cramps, flatulence and diarrhoea with mucus, sometimes with streaks of blood and the stools often have an offensive odour. Periods of diarrhoea alternating with constipation are common. Painful spasms of the anal sphincter usually indicate the presence of amoebic rectal ulceration.

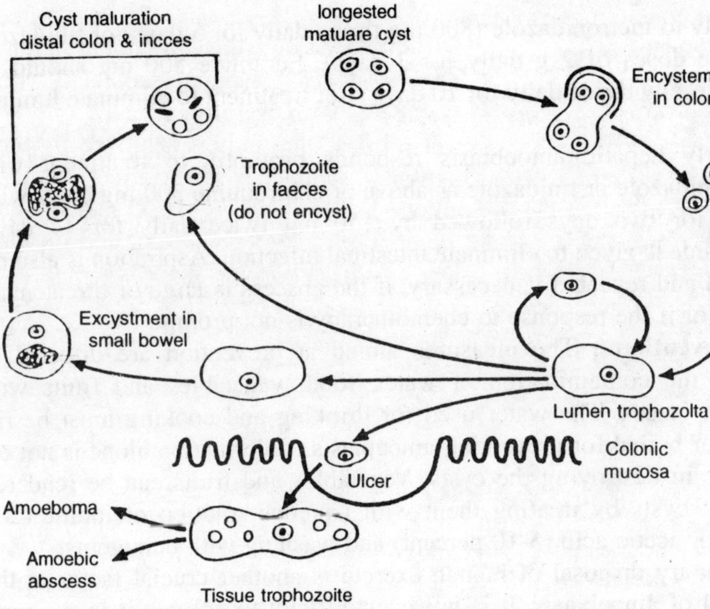

Fig. 8.2 Life Cycle of Entamoeba histolytica

Hepatic amoebiasis : Right upper quadrant pain, hepatomegaly and liver tenderness with referred pain to the left or right shoulder usually suggest an amoebic liver abscess which is generally found in the right hepatic lobe. Liver abscesses from the right lobe can spread to the lungs and pleura. A large abscess may penetrate the diaphragm and rupture into the lung from where its contents may be coughed up. Rupture into the pleural cavity, the peritoneal cavity or pericardial sac is less common but more serious.

Mode of Transmission : Amoebiasis is mainly transmitted by the faecal-oral route usually through ingestion of food or water contaminated with faecal matter containing the cysts of **E. histolytica**. Epidemic water-borne infections can occur if there is heavy contamination of fresh water supply. Vegetables, specially those eaten raw, from the fields irrigated with sewage polluted water can readily transmit the infection. Viable cysts have been found on the hands and under the finger nails. They may lead direct person to person or direct hand to mouth transmission. Infected food handlers in the restaurants, hostels and community kitchens can spread infection through their unhygienic habits and practices.

Management : There is no single drug that is totally effective against all forms of the disease. Invasive intestinal amoebiasis responds quickly to metronidazole (800 mg thrice daily for 5 days) or tinidazole (single doses of 2 g daily for 3 days). Furamide 500 mg should be given orally thrice daily for 10 days after treatment to eliminate luminal cysts.

Early hepatic amoebiasis responds promptly to treatment with metronidazole or tinidazole as above or chloroquine 300 mg base twice daily for two days followed by 150 mg twice daily for 14 days. Furamide is given to eliminate intestinal infection. Aspiration is also required and repeated if necessary, if the abscess is large or threatens to burst, or if the response to chemotherapy is not prompt.

Prevention : The measures aimed at prevention are directed to check the contamination of water, food, vagetables and fruits with human faeces. The water used for drinking and cooking must be filtered or boiled for preventing amoebiasis. Chlorination alone is not effective in destroying the cysts. Vegetables and fruits can be rendered free of cysts by treating them with aqueous solution of iodine (200 ppm) or acetic acid (5-10 percent) and washing with detergents.

Sanitary disposal of human excreta is another crucial factor in the control of amoebiasis. It is however difficult to enforce it in the rural areas of many developing countries.

The periodic examination of food handlers and their education in matters of personal hygiene and proper toilet habits such as washing of hands after defecation can significantly control the spread of amoebiasis.

All these measures require effective health education.

C. ARTHROPOD BORNE INFECTIONS

PLAGUE

Epidemics of plague have attacked man since ancient times. Now the disease is confined to rodents in the wild with occasional sporadic human cases or local outbreaks. The causative organism is a small gram-negative bacillus **Yersinia pestis.** It is spread between rodents by their fleas and when the domestic rats become infected their fleas may bite man and spread the disease in the human population. In the later stages of human plague **Y. pestis** may be expectorated and inter-human spread may occur by droplets. (Fig.8.3).

Pathology: Organisms that are inoculated by fleas through the skin are phagocytosed and taken rapidly to the draining lymph nodes where they produce a severe inflammatory response that may be haemorrhagic. If the infection is not controlled septicemia may follow and necrotic purulent or hemorrhagic lesions develop in many organs.

Vascular damage and fluid loss may lead to oliguria and shock and disseminated intravascular coagulation may result in widespread hemorrhage. Inhalation of **Y. pestis** may cause alveolar damage and copious exudation. The incubation period is short e.g., 3-6 days, which may even be shorter in pneumonic plague. Three forms of plague are usually prevalent.

Bubonic plague: This is the most common form of plague. It can be cured if detected early enough. It is characterized by a sudden onset, rigor, high fever, severe headache, dry skin, aching and swelling at the site of the affected lymph nodes. The most common site of the bubo, made up of the swollen lymph nodes and surrounding tissues is one groin. In the majority of patients toxaemia rapidly increases with a rapid pulse rate, hypotension and mental confusion. The spleen becomes palpable. This is not so fatal form but it can pass on to the more severe septicemic plague and then to the highly fatal and contagious, pneumonic or tonsillar form.

Septicaemic plague: Thirty percent of bubonic cases may lead to a stage when bacilli show up in the blood. Meningitis, pneumonia and expectoration of blood stained sputum containing **Y.pestis** may appear as complications of bubonic or septicaemic plague.Septicemia starts with overwhelming infection and leads to weak defense mechanism which can then affect lungs and bacilli begin to appear in the sputum. From this lung involvement it develops into the pneumonic form which spreads rapidly through droplet and air and spreads from patients with primary pneumonic plague and from patients with primary bubonic plague and secondary pneumonic plague.

Pneumonic plague: Pneumonic plague is characterized by very sudden onset with cough and dyspnea. The patient soon starts expectorating copious, blood stained, frothy, highly infective sputum; becomes cyanosed and dies. X-ray examination of lungs show a lobar opacity. Pneumonic plague is highly contagious and can lead to serious epidemics resulting in large scale fatalities.

Management : When the diagnosis of plague is made on clinical or epidemiological grounds, treatment must be started at the earliest possible. The drug of choice is tetracycline 10 mg/kg every 6 hours orally or i.v. is given for 10 days. Alternatively, streptomycin is given by i.m. or i.v. injection every 6 or 12 hours at a daily dose of 30mg/kg for 10 days. Adequate treatment may also be necessary for acute circulatory failure, disseminated intravascular coagulation or hypoxia. Co-trimoxazole is also effective and is preferred for use in pregnant women. Other drugs like chloramphenicol, and sulphadiazine can also be used if tetracycline is not available. It is the failure to detect the infection early and treat it immediately that leads to fatalities.

Prevention: Effective prevention depends on controlling the biting by fleas which carry plague. Powder containing 1.5% of Dieldrin or 2% Aldrin is applied to the floors and blown into rat holes to kill all the fleas. In endemic area people should avoid handling and skinning wild animals. Patients are isolated and attendants must wear gowns, masks and gloves. Contacts should be protected by tetracycline 2 g daily for a week.

Vaccination : Immunization with plague vaccine is a valuable preventive measure. To be effective, vaccination should be carried out at least a week before an anticipated outbreak and the vaccine should be given in two doses of 0.5 and 1.0 ml subcutaneously at an interval of 7 to 14 days. Booster doses are recommended six monthly for persons at continuing risk of infection.

The vaccine used in India has been manufactured by Haffkine Institute, Bombay. It is a formalin killed vaccine, Virulent strains of **Y.pestis** are grown in casceine hydrolysate broth for 2 weeks at 27° C and killed by 1% formalin for 3 days at 37°C. The final vaccine is a suspension of 2000 millions organisms per ml.

Chemoprophylaxis is a very effective preventive measure for all plague contacts, medical, nursing and public health personnel exposed to the risk of infection. The drug of choice is tetracycline, 500 mg, 6 hourly for 5 days.

The 1994 Plague Epidemic in India :

On September 2, 1994, 25 years after the disease was believed to have been conquered in the country four cases of bubonic plague were detected in Beed district of Maharashtra about 100 km from the earthquake hit Latur District. The number rose to 38 within a week but none of the patient died there. On September 23,1994 the disease was discovered to have spread to Surat in Gujarat in its highly contagious pneumonic form and till the end of September more than 50 patients had died there and the disease had spread to other towns like Baroda, Ahmedabad and New Delhi. Extensive immediate measures had been taken to control the epidemic but by then it had already created a world-wide scare.

Plague contrary to general belief, has not been eradicated because of its peculiar chain of transmission from animals (rodents) to man through rat flea bites (Fig. 8.3). It has been effectively contained by breaking the chain of contact between rodents and human beings through suitable measures. Pockets of rat population, particularly the wild rodents who harbour the infection and getting rid of endemic rat population worldwide is not feasible. What is possible is to prevent carriers of the infection, the rat flea **Xenospylla cheopis** from coming into contact with humans. Further, in areas where natural plague foci exist or where there is past history of infection surveillance is indispensable. The W.H.O. has recommended serological surveys as a dependable means of mapping natural foci and this is done by detecting plague antibodies in rodent sera and bacteriological confirmation of the disease. One such Plague Control Unit operational in Pune was closed down in 1987 as there was no detectable case of human plague after 1960s.

Ecological disturbances like earthquakes, floods etc. are major causes of migration of plague carrying rodent populations towards human habitations. Indeed after the earthquake in the Latur region exactly an year ago the National Institute of Communicable Diseases pointed out that surveillance of rodent borne human infections is warranted in the area. The possibility of rodent population migrating from endemic sylvatic foci in Karnataka and infecting domestic and peridomestic rats warranted to get the Control Unit in Pune functional again and it was so emphasized by the N.I.C.D. also but it was not done. The earthquake ruins converted into granaries and provided haven for the infected rats and this resulted in the sudden spurt of plague cases in Maharashtra from where the migrant population is likely to have carried it to Surat and elsewhere. The constant surveillance could have prevented this and it is abvious from the fact that the continued surveillance programmes in Tamil Nadu and Karnataka have been effective in containing the infection even though there are pockets of wild rodent populations carrying the disease in these states at Salem and Kolar.

MALARIA

Malaria is caused by **Plasmodium falciparum, P.vivax, P.ovale and P.malariae.** It is transmitted by the bite of anopheline mosquitoes in which the parasite undergoes a temperature dependent cycle of development. It is therefore a disease of hot wet climates. It may also be transmitted by blood transfusion or inoculation. It is endemic or sporadic throughout most of the tropics and subtopics below an altitude of 1500 m excluding **mediterranean littoral,** the U.S.A. and Australia. One hundred million people are attacked by malaria every year of whom about 1%, mostly children, die. Following the WHO sponsored campaigns of prevention and more effective treatment, the incidence of malaria was significantly reduced in 1950-60 but since 1970 there is resurgence. In the 1980s **P.falciparum** became resistant to chloroquine. Malaria due to this parasite is now more severe than that due to the other sensitive parasites.

Pathogenesis : The female anopheline mosquito becomes infected when it sucks the human blood containing gametocyte, the sexual forms of malarial parasite. The development in the mosquito takes from 7-20 days. The infected mosquito inoculates sporozoites into the human blood which disappear within 30 min from the blood and enter the liver. After some days merozoites leave the liver and invade the RBCs where further asexual cycles or multiplication takes place, producing schizonts (Fig.8.4). Rupture of schizonts releases more merozoites into the blood and causes fever, whose periodicity depends on the species of parasite (Table 8.9).

P.vivax and **P.ovale** may persist in the liver as dormant forms, hypnozoites, which can develop into merozoites months or years later. Thus the first attack of malarial fever may occur long after the patient has left the endemic area and the disease may relapse after the treatment with drugs which kill only the erythrocytic stage of the parasite. **P.falciparum** and **P.malariae** have no persistent exo-erythrocytic phase but recrudescence of fever may result from multiplication in the red cells of parasites which have not been eliminated by treatment and the immune process.

Malaria is always accompanied by hemolysis and following a severe or prolonged attack anaemia may be profound. Hemolysis is most severe with **P.falciparum** which invades. RBCs of all ages but in particular the young cells. **P.vivax** and **P.ovale** invade reticulocytes and **P.malariae** normoblasts so that the infections with these species remain lighter. In **P.falciparum** malaria the RBCs containing schizonts adhere to the lining of capillaries in brain, kidney, liver, lungs and gut. The vessels become congested and the organs anoxic. Rupture of schizonts liberates toxic and antigenic substances which may cause additional damage. Thus the main effects of malaria are hemolytic anemia and with **P.falciparum** a widespread organ damage can take place.

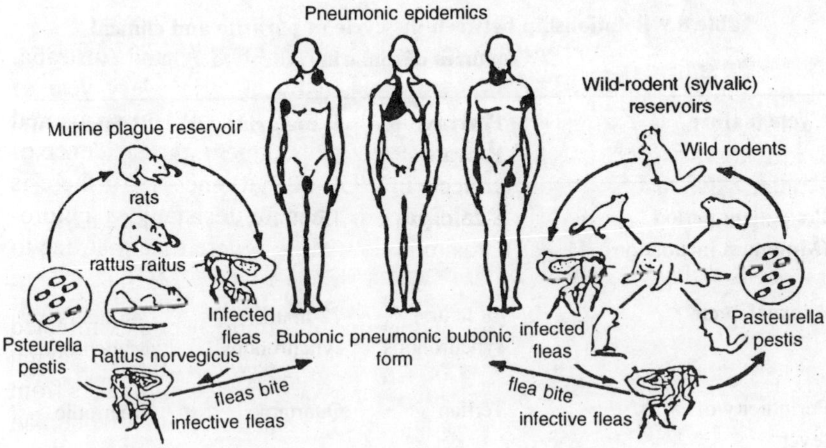

Fig. 8.3 Life Cycle of Pasteurella pestis in wild and murine rats and pathogenesis of plague in man

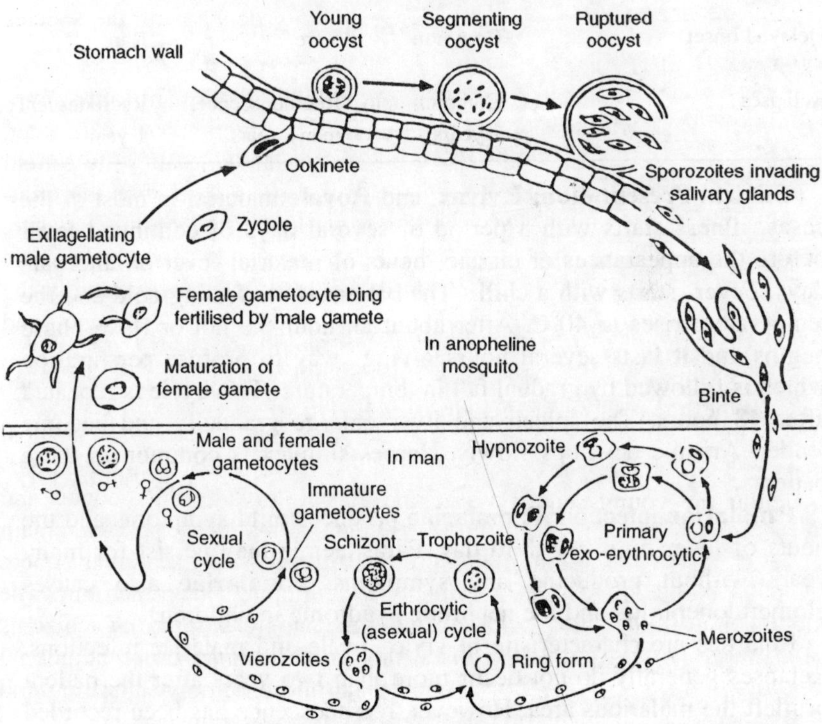

Fig. 8.4 Life Cycle of Malarial Parasite

Table 8.9 Relationship between the cycle of parasite and clinical features of malaria

Cycle feature	P. vivax, P. ovale	P. malariae	P. falciparum
Pre-patient period (Minimum incubation)	8-25 days	15-30 days	8-25 days
Asexual cycle	48 hours, synchronous	72 hours synchronous	48 hours asynchronous
Periodicity of fever	Tertian	Quartan	Aperiodic
Exoerythrocytic cycle	Persistent as hypnozoites	Pre-erythrocytic only	Pre-erythrocytic only
Delayed onset	Common	Rare	Rare
Relapses	Common upto 2 years	Recrudescence, many years	Recrudescence, 1 year

Clinical Presentation: P.vivax and **P.ovale** malaria: In most of the cases, illness starts with a period of several days of continued fever before the appearances of classic bouts of malarial fever on alternate days. Fever starts with a chill. The patient starts feeling cold and the temperature rises to 40°C. After about an hour the hot or flush phase begins and it lasts several hours giving way to profuse perspiration which is followed by gradual fall in temperature. This cycle is repeated after 48 hours. The spleen and liver enlarge gradually and become tender. Anemia develops slowly. Herpes simplex is common in these patients.

P.malariae infection: **P. malariae** produces mild symptoms and the bouts of fever on every third day. Parasitaemia may persist for many years without producing any symptoms. **P.malariae** also causes glomerulonephritis and the nephrotic syndrome in children.

Relapses are characteristic of vivax, ovale and malariae infections. Relapses generally do not occur more than two years after the patient has left the malarious area. However, recrudescence has been recorded many years after **P.malariae** infection.

P.falciparum infections : Falciparum malaria is more dangerous than the other forms. The onset, particularly of primary attacks is generally insidious with malaise, headache and vomiting. Cough and mild diarrhoea are often suggestive of influenza. The fever has no particular pattern and hyperpyrexia is usually not so high as in the other forms. The cold, hot and sweating stages are seldom seen. Jaundice is common due to hepatitis and hemolysis. The liver and spleen enlarge and become tender. Anemia also develops rapidly.

A patient of falciparum malaria though not seriously ill, may develop serious complications. Children with hyperpyrexia die rapidly without developing any other symptoms.

Mixed infections: Mixed infection with more than one species of plasmodium may occur in certain cases.

Complications of falciparum malaria: Important complication secondary to P.falciparum maria have been summarized in Table 8.10.

Table 8.10 Complications of falciparum malaria

	Severe anemia	
	Organ damage due to anoxia	
	Brain	Confusion
		Coma
	Kidney	Oliguria
		Uraemia
	Lungs	Cough
		Pulmonary oedema
	Intestine	Diarrhoea
		Congestion
	Liver	Jaundice
Intravascular hemolysis		
Blackwater fever		
Hypoglycemia		
Septicemia		
Metabolic acidosis		
Splenic rupture		
In pregnancy—maternal death, abortion.		

Of these cerebral malaria is the most dangerous complication and is manifested by confusion or coma. Blackwater fever has been associated with chronic falciparum disease and it is generally seen in those patients who have taken antimalarial treatment irregularly or who are deficient in glucose-6-phosphate dehydrogenase. Hemolysis is unpredictable and severe. It destroys normal as well as parasitised cells. The urine is dark and black.

Management:

Acute attack : The drug of choice for treating acute attack is chloroquine. The usual course is 600 mg of the base (4 tablets) followed by 300 mg base in 6 hours and then 150 mg base twice daily for 3-7 days.

Infections with falciparum malaria from a chloroquine resistant area are treated with Quinine dihydrochloride or sulphate 600 mg salt (10 mg/kg) 3 times daily for 5 days by mouth followed by a single dose of sulfadoxine 1.5 g combined with pyrimethamine 75 mg i.e., 3 tablets of Fansidar. If quinine is not tolerated amodiaquine can be used in the same dose as chloroquine or mefloquine can also be used as an alternative to quinine. If sulphonamide sensitivity is suspected, quinine may be followed by tetracycline 250 mg 6 hourly for 7 days.

Artemisia annua : With malaria on the upsurge, and chloroquine proving ineffective in several parts of the country for containing the disease, a great hope is placed on a Chinese wonder plant **Artemisia annua** for controlling the disease in those so far considered incurable. This plant, which is now also cultivated in India, has in its ariel parts, minute quantities of a chemical compound artemisinin, which after extraction and processing can be used to treat the deadly **P.falciparum** cases of malaria. Clinical trials on - arteether (artemisinin) undertaken by the Central Drug Research Institute at the Rourkela Ispat Hospital have established that artemisinin can be used to treat serious and resistant cases of malaria that do not respond to other drugs.

Falciparum malaria complications : Cerebral malaria is treated as a medical emergency. Chloroquine 5 mg/kg is administered by slow i.v. infusion over 2-4 hours every 12 hours till the patient can take the drug orally. In chloroquine resistant cases quinine 10 mg/kg is given in the same way. Severe anemia requires transfusion with packed red cells. If oliguria develops furosemide or an i.v. infusion of mannitol can forestall renal failure. Exchange blood transfusion is life saving in complicated very heavy infections.

Radical cure of P.vivax and P.ovale malaria: Radical cure is achieved in most patients by a course of primaquine 15 mg daily orally for 14 days which destroys hyponozoites phase in the liver.

Chemoprophylaxis: Acute attacks of malaria can be prevented by drugs such as proguanil which attack the pre-erythrocytic form (causal prophylaxis) or after it has entered the erythrocyte (suppression). Maloprim (Pyrimethamine 12.5 mg + Dapsone 100 mg) and Fansidar (Pyrimethamine 25 mg+ Sulfadoxine 500 mg) contain two compounds which block two successive enzymes in the parasite's folate pathway.

Prevention : Spraying of the houses by residual insecticides lethal to anopheline mosquitoes significantly reduces or even abolishes the risk of malaria in many areas. However, unless the malaria is completely eradicated, all visitors to endemic areas should take the regular prophylactic drugs. Chemoprophylaxis alone may not be sufficient to prevent malaria. It is equally important to avoid anopheline mosquitoes which usually bite during the nights. Persons moving outside the houses should put on long sleeves and trousers. Mosquito repellent creams and sprays can be useful. Other prophylactic measures include screened windows in the houses, use of mosquito nets and burning of pyrethrum based mosquito coils.

FILARIASIS

Etiology: Filariasis is a disease state due to the infection with the filarial worm **Wuchereria bancrofti**. It is conveyed to the man by the bites of infected mosquitoes of **Culex fatigans** species. The adult worms 4-10 cm in length live in the lymphatics and the females produce microfilariae which at night circulate in large numbers in the peripheral blood. In the mosquito, ingested microfilariae develop into infective larvae. As **Culex fatigans** bites at night the nocturnal periodicity of microfilariae facilitates the spread of infection. The microfilariae are chiefly in the capillaries in the lungs when not circulating in the peripheral blood and may cause pulmonary eosinophilia. (Fig. 8.5).

Pathology: The presence of adult filarial worms in the lymphatics causes allergic lymphangitis. Recurrent episodes may lead to intermittent lymphatic obstruction and transient lymphoedema which may later become permanent in the leg, arm, genitalia or breast, and hydrocele. Obstructed lymphatics may become dilated and tortuous and rupture. Rupture into the tissues leads to cellulitis, fibrosis and elephantiasis. As the lymphatic pressure increases, it may cause retrograde flow or rupture, in turn causing chyluria, chylous ascites and chylous pleural effusions. The incubation period is not less than 3 months.

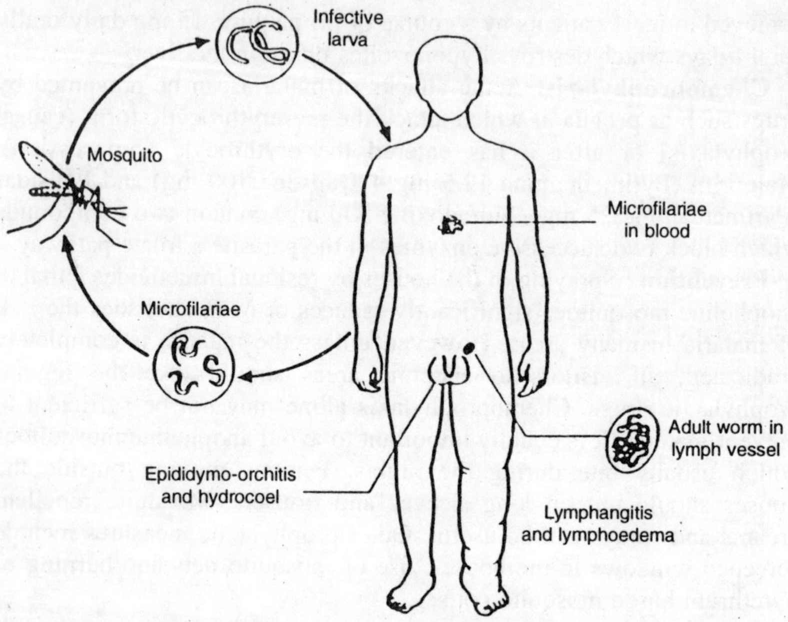

Fig. 8.5 Life cycle and pathogenesis of Lymphatic filariasis caused by W. bancrofti

Clinical Presentation: The symptoms of filariasis may start with bouts of fever accompanied by pain, tenderness, erythema along the course of inflamed lymphatic vessels. Inflammation of the spermatic cord, epididymitis and orchitis is common. The fever gradually abates after a few days and the initial signs and symptoms subside.

Further attacks follow, temporary oedema becomes more persistent and regional lymph nodes enlarge. This is followed by progressive enlargement, coarsening, corrugation and fissuring of the skin and subcutaneous tissue with warty superficial excrescences leading gradually to irreversible elephantiasis. The scrotum may reach an enormous size. Chyluria and chylous effusions are milky and opalescent; on standing fat globules rise to the top. Eventually the adult worms may die but lymphatics remain obstructed. The interval between infection and the onset of elephantiasis is usually not less than 10 years and elephantiasis develops only in association with repeated infections in highly endemic areas.

Management: The most effective single drug used in the management of filarisis is diethylcarbamazine (Hetrazan, Banocide). It kills both the microfilariae and adult worms. The dose is 9-12 mg/kg daily administered orally in 3 divided doses for 14 days. This course may be repeated twice at intervals of 4-6 weeks. Antihistaminics or corticosteroids may be necessary for controlling the allergic phenomena. Established elephantiasis may require plastic surgery. A significant relief can be obtained by the removal of excess tissue but recurrences are possible unless new lymphatic drainage is established. Tight bandaging, or bed rest with suspension or raising of the affected part or the nightly use of pneumatic stockings may also control swelling to some extent.

Prevention: Treatment of the entire population in the endemic areas with diethylcarbamazine (100 mg three times a day for 7 days in adults and 50 mg 3 times daily for 7 days in children) can reduce the incidence of filariasis. Children are also given such a course on starting and before leaving school. This mass treatment should be combined with control of the vector by insecticides. It should be remembered that the early chemotherapy prevents later elephantiasis.

D. SURFACE INFECTIONS

RABIES

Etiology :

Rabies is caused by a rhabdovirus which infects the central nervous tissue and salivary glands of a wide range of mammals and is usually conveyed by saliva through bites or licks on abrasions or on intact mucous membranes. Man is most frequently infected from dogs.

The incubation period, during which the virus spreads centripetally along axons to the brain, varies in man from a minimum of 9 days to many months but it usually lies between 4 to 8 weeks. Severe bites especially if on the head or neck are associated with short incubation periods.

Clinical presentation:

Not all the individuals bitten by a rabid animal develop the disease, but once manifest, rabies is almost invariably fatal. At the onset there may be only fever and paraesthesia at the site of the bite. What follows then, comprises the most characteristic feature of this disease. A prodromal period of 1 to 10 days during which the patient is increasingly anxious, leads to the characteristic fear of water, "hydrophobia". Although the patient feels thirsty, attempts at drinking provoke violent contractions of the diaphragm and other inspiratory muscles and thereafter, even the sight or sound of water may precipitate distressing spasms and attacks of panic. Delusions and hallucination may develop accompanied by spitting, biting and mania with lucid intervals during which the patient is acutely anxious. Cranial nerve lesions develop and terminal hyperpyrexia is common. Death ensues within a week of the onset of symptoms.

Management:

Only a few patients with rabies have survived. All received some post-exposure prophylaxis and needed intensive care with facilities to control cardiac and respiratory failure. Otherwise, only palliative treatment is possible after the symptoms develop. The patient needs to be heavily sedated with diazepam 10 mg, 4-6 hourly supplemented by chlorpromazine 50-100mg, if necessary. Nutrients and fluids are generally administered intravenously.

Prevention:

Rabies vaccine, which is a sterile lyophilized preparation of the Wistar rabies virus strain PM-1503-3 M grown on human diploid cell cultures and inactivated with Beta-propiolactone (BPL) is used for the prevention of rabies. Two vaccines one for intramuscular use and the other for intradermal use are available.

Both vaccines are indicated for active immunization in pre-exposure situations for veterinarians, animal handlers, research workers or other similar personnel working in laboratories, hospitals etc. whose pursuits bring them in contact with potentially rabid animals or with the handling of rabies virus or potentially contaminated materials or for people who live at special risk in rabies endemic areas. Protection is afforded by two intradermal injections of 0.1 ml human diploid cell strain vaccine or two intramuscular injections of 1.0 ml given 4 weeks apart, followed by yearly boosters.

Post-exposure prophylaxis: The wounds should be thoroughly cleaned with a quaternary ammonium detergent or soap, damaged tissues should be excised and the wound left unsutured. Rabies can be prevented if treatment is started within a day or two of biting. Delayed treatment may still be of value in some cases. For maximum protection hyperimmune serum (Rabies Immune Globulin: Human) and the rabies vaccine, both are required.

Rabies Immune Globulin (Human) is used in the dose of 20 IU/kg.

Half of this dose should be used to infiltrate the wound and the other half be administered intramuscularly preferably in the gluteal or deltoid region and at a different site from the vaccine. The human diploid cell strain vaccine, 1.0 ml is given intramuscularly on days 0, 3,7,14,30 and 90. In developing countries, where human rabies globulin may not be available, 0.1 ml of Rabies vaccine should be given intradermally into 8 sites on day 1, with single boosters on day 7 and 28.

The biting animal should be confined, if possible. If it rcmains healthy after 5 days, if does not have rabies and the treatment can be then stopped.

Control of spread:

Human rabies is an infrequent disease even in the endemic areas. Its fearful manifestations and fatal prognosis, however, justify stringent measures being taken to limit its spread. Measures to control rabies include: a) Licensing and vaccination of all domestic dogs, b) killing of stray dogs,c) monitoring of reservoir hosts, d) control and quarantine of imported animals, and e) vaccination of at risk animals and man.

TRACHOMA

Etiology:

Trachoma is a specific communicable keratoconjunctivitis caused by **Chlamydia trachomatis**. It is usually transmitted by contact or from fomites in unhygienic surroundings. Infections may also occur in neonates during birth from infected genital passages.

Incidence:

Vast populations of inhabitants suffer from trachoma in the hot, dry and dusty areas of subtropics and tropics. The disease varies markedly in its incidence and severity in different geographical areas. In the endemic areas the disease is most common among the children.

Pathology:

Trachoma is a chronic infection lasting for years. It may be latent over long periods and may recrudesce. The conjunctiva of the upper lid is first affected with vascularization and cellular infiltration. Pannus spreading to the cornea usually causes opacity and impairment of the vision.

Clinical Presentation:

The onset of trachoma is usually insidious and infection may not be apparent to the patient. Early symptoms include conjunctival irritation and blepharospasm, but the problem may not be detected until the vision appears to fail. It may also be present as an acute ophthalmia neonatorum. The early follicles of trachoma are quite characteristic but clinical differentiation from conjunctivitis due to other viruses may be difficult at this stage. Scarring of the lid causes entropion.

Management:

Ophthalmic ointment or drops of 1-3% tetracycline should be applied twice daily for 3 months. As mass therapy in the endemic areas, topical application twice daily for 3-6 consecutive days each month for 6 months has given good results. Oral tetracycline, doxycycline or sulfonamide given for 3 weeks are equally effective. Deformity and scarring of lids, corneal opacities, ulceration and scarring often require surgical treatment after the control of local infection.

Prevention:

Improvement in the personal and family cleanliness and proper care of the eyes of new born and young children are essential for adequate prevention of this contagious disease. Family contacts should also be examined and treated if necessary. General population surveys e.g. in the schools and offices may lead to discovery and treatment of asymptomatic infections. Trachoma clinics are necessary in the highly endemic areas.

TETANUS

Etiology :

Tetanus results from infection with **Clostridium tetani** which exists as a commensal in the gut of man and domestic animals and is found in the soil. Infection enters the human body through wounds which may often be trivial such as those caused by a splinter, a nail in the shoe, a garden fork or following septic infection such as a dirty abrasion. The disease is common in the developing countries where dust contains spores derived from animal and human excreta. If childbirth takes place in an unhygienic environment, **Tetanus neonatorum** may result from infection of the umbilical stump or the mother may develop the disease.

Pathology :

If the circumstances are not favorable to the growth of the organism, spores are formed and these may remain dormant for years in the soil. Spores germinate and bacilli multiply only in the areas of tissue necrosis or if the oxygen tension is low due to the presence of other organisms particularly the aerobic ones. The bacilli generally remain localized and produce an exotoxin which has an affinity for motor nerve endings and motor nerve cells. The anterior horn cells are affected after the exotoxin has passed into the blood stream and their involvement leads to rigidity and convulsions. The incubation period may vary from 2 days to several weeks. However, a shorter incubation period of few days may produce more severe attack and the outcome may often be fatal.

Clinical presentation:

The most important early symptom of tetanus is trismus-spasm of masseter muscles, which causes difficulty in opening the mouth and in masticating, hence the name "lock jaw". This tonic rigidity soon spreads to involve the muscles of face, neck and trunk. Contraction of the frontalis and the muscles at the angles of the mouth gives rise to the "risus sardonicus". There is rigidity of the muscles of the neck and trunk of varying degree. The back is usually slightly arched and there is board-like abdominal wall. Violent spasms lasting for few seconds to 3 to 4 minutes occur spontaneously in very serious cases or can be induced by stimuli such as movement of the patient or noise. Such convulsions are painful, exhausting and of very serious significance particularly if they occur soon after the onset of symptoms. They gradually increase in frequency and severity for about one week and the patient may die due to exhaustion, asphyxia or aspiration pneumonia. In less severe illness convulsions may appear after about a week of the first signs of rigidity. In very mild infections convulsions never appear. Autonomic involvement, if present, may cause some cardiovascular complications like hypertension. Rarely the only manifestation of the disease may be confined to local tetanus which is characterized by stiffness or spasm of the muscles near the infected wound and it indicates a good prognosis if the treatment is started at this stage. Nevertheless, tetanus is still considered as one of the major killers of adults, children and neonates in the tropics where mortality rate can be close to 100% in the newborn and around 40% in others.

Management:

This must be done as soon as possible after the first sign of tetanus becomes apparent. It essentially comprises of

(a) Prevention of further toxin production by the debridement of wound and treatment with benzylpenicillin 600 mg, q.i.d., i.v.

(b) Controlling the spasms if present by nursing in a quiet room and by avoiding unnecessary stimuli. I.V. diazepam may be used if spasms continue.

(c) Taking general measures like maintaining the patient in the state of adequate hydration and nutrition and treating secondary infections if present.

Prophylaxis:

Tetanus Toxoid Adsorbed is used for active immunization against tetanus in adults and children. In children less than 1 year, 3 injections of 0.5 ml are given, 4-8 weeks apart followed by a fourth, re-inforcing dose of 0.5 ml, 6-12 months later. This is followed by a booster of 0.5 ml given at 4 to 6 years preferably prior to entrance into kindergarten or elementary school. It is commonly administered for routine prophylaxis in the form of Diphtheria and Tetanus Toxoids and Pertussis Vaccine Adsorbed (DTP) to children under 7 years.

LEPROSY

Etiology and Incidence:

Leprosy is the commonest cause of peripheral neuritis in the world. It is a chronic granulomatous disease caused by **Mycobacterium leprae**, an acid and alcohol fast bacillus. Leprosy is one of the most seriously disabling and economically important diseases of the world and it is estimated that 20 million people are affected. The most important mode of transmission of **M.leprae** is by droplets from the sneezes of lepromatous patients whose nasal mucosa is heavily infected. The organism may enter the body through the nasal mucosa or by inoculation through the skin.

Pathology:

The **M. leprae** organisms show a predilection for peripheral nerves, skin and mucosa of the upper respiratory tract. The early infection, usually transient and self healing, is called indeterminate. If the infection does not heal, it develops into one of the determinate types:

Tuberculoid leprosy: it is characterized by a marked response of epithelial cells, lymphocytes and giant cells around nerves, sweat glands and hair follicles. Caseation does not occur except occasionally in a nerve. Organisms are scanty and difficult to find.

Lepromatous leprosy: In the infective form of this disease there is no cell mediated immune response to **M.leprae.** Organism are present in great abundance in the dermis and at other sites. They are carried in the blood stream to the peripheral nerves, eyes and mucosa of the nose and upper respiratory tract, the testes and small muscles and bones of the hands, feet and face, in which they multiply.

Borderline or dimorphous leprosy : Between these two polar types of leprosy, there is a spectrum of manifestations grouped under the terms borderline or dimorphous. **M.leprae** are demonstrable in varying numbers. The host reaction may vary from near-lepromatous to near-tuberculoid. Immunity may diminish in untreated patients and may increase in response to successful chemotherapy. The disease may become mere tuberculoid after adequate chemotherapy.

Lepra reactions: Any determinate form of leprosy may undergo an acute exacerbation or reaction which is caused by an episode of acute allergic manifestation. In lepromatous disease the reaction, lepra reaction type 2 is due to immune complex mediated vasculitis. In borderline and tuberculoid disease the reaction, lepra reaction type 1 is due to sudden increase in cellular hypersensitivity. Leprosy can damage the body in three main ways.

Peripheral neuritis: This leads to loss of sensory, motor and autonomic functions. The important manifestations of peripheral neuritis include trauma from pressure, friction, burns and cuts; dry skin which cracks easily and heals slowly. A combination of fifth and seventh cranial nerve damage exposes an anesthetic cornea to trauma and sepsis leading to blindness.

Lepromatous leprosy: In this condition bacillary growth insidiously damages the infiltrated organs and renders them liable to type 2 lepra reactions. Bones of hands and feet are easily fractured.

Acute lepra reactions: These may destroy nerves overnight or cause severe damage to the eye.

Clinical presentation:

The onset is usually gradual. The most common first symptom is a small but persistent area of impaired sensation or numbness.

Tuberculoid leprosy is characterized by a few solitary lesions on skin and peripheral nerves. Lesions are macular or raised and hypopigmented. They occur anywhere in the body especially on the outer surface of arms, legs or buttocks. Tuberculoid leprosy tends spontaneously to heal slowly and often without residual disability.

Lepromatous lesions of the skin are initially macules. They are small numerous, hypopigmented, erythematosus, and widely scattered on the body. As the disease advances, the macular lesions become infiltrated and succulent, nodular lesions appear on ears and face and eyebrows are lost. Clinical evidence of nerve damage appears late in lepromatous leprosy. Untreated lepromatous leprosy gradually gets worse.

Borderline or dimorphous leprosy presents with lesions that are intermediate in character between lepromatous and tuberculoid or as a mixture of them. Skin lesions are often bizarre. Nerve lesions are more numerous than in tuberculoid disease. In Asia, the majority of patients have borderline lepromatous leprosy.

Lepra reactions are defined as episodes of acute inflammation in pre-existing lesions of leprosy. One half of patients with lepromatous leprosy and one quarter with borderline lepromatous disease will suffer type 2 lepra reactions usually in the second year of treatment. These reactions are characterized by fever and the appearance of crops of painful red papules or nodules, called erythema nodosum leprosum- which may necrose and discharge sterile pus before subsiding. Type 1 lepra reactions are especially common in borderline tuberculoid patients. They occur either spontaneously or may be precipitated by treatment. Nerve function is rapidly lost. It may be irretrievable unless the reaction is promptly treated.

Management:

Treatment of leprosy is quite long and often complicated. The patient must learn to understand the disease and its complications, comply and persevere in the treatment. Patient should also be able to look after anesthetic limbs, control fear and cope with any stigma that exists in the community.

Patients with multi-bacillary disease (Lepromatous and borderline lepromatous): Ideally they should be treated with three drugs: rifampicin, clofazimine and dapsone to prevent the emergence of drug resistance. Rifampicin is given monthly on two consecutive days in a daily dose of 600 mg. Clofazimine is given 50 mg daily or 100 mg 3 times in a week. Dapsone is given 2 mg/kg daily not exceeding 100 mg. Treatment should continue for two years.

Patients with pancibacillary disease (Intermediate, tuberculoid or borderline tuberculoid): These are treated with rifampicin once monthly and dapsone daily for one year. Patients should be followed up for 5 years.

Prevention:

In the endemic areas the disease is commonest among intimate contacts of patients. Children and young adults are most susceptible. Leprosy is easily spread and two-thirds of contacts undergo subclinical immunising infections with 2 years of regular exposure. BCG vaccination is of some value and should be given to all child contacts of lepromatous patients. Dapsone and rifampicin may be given as for pancibacillary disease for 6 months to child contacts of lepromatous patients. All contacts must be subjected to medical check-up for possible infections every six months.

Mass prophylaxis is impossible but treatment and follow up of all cases identified during a population survey can reduce deformity and lower the incidence of leprosy. With improvement of socio-economic condition and spread of health education the disease tends to disappear.

SCABIES AND PEDICULOSIS

Scabies is produced by the mite **Sarcoptes scabei** and it is common all over the world. The 0.3 mm by 0.4 mm female mite, after being fertilized burrows into the stratum corneum where she can lay upto 40 eggs. The mite can travel upto 5mm per day and can live for one to two months. The burrows appear as irregular greyish-black lines which may be '5' shaped and generally have a papule at one end indicating where the mite is. The most common sites for scabies are interdigital spaces, elbows, wrist, feet, buttocks, åxillary folds, penis and nipples in famales.

Clinical presentation:

There is itching, initially between the fingers or on the buttocks or genitals where the mite burrows and later all over the body. The severe pruritis which occurs predominantly at bed time, is generally not apparent for two to four weeks after infestation and probably represents a hypersensitivity reaction to the organism, eggs and the feces of the mite that is deposited in the burrows. Secondary streptococcal infection is an important cause of glomerulorephritis in the tropics.

Transmission:

Transmission of scabies most frequently occurs by direct person to person contact but can also be transmitted via infested clothing,linens or towels.

Treatment

Scabies is treated by a single application of gammabenzene hexachloride (GBH) 1% to the whole body below the neck. Patients should bathe prior to application of GBH. The GBH cream or lotion should then be applied to the entire body from the neck down. All exposed areas must be covered. Approximately 60 ml of GBH lotion is required for total body application and it should be left in place for 24 hours before washing it off. Transmission is unlikely after 24 hours. A second application may be applied one week later to destroy any recently hatched larvae or nymphs. Alternative treatments of scabies include, a) 20 to 25% benzylbenzoate in an alcoholic vehicle applied daily for 3 days b) Crotamiton applied as cream twice during a 48 hour period, or c) 6-10 percent precipitated sulphur in water washable base applied on 3 subsequent nights. The pruritis accompanying scabies can be effectively controlled by hydroxyzine hydrocholoride 25-50 mg given orally or by topical steroids.

Pediculosis

Pediculosis or infestation with lice is caused by the 1-4 mm long blood sucking louse, **Phthirus humanus. P. humanus** causes head and body infestation but its occurrence is not so common. The head louse **P.capitis** is cosmopolitan and is increasing in prevalence in the school going children. It makes the child itch and alarms the parents and teachers. Tiny white oval egg nits are seen attached to the base of hairs on the scalp and they confirm the diagnosis. Lice are transmitted through shared clothing, combs, brushes or bedding. They are completely dependent on blood for survival and cannot survive away from their host for more than 24 hours. As the lice burrow their way through the scalp and skin, they inject their digestive juices and fecal material into the skin which contributes alongwith the punctured wound to the pruritis which the patient experiences. The pruritis caused by lice seems to bother the patients more during the day than at night.

Treatment

A single treatment with gammabenzene hexachloride (GBH,BHC) shampoo or lotion is usually curative. One ounce of GBH shampoo should be worked into a lather and left on the scalp for five minutes.

The hair should be thoroughly rinsed, and a fine tooth comb used for removing the 'nits'. In rare cases a repeat shampoo may be required within 24 hours. In some countries where resistance is developing to GBH/BHC, malathion or carbaryl is being preferred to treat head lice.

Prevention

In order to prevent the incidences of scabies and pediculosis, all close contacts and family members should be treated to avoid reinfestation. All recently worn clothing, bedding, towels should be washed in hot water. Ironing with a hot iron is also effective in destroying the lice and scabies. Care should be taken not to share personal items. Good personal hygiene should be encouraged. Toilets should be cleaned with hot water and disinfected.

E. SEXUALLY TRANSMITTED DISEASES

After being beaten in the early 1950s, the sexually transmitted diseases have staged a phenomenal comeback and some are now a epidemic or pandemic in most countries. The primary reasons for this are largely social, not medical. Popularization of pre- and extra-marital sex, a proportion of which is always promiscuous, and the decline in the popularity of the condom have probably facilitated the spread of organisms concerned, which have overwhelmed the epidemiological defences in many countries. Moreover, it is important to note that for every case reported about 8 go unreported and hence the actual incidence is much higher than the reported demographic figures tell us. This alarming increase is therefore a matter of great concern for the medical personnel and health official of any country.

The five official venereal diseases comprise of gonorrhoea and syphilis and their three topical counter parts, chancroid, lymphogranuloma venereum and granuloma inguinale. There is strong epidemiological evidence that nongonococcal urethritis is also transmitted by sexual activity. Other conditions, the transmission of which can be linked to sexual contact but not confined to it, and which have become common again comprise AIDs, two vaginitides (trichomoniasis and candidiasis), three viral infections (herpes genitalis, genital warts, mollusca contagiosa) and two parasitic infections (public lice and scabies). The increased prevalence of sexually transmissible conditions is especially true of gonorrhoea and syphilis. Gonorrhoea with its short incubation period and large carrier reservoir, particularly in women, has increased.With syphilis, the position is slightly better as its long incubation period facilitates contact tracing and thus epidemiological control. Despite this, its incidence has risen in practically all the countries. Apart from this classical pair, which heads the list of five official venereal diseases, the biggest problem is nongonococcal urethritis, which in most countries has increased at a rate faster than gonorrhoea to a position where it is probably the most common sexually transmissible condition encountered in clinical practice.

Effective control of sexually transmissible diseases is aimed at reducing the silent reservoir of infection and in further preventing the disease. This requires a major team effort and depends upon accurate diagnosis, specific and curative treatment regimens, contact tracing, post treatment surveillance, education and other social and medical awareness programmes.

SYPHILIS

Etiology:

Treponema pallidus, a spirochete, is the causative organism of syphilis. It can invade any tissue or organ of the body causing acute, chronic or contagious syphilis. Infection usually occurs through sexual activity, but a fetus may get infected during birth if the mother has syphilis (congenital syphilis) or a patient may become infected if he receives donated blood contaminated with **T. pallidum.** The only naturally occurring host for **T.pallidum** is man.

Epidemiology:

The peak incidence of syphilis occurs in the age group of 20-24. Syphilis is more common in men than women; twice as many males as females are reported to have syphilis, a reflection of the high incidence among male homosexuals and bisexuals. In addition to being highly contagious, syphilis is of major concern because untreated, it can progress to a chronic systemic disease which can be fatal or seriously disabling.

Pathophysiology:

Trepanoma palladium can rapidly penetrate intact mucous membranes or abraded skin and within a few hours enters the lymphatics and blood to produce systemic infection and metastatic foci before the appearance of a primary lesion. The average incubation time for syphilis is 21 days, however, it ranges from 10-90 days depending upon the size of the inoculum. Primary syphilis is manifested by a single, usually raised and indurated lesion which appears at the site of inoculation. The lesion is known as a chancre and heals spontaneously in 2-6 weeks. The chancre is an infectious lesion. Secondary syphilis appears approximately 6 weeks after the chancre has healed and is manifested by a symmetrical maculopapular rash and nontender generalized lymphadenopathy. The rash subsides in 2 to 6 weeks and the patient enters the latent stages, which can be detected only by serological testing. About one-third of the untreated patients develop tertiary syphilis which is characterized by the presence of gummas in any part of the body or degeneration of central nervous system or cardiovascular system.

Clinical Presentation:

The typical primary chancre begins as a papule which rapidly becomes eroded and forms an ulcer. The chancre is most commonly found on the external genitalia or the anal canal but can be found anywhere. It is painless, if located on the genitals. Atypical primary lesions are common.

Secondary syphilis is characterized by appearance of nonpruritic red or pink macules on the trunk and proximal extremities. In about 1-2 months, red papular lesions also appear that may progress to pustular or necrotic lesions. The lesions are widespread and may involve the palms, soles, face and scalp. In warm, moist, intertriginous areas including the perianal region, vulva, scrotum and inner thighs, axilla and skin under the pendulous breast, papules enlarge and become eroded to produce broad, moist, pink or gray white highly infectious lesions called condyloma lata. Superficial mucosal erosions called mucous patches occur and may involve lips, oral mucosa, tongue, palate, pharynx, vulva, vagina, glans penis or inner prepuce in about one third of patients.

Tertiary syphilis may involve the CNS in one of three ways and is seen in 4 to 6.5% of patients. **Meningovascular syphilis** may occur 5-10 years after the primary infection and involves inflammation of the pia and the arachnoid. There may be either focal or widespread symptoms. **General paresis** reflects widespread parenchymal damage to brain and results in changes in personality, changes in affect, hyperactive reflexes, a small irregular pupil which accommodates but does not react to light, changes in sensorium including illusions, delusions and hallucinations, changes in intellect, decreased recent memory, impaired orientation, judgement and insight and an inability to perform simple calculations and difficulty with speed. General paresis is seen about 20 years after infection. **Tabes dorsalis** is due to demyelinization of the posterior columns, dorsal roots and dorsal-root ganglia of the spinal cord. Signs and symptoms include ataxia, wide-based gait, foot-slap, paresthesias, bladder disturbances, importance and loss of position, deep pain and temperature sensations. Trophic degeneration of joints and ulcers of the feet may develop as a result of loss of pain sensation. Tabes dorsalis occurs 25-30 years after infection.

Prevention : The pharmacists can play an active role in the prevention of syphilis, gonorrhoea and other sexually transmitted diseases. They can disseminate accurate and factual information about these diseases and propagate the necessary prophylactic measures. For example the condom is an effective mechanical barrier to the acquisition and spread of venereal diseases and also a highly effective contraceptive device.

Similarly, having known the diagnosis of the patients, pharmacists can advise them on the importance of compliance and follow-up examinations. Similarly, few people are aware that washing the genitals and urinating after intercourse can help to reduce the possibility of infection. The soap and water simultaneously dilute the bacteria and act as antiseptic too. Urination helps to wash the bacteria from urethra. Careful douching may also help in preventing the spread of organisms.

GONORRHOEA

Etiology:

Gonorrhoea is caused by the nonmotile, nonspore-forming gram-negative diplococcus, **Neisseria gonorrhoeae**. There are no nonhuman reservoirs of gonorrhoea.

Epidemiology:

The highest incidence is in persons aged 15 to 24 years and is more common in men. City dwellers have a higher incidence than those living in the thinly populated rural areas. The incidence and prevalence of gonorrhoea relate to age, sex, race, socioeconomic status and marital status. These factors correlate with sexual activity, the motivation to seek medical attention and accessibility to health care.

Pathophysiology:

Gonococci are inoculated onto mucous membranes by an infected person. Common sites for inoculation include the pharynx, urethra, cervix and anus. The incubation period for gonorrhoea is 3 to 5 days. After getting inoculated in the genital tract, the infection usually ascends in the female. In the male the infection may extend into seminal vesicle, epididymis and prostate. In the female the gonococcus does not survive well in the uterus but infects the fallopian tubes in about 15% of cases. This may lead to scarring and later sterility. Upto 3% of infected adults develop gonococcemia and about two thirds of them are females. Infection may also extend to distant sites like the joints, meninges and the heart valves.

Clinical Presentation :

Clinical manifestations depend largely on the site and duration of infection and also whether the infection is localized or systemic. Gonorrhoea is characterized by a profuse, purulent, yellow urethral discharge associated with dysuria and urinary urgency in 90-95% males. Anorectal and pharyngeal gonococcal infections are common in homosexual men but they mostly remain asymptomatic.

Upto 10% of infected females are symptomatic. Gonorrhoea in females is characterized by dysuria, frequency, increased vaginal discharge, abnormal menstrual bleeding and anorectal discomfort. Pelvic inflammation may occur as a complication of gonorrhoea and it may be responsible for infertility, sterility and ectopic pregnancy.

Gonococcemia usually appears as the first sign of disseminated infection which is more common in females. The symptoms include fever, polyarthralgias and hemorrhagic rash. The joint infection leads to septic arthritis of a single, large joint or several joints. Seventy percent cases of arthritis in young sexually active patients are secondary to gonococcal disease.

ACQUIRED IMMUNODEFICIENCY SYNDROME (AIDs)

The acquired immunodeficiency syndrome (AIDs) was initially recognized in the late seventies but formally introduced to the medical community as a distinct clinical entity in 1981. This syndrome is a condition characterized by the development of life-threatening multiple opportunistic infections and/or uncommon forms of malignant neoplasms in patients with severe depression of the T-cell mediated immune system caused by human immunodeficiency virus (HIV) which has been firmly implicated as the cause of AIDs.

Various means are now used to characterize patients with manifestations of HIV infection and to describe their signs, symptoms and laboratory phenomena. A large number of persons with serologic evidence of HIV infection may not manifest symptoms, neurologic disease or overt AIDs (defined by the appearance of an opportunistic infection or related malignancy). Several populations at risk for HIV infection have been identified including homosexual males, intravenous drug abusers, hemophiliacs and sexual partners of persons in these groups. Evidence strongly suggests that this retrovirus is transmitted by sexual contact or contact with contaminated blood or blood related products. Transmission of HIV between heterosexuals has been observed. The number of sexual partners may be an important factor in the identification of either male or female patients at risk for HIV infection. Fear of catching AIDs and a lack of understanding of the disease have precipitated a general alarm throughout the world both in general population and in medical communities. The availability of blood tests to detect the presence of antibodies to HIV is a major achievement. The terminologies and criteria for diagnosis of HIV infection are changing; consequently, caution should be used when a patient is given a diagnosis of HIV infection. It must be emphasized that not all patients with HIV infection have AIDs or will develop the disease in future.

Etiology:

AIDs has been recognized by different research groups to be caused by infection with HIV, one of five distinct but related retroviruses known to cause human disease. These have been referred to collectively as human T-cell leukemia viruses (HTLV). HTLV1 has been associated with acute T-cell leukemia in adults. HTLV2 infection is associated with chronic forms of T-cell leukemia. HTLV-3 is now referred to as HIV-1. Similarly, another recently described AIDs-causing virus which would have been named HTLV-4 in the previous classification is referred to as HIV-2. HTLV-5, also described recently is associated with the skin malignancies, mycosis fungoides and cutaneous T-cell lymphoma.

The pathogenesis of this disease is not completely understood, although our understanding is gradually increasing. It would appear that HIV begins its assault on the host's immune system through direct attachment to specific CD4 receptors on a subpopulation of T-lymphocytes (T-4), Monocytes/macrophages may also become infected. Upon entering the lymphocyte, the virus is uncoated and viral RNA is acted on by reverse transcriptase, an enzyme located in the core of the virus and a single-stranded DNA is formed. Once a cell is infected, the cell may evolve into cancer cells or lead to changes in the expression of other cellular genes resulting in the pathogenic effect of the virus.The depletion of T4 lymphocytes leads to a multitude of abnormalities which collectively undermine the immune response to infections. The infections often are lethal.

Other cells with CD4 receptors may also be infected, including monocytes and macrophages. The monocytes are important in the pathogenesis of AIDs as unlike T4 lymphocytes they are not rapidly killed by the virus. They harbor HIV and disseminate it to brain, bonemarrow and other organs.

Clinical Presentation : HIV infection attacks the immune system and a wide number of immunologic abnormalities have been described in persons with full blown AIDs. Although the diagnosis of AIDs cannot be made solely on immunologic evidence, a distinct immunologic pattern has emerged especially in patients with the full blown syndrome. A persistent quantitative decrease in the T4 lymphocyte subpopulation and functional depression in other lymphocyte populations have been observed. The clinical manifestations of AIDs are now recognized to include a broad spectrum of conditions, including an asymptomatic state, an acute mononucleosis-like syndrome, persistent generalized lymphadenopathy (PGL) and severe cellular immunodeficiency complicated by multiple infections and malignancies..

Infection by HIV usually is followed in a few days by a minor illness lasting 2-3 weeks. Symptoms generally include fever, weakness, rash, myalgia and headache. The patient is then asymptomatic for several months to several years. During this period antibodies to HIV can be detected in almost all the patients but the disease is considered to be in a period of latency. When HIV is activated and replicates, the number of T4 lymphocytes declines and signs and symptoms begin to appear. Most of the patients first experience fatigue, anorexia, rapid unexplained weight loss, fever and night sweats. Chronic lymph node enlargement particularly in the neck is common. Diarrhoea often ensues. Nonproductive cough and unusual shortness of breath often herald the presence of opportunistic pneumonia. A number of neuropsychiatric symptoms including confusion, headache, seizures, personality changes and impairment of memory may also appear.

Most of these clinical manifestations of AIDs result from opportunistic infections. Dementia in AIDs patients is fostered or caused by cytokines released from HIV infected macrophages or monocytes. Kaposi's sarcoma appears to be due to the release of tumor-promoting factors from infected cells.

Kaposi's Sarcoma: Kaposi's sarcoma is the most prevalent neoplasm associated with AIDs. A malignant tumor primarily manifested by multiple vascular nodules, it initially appears on the skin of lower extremities but can progress to involve the lymph nodes and other organs. Until recently, Kaposi's was a relatively rare cancer usually occurring as a chronic, indolent generally nonfatal disease in elderly men. However, it can also cause a more fulminant, rapidly fatal disease in patients who had renal transplants, in those with lupus erythematosus, who are receiving immunosuppressive therapy and in individuals treated with corticosteroids for other diseases. The clinical features, history and mortality of the disease in AIDs victims are similar to those seen in immunospressed patients.

Diagnosis of AIDs : The WHO's criterion for the clinical diagnosis of AIDs envisages the presence of at least two major signs associated with at least one minor sign in the absence of other known causes of immunosuppression such as cancer or severe malnutrition etc.

Major signs :

(a) Weight loss (10% of body weight).
(b) Chronic diarrhoea of more than a month's duration.
(c) Prolonged fever (either intermittent of constant) of more than a month's duration

Minor Signs :

(a) Persistent cough of more than a month's duration.
(b) Geernalized pruritic dermatitis.
(c) Recurrent herpes zoster infection.
(d) Oropharyngeal candidiasis.
(e) Chronic progressive and disseminated herpes simplex.
(f) Generalized lymphodenopathy.

The presence of generalized Kaposi's sarcoma or cryptococcal meningitis are sufficient by themselves for the diagnosis test.

The diagnosis of HIV infection is confirmed by the demonstration of serum antibodies to the virus. Current knowledge suggests that the virus persists in the body for life and a patient who is HIV antibody positive must therefore be considered to be infectious.

Management : There is no specific therapy for HIV infection. However, several clinical trials had earlier established the efficacy of zidovudine (azidothymidine) as the first line agent in the treatment of patients with advanced HIV infection or AIDs related complex. It has now been shown that ziodovudine only delays the onset of AIDs, it does not prolong the survival time of an HIV positive person. Its side effects are so severe that the often offset any benefit of delayed AIDs onset. The management of AIDs therefore depends on supportive measures and the treatment of secondary infection. No vaccine is yet available.

Other opportunistic malignancies and infections commonly occuring in patients with AIDs are summarized in the Table 8.11.

Table. 8.11 Opportunistic Infections and Malignancies in Patients with Aids

Pulmonary infections:	
	Pneumocystis carinii
	Mycobacterium aviam-intracellulare
Neurologic infections:	
	Toxoplasma gondii
	Cryptococcus neoformans
	Herpes simplex virus.
	Cytomegalovirus retinitis
Gastrointestinal infections:	
	Candida albicans
	Salmonella typhimurium
	Cryptosoporidium sp.
	Isospora belli
Disseminated viral diseases:	
	Herpes simplex and Varicella zoster viruses
	Cytomegalovirus
	Epstein- Barr virus
	Hepatitis B virus
AIDs related malignancies	
	Kaposi's sarcoma
	Lymphomas (Hodgkin's and Non-Hodgkin's)

Control of AIDs: Prevention of transmission of infection depends on:

(i) Modification of sexual practices particularly with regard to promiscuity and anal intercourse.
(ii) Screening of donated blood and blood products for HIV antibody.
(iii) The counselling of persons found to be antibody positive.

To achieve effective prevention of AIDs, the following precautions are necessary and adequate health education can significantly contribute to their adoption by the general population. The most important precautions are avoiding indiscriminate sex, use of shared razors and tooth brushes and sharing of needles and syringes by intravenous drug users. Women suffering from AIDs or even those who are HIV positive, should avoid becoming pregnant since the infection can be transmitted to the fetus or new born.Educational material and guidelines for the prevention should be freely distributed and all the mass media e.g. news paper, radio and television should be actively involved in educating the people about AIDs, its nature, transmission and prevention. Blood donors and other persons who come into the high risk groups must be refrained from donating blood or other body organs like kidneys, eyes, sperms etc. Pre-sterilized and disposable syringes should only be used for injections as far as possible.

9

NON-COMMUNICABLE DISEASES

Causative agents, prevention, care and control of cancer, diabetes, blindness, cardiovascular diseases (hypertension, angina, congestive heart failure, myocardial infarction), epilepsy, management of pain, rheumatoid arthritis, gout, and peptic ulcer disease.

CANCERS

Cancer is a term that is used to describe a wide variety of malignant diseases, the management of which involves several medical disciplines. Cancer may best be regarded as a group of neoplastic disorders characterized by

(*i*) an abnormal growth of cells.

(*ii*) ability to invade adjacent tissues and even distant organs (metastases).

(*iii*) eventual death of the patient if the tumor has progressed beyond the stage when it can be successfully removed.

Cancer can occur at any site or in any tissue of the body and may involve any type of the cells. Cancers are generally classified into two major categories: a Solid tumors and b. Leukemias and lymphomas. The latter are often disseminated right from the initial stages.

Cancer ranks second only to coronary heart disease as being the commonest cause of death in the developed countries, the U.S.A. and U.K. Fortunately approximately one third of diagnosed patients can be cured with surgery, irradiation or chemotherapy. Those who are less fortunate will develop a constellation of signs and symptoms consistent with advanced disease.

Most patients seek medical attention when symptoms such as pain, weight loss, bleeding, malaise or an abnormal tissue growth initiate such action. The ability of today's clinician to diagnose cancer has improved dramatically in recent years with the advent of newer radiological techniques, tumor markers and other diagnostic tests.

The patient with an abnormal mass will usually undergo a basic examination that includes a physical examination, a chest X-ray, blood examination that includes a physical examination, a chest X-ray, blood chemistry panel and an evaluation of the pathology of the tumor from a biopsy specimen. Other tests will be included depending on the normal pattern of metastatic spread.

The results of these tests assist in the staging of the disease and the pathologic or histologic grading of the tumor. Table-1 lists some common cancers and their usual sites of metastases.

Table9.1 Common cancers and sites of their metastases

Cencer	Sites of Metastases	
	Primary	**Secondary**
Breast	Liver, lung, bone, Soft tissue	Brain, lung
Colon	Liver	Lung, brain
Pancreas	Liver	Adrenal gland, lung
Hodgkin's	Lymph nodes, stomach, liver	Bone marrow, lung
Lung	Liver, bone	Brain

The staging of tumor determines the aggressiveness of the tumor cell type, whether it has invaded other sites, if so, the location of metastases and its prognosis. A cancer which is more advanced (stage IV) at the time of diagnosis carries a poor prognosis as compared to the one which is diagnosed at an early stage.

The Cancer problem:

Different types of cancers are responsible for causing about 9% of the total deaths throughout the world. In the developed countries cancer is the second leading cause of death and accounts for 19% of all mortality whereas it ranks fourth as a cause of death and accounts for 6% of all the deaths in developing countries. According to one estimate cancer kills 8,00,000 Indians every year.

The incidence of cancer is rising in India with the rise in life expectancy and the control of communicable diseases. According to the foremost cancer expert of the country Dr. D.J. Jussawala, cancer is one of the ten leading causes of death in the country and its rank is advancing year by year. The incidence of cancer is bout 70 per 1,00,000 population in India as compared to 289 per 1,00,000 population in the developed countries. The hospital data show that in our country cancer affects two organ sites most commonly, the uterine cervix in women and the oropharynx in both the sexes. Other prominent types of cancers in females include the cancer of the breast, ovary, oesophagus, stomach and rectum and in the male they comprise of cancer of prostate, lung, oesophagus, stomach, large intestine and rectum.

Aetiology

Cancer has a multifactorial aetiology. It has been estimated that 90% of all cancer deaths could be attributed to potentially avoidable factors namely tobacco, alcohol, diet, reproductive and sexual behaviour, occupation, pollution and geographical features.

Tobacco. Tobacco, either smoked or chewed is the major environmental cause of cancers of the lung, larynx, mouth, pharynx, oesophagus, bladder, pancreas and kidney. It is estimated that in the world as a whole, cigarette smoking is now responsible for more than one million premature deaths every year. The public health campaigns emphasizing the indisputable association between cigarette, tobacco and lung cancer are beginning to prove successful, and there are indications that cigarette consumption has at last started to decline. There is, however, still a continuing need for such education which is aimed particularly to the young to warn them against the dangers of tobacco and cigarette smoking.

Alcohol. Excessive intake of alcoholic beverages has been associated with the cancers of oesophagus and liver. Recent studies have indicated that beer consumption may be associated with rectal cancer.

Diet. It appears easier to influence dietary habits but studies are needed to identify the specific agents responsible for the development of tumours where diet plays a role such as gastrointestinal carcinomas. There exists some association between smoked fish to stomach cancer, dietary fibre to intestinal cancer, beef to bowel cancer and a high fat diet to breast cancer. Other dietary factors such as food additives, coloring agents and flavours are under suspicion as causative agents.

Occupational factors. Exposures to chemicals in the form of their vapors and dusts has been known to produce cancers. These include benzene, arsenic, cadmium, chromium, vinyl chloride, asbestos and polycyclic hydrocarbons. The risk of cancers following exposure to these agent is further increased if the individual also happens to be a smoker.

Viruses. It is now known that some viruses are involved in the pathogenesis of human neoplasms. Hepatitis-B virus is causally related to hepatocellular carcinoma. The Epstein-Barr virus (EBV) is associated with Burkitt's lymphoma and nasopharyngeal carcinoma. Cytomegalovirus (CMV) has been suspected as a causative agent of the Kaposi's sarcoma. Human Papillo Virus (HPV) is the chief suspect in cancer cervix.

Sexual behaviour. The incidence of the carcinoma of the uterine cervix has increased in recent years particularly amongst younger women. This coincided with the changing social patterns of greater sexual freedom and use of oral contraceptives, suggesting that a sexually transmissible agent may be the aetiological factor responsible.

Geographical distribution. The incidence of carcinoma of oesophagus is particularly high in Afganistan, Soviet and Central Asia, Mongolia, Northern China and Iran. Diet or cooking practices may be responsible for this higher incidence. The incidence of carcinoma of pancreas is relatively rare in Japan as compared to most developed countries, whereas the reverse is true for stomach cancer which is particularly prevalent in Japan. The incidence of malignant melanoma is high in countries closer to equator which supports the contention that exposure to sunlight is involved in the genesis of this carcinoma.

Prevention of cancer.

Prevention of cancer encompasses a series of measures based on the present status of knowledge. It aims at significant reduction in the number of new cases, increasing the cure rate and reducing the invalidism of cancer patients. It is estimated that at least one third of all cancers are preventable. The methods of prevention can be considered under the headings of primary and secondary prevention.

Primary prevention. This consists of the control of important causative factors in the general population and in particular occupational groups.

(*i*) **Control of tobacco and alcoholic beverages.** Tobacco and alcohol related cancers can be significantly reduced by controlling smoking, tobacco chewing and more than moderate level of drinking.

Approximately 90% of oral and lung cancers have been linked to tobacco chewing and smoking. WHO has evolved a detailed strategy for the control of tobacco menace. Alcohol also plays an important role in the genesis of oral cancers and is supposed to have a synergistic carcinogenic action in tobacco users.

(*ii*) **Personal hygiene.** Improved personal hygiene and birth control has shown significant decline in the incidence of cancer of uterine cervix.

(*iii*) **Radiation.** Level of radiation including the medical radiation received by each individual should be reduced as radiation has been associated with malignant melanoma and other cancers.

(*iv*) **Occupational exposures.** The workers employed by industrial units must be protected against the exposures to chemical carcinogens. Necessary measures for their protection and frequent medical check-ups for early detection must be taken in high risk areas.

(*v*) **Immunization.** Immunization against Hepatitis B virus has great prospect of reducing the liver cancer.

(*vi*) **Food, Drugs & Cosmetics**. These items must be regularly checked for the presenc of carcinogenic materials.

(*vii*) **Treatment of precancerous lesions.** Early detection and prompt treatment of precancerous lesions such as cervical tears, warts, chronic gastritis and chronic cervicitis can help in the prevention of cancers of these organs.

(*viii*) **Cancer education**. Cancer education can go a long way in the early detection and prevention of cancers, e.g. self examination of breast has helped in very early detection of breast cancer and saved many women from the suffering. Voluntary organizations and cancer hospitals in many countries remind the public of early warning signs of cancers. These are:

(*a*) a lump or hard area in the breast.
(*b*) a change in a wart or mole.
(*c*) a persistent change in digestive or bowel habits.
(*d*) a persistent cough or hoarsenes.
(*e*) excessive loss of blood at the monthly period or bleeding outside the dates.
(*f*) blood loss from any natural orifice.
(*g*) a swelling or sore that does not get better.
(*h*) unexplained loss of weight.

Secondary Prevention.

Secondary prevention consists of the following measures:

(*a*) **Cancer registration.**

It is a must for any successful cancer control programme. It is essential for assessing the magnitude of the problem and for planning the necessary services. There are two types of cancer registration.

(*i*) **Hospital based registries.** These include uniform and minimum set of data recommended by the WHO Handbook for Standardized Cancer Registers.

(*ii*) **Population based registries.** These registries cover the complete cancer information of a given geographic area. The optimum size of base population for such registry is 2-7 million. Population based cancer registries have been operational in Bomaby, Bangalore and Madras under the National Cancer Registry Project of the Indian Council of Medical Research.

(*b*) Early detection of cases.

Cancer screening is the most important weapon for early detection of cancer at a pre-invasive or pre-malignant stage. Such programmes have been developed for cervical cancer, breast cancer and oral cancer. Such cases must be treated immediately after the diagnosis is made.

(*c*) Treatment.

Treatment must be provided to all the cancer patients. Some of the cancers can be surgically removed while certain others may respond to radiation or chemotherapy or combination of both the modalities. For such patients who cannot be cured by any of the available modality or their combination, the goal must be to provide the relief from pain. The WHO has developed guidelines on the relief of cancer pain. Freedom from cancer pain is now considered a right for cancer patients and it is permissible to use some extremely potent and controlled drugs like heroin for this purpose.

Notes on Selected Cancers.

Oral cancer. Oral cancer is one of the ten most common cancers in the world. It is a major problem in India and accounts for 50-70 percent of all diagnosed cancers. Approximately 90 per cent of oral cancers are linked to tobacco chewing and smoking. They are almost always preceded by some types of precancerous lesion. Cancer always occurs on the side of mouth where tobacco quid is placed and the risk is 36 times higher than for nonchewers if the quid is left in the mouth during sleep.

Cancer of the cervix. Cancer of the cervix is the most prevalent form of cancers in developing countries. It accounts for 25-50 percent of all cancers in Indian women. It follows a progressive course from epithelial dysplasia to carcinoma in situ to an invasive carcinoma of cervix. It may take 15-20 years for the conversion of the preinvasive stage to invasive carcinoma. Once the invasive stage is reached the disease spreads by direct extension into the lymph nodes and pelvic organs.

There is some evidence pointing to the sexually transmitted Human Papilloma Virus (HPV) as the cause of cervical cancer. Cancer cervix affects relatively young women with incidence increasing rapidly from the age of 25 to 45 years. The risk factors includes genital warts, early marriage, early coitus, early childbearing, repeated childbirths, oral contraceptive pills and lower socio-economic status.

Breast Cancer. Breast cancer is one of the commonest cause of death in many developed countries and its incidence is increasing in developed countries also. Breast cancer generally occurs between the ages of 35 and 50. A bimodal trend in the age distribution has been observed with a secondary rise in the incidence after the age of 65. The risk is high in those women who have a positive history of breast cancer in the family, particularly if mother or sister had developed breast cancer before menopause. An early first fullterm pregnancy seems to have a protective efect. Those who bear their first child in late thirties are at a higher risk. Early menarche and late menopause have also been associated with breast cancer. Recent evidence suggests that both elevated estrogen as well as progesterone are important factors and increase the risk of breast cancer. Higher socio-economic status, obesity and high fat diet have also been associated with breast cancer.

Lung Cancer. Lung cancer is the leading cause of death in men in many developed countries. Its incidence in western women is also increasing at very fast rate. Studies in India have shown that the lung cancer risk for smokers is 8.6 times higher than that for the nonsmokers. The risk is related to the number of cigarettes smoked in a day, the age of starting the habit, extent of inhalation of smoke and the nicotine and tar content of cigarettes. Those, who are highly exposed to passive smoking are at an increased risk of developing lung cancer. Other factors implicated in the etiology of lung cancer are radiation, air pollution and occupational exposure to asbestos, arsentic compounds, particles containing polycyclic aromatic hydrocarbons and nickel bearing dusts.

In lung cancer control, primary prevention is of greatest importance and the most promising approach is to control smoking which is responsible for 80-90 percent of all cases of lung cancers. WHO has also laid a great emphasis on controlling the smoking epidemic.

Efforts to find effective treatment of lung cancer have not been very successful. The untreatd patients survive for 2-3 months whereas the patients receiving combined chemotherapy may survive for 10-14 months. An important part of the treatment is producing relief from the severe terminal pain in these patients. Considering these problems, the primary prevention of lung cancer merits greater attention.

Blood Cancer (Leukemias). The leukemias are a group of related malignant diseases characterized by quantitative and morphological alterations in the peripheral blood white cells and in the precursors of the affected white cell series in the bone marrow and by secondary anemia, granulocytopenia and thrombocytopenia due to leukemic cell infiltration of the bone marrow and competition with normal myeloid elements.

Luekemia may be present in either acute or chronic form for each main type of white cell and their varying histories and clinical courses indicate that each may have a different pathogenesis. No definite etiology other than high dose of radiation exposure has been proved for any of the leukemias.

The term acute and chronic leukemia refer to expected prognosis in the natural course of the condition if left untreated. The prognosis of untreated acute leukemias is a life span of 2-3 months or less. Chronic leukemias, in contrast, would be expected to permit a life span of 2-5 years if untreated and the predominant white cell would be a more mature form. Proper treatment prolongs the symptom free and useful life of leukemia patients for periods many times the expected survival if left untreated.

DIABETES

Diabetes mellitus is a clinical syndrome characterized by hyperglycemia due to absolute or relative deficiency of insulin. Lack of insulin affects the metabolism of carbohydrate, protein, fat. water and electrolytes.

Diabetes is by far the most common amongst the endocrine diseases. It is world wide in distribution. There are two major clinical presentations of diabetes. Incidence of both types of primary diabetes, that is Insulin Dependent Diabetes Mellitus (IDDM) and Non-Insulin Dependent Diabetes Mellitus (NIDDM) is rising throughout the world.

IDDM (Type I Diabetes, Juvenile Diabetes)

Approximately 5-10% of the diabetic population has Type-1 diabetes. These patients have no pancreatic reserve, have a tendency to develop ketoacidosis and are dependent on exogenous insulin to sustain life. The mean age of onset is 12 years although it is also observed in adults. The onset of disease may occur slowly over 1-2 months or abruptly over a few days. This type of diabetes has some genetic predisposition and is closely associated with certain histocompatibility antigens and presence of circulating islet cell antibodies early in the disease. It has been proposed that in genetically predisposed individuals autoimmune destruction of islet cells is triggered by viruses, chemicals and other unknown environment factors. Type-1 diabetes is also known as juvenile, unstable, ketosis prone or brittle diabetes.

NIDDM (Type-II Diabetes, Maturity onset Diabetes).

Type-II diabetics comprise approximately 90% of the diabetic population. It is characterized by the presence of endogenous insulin, an absence of ketosis, an absence of circulating islet cell antibodies and a lack of association with histocompatibility antigens. Unlike IDDM, symptoms are relatively mild and gradual in onset and are generally easily controlled with diet, oral sulphonylureas or insulin. The diagnosis is generally made after the age of 40, but can occur during childhood and young adulthood also. There is also a stronger family history of diabetes in this group of diabetics than in Type-I insulin dependent diabetics. Type-II diabetics may release high, low or normal amounts of insulin in response to a glucose challenge and exhibit varying degrees of tissue insulin resistance. Subclasses of these patients have been suggested based upon weight , age of onset, insulin levels, and the presence or absence of a chlorpropamide alcohol flush. Type-II diabetes has also been described as ketosis resistant or stable diabetes.

Carbohydrate metabolism. An understanding of the signs and symptoms of diabetes mellitus is based upon a knowledge of the multiple metabolic effects of insulin as well as glucose metabolism and homeostasis in diabetic and nondiabetic subjects during the fed (postprandial) and fasting states. The homeostatic mechanisms in the body are tuned to maintain a blood glucose concentration within a range of 40-160 mg/dl. A minimum concentration of 40 mg/dl is required to provide adequate fuel for the brain which is heavily reliant on glucose as the principal source of energy and is not dependent upon the presence of insulin for its utilization. When the concentration of blood glucose exceeds the reabsorptive capacity of the kidneys (approximately 180 mg/dl), glucose spills into the urine resulting in the loss of energy and water. Muscles and fat also use glucose as major energy source but they need the presence of insulin. If glucose is not available in adequate amount, these tissues are able to use alternative substrates such as aminoacids and fatty acids for fuel.

Postprandial glucose metabolism. After the ingestion of food blood glucose concentrations rise and stimulate the release of insulin which is the key to efficient glucose utilization. It promotes the uptake of glucose, fatty acids and amino acids and facilitates their conversion to storage forms in most tissues. As a result it also maintains the blood glucose within normal range so that none will be wasted in the urine. In muscles insulin promotes the uptake of glucose and its storage as glycogen. It also stimulates the uptake of amino acids and their conversion to proteins. In adipose tissue, glucose is converted to free fatty acids and stored as triglycerides. Insulin also prevents the breakdown of these triglycrides to free fatty acids which may be transported to other tissues for utilization. The liver does not require insulin for glucose transport but the presence of insulin facilitates the conversion of glucose to glycogen. Glycogenolysis is the major source of glucose during fasting state.

Fasting Glucose Metabolism. During the fasting state hypoglycemia inhibits the release of insulin and promotes the release of other hormones like glucagon, epinephrine, glucocorticoids and growth hormone which antagonise the effect of insulin and thus promote an increse in blood glucose. Due to the lack of insulin several processes occur which maintain and conserve a minimum blood glucose level for the brain. Glycogen in the liver is broken down to glucose (glycogenolysis), aminoacids are converted to glucose through gluconeogenesis, there is diminished uptake by insulin dependent tissues in order to conserve glucose for the brain and the triglycerides are broken down to free fatty acids and used as fuel by muscles and fat which are unable to use glucose in the absence of insulin.

Clinical Presentation. In a patient of diabetes, blood glucose concentrations remain high after a meal because the uptake, utilization and storage of glucose by adipose tissue, and muscle are diminished due to the absence of insulin or tissue resistance to insulin's effects. Because glucose is not accessible to the cells in spite of high blood glucose concentration, fasting metabolism, which further increases blood glucose concentaration through glycogenolysis and gluconeogenesis, is triggered. If glucose concentrations surpass the renal threshold, glucose spills into urine taking water with it by the process of osmotic diuresis. Due to the loss of the calories and water, patients experience symptoms of polyuria, polydipsia, fatigue and weight loss despite normal or excessive food intake. High glucose levels provide an excellent medium for bacterial growth, and hence diabetics may frequently suffer from recurrent respiratory, vaginal and other infections. Muscle begins to metabolize stored glycogen for fuel and the liver metabolizes free fatty acids which are released in response to epinephrine and low insulin levels. An absolute lack of insulin can cause excessive mobilization and metabolism of FFAs which results in elevated blood and urinary ketones, the metabolic products of fatty acid metabolism. These ketone bodies may ultimately produce metabolic acidosis. Patients with high blood glucose may also complain of blurred vision which may be due to osmotically induced changes in the lens.

It is important to note that weight loss and ketoacidosis primarily occur in poorly controlled Type-I diabetics. Type II diabetics frequently have mild symptoms related to hyperglycemia such as fatigue, polyuria, polydipsia and vaginal infections, but they rarely develop ketoacidosis bacause of the presence of insulin which suppresses lipolysis. Weight loss is also uncommon in these patients because endogenous insulin levels promote lipogenesis. Type II diabetes is primarily a disease of tissue unresponsiveness to insulin with high blood glucose concentrations resulting from poor utilization as opposed to the combination of poor utilization plus glucose production via fasting metabolic processes in Type I diabetes.

Complications. Complications secondary to long standing disease account for the morbidity and mortality in the diabetic population. However, it is not possible to predict which diabetics will develop long term complications. Some Type I and Type II diabetics progress through the disease for 30-40 years without major complications while others pass through an apparently relentless course of widespread complications. This observation is further evidence of the heterogenous nature of the disease and has led to the theory that a predisposition to these complications may be, to some extent, genetically linked to diabetes.

Cardiovascular disease. Diabetics appear to have more widespread and rapid progression of cardiovascular disease and show a greater disposition to hypertension, congestive heart failure and coronary artery disease. A significant percentage of diabetics have been shown to die of atherosclerotic disease in different studies. Hence, it is all the more important to minimize or eliminate all other preventable risk factors for cardiovascular disease in diabetics such as smoking, hypertension, hyperlipedemias and obesity.

Peripheral vascular disease. In diabetics peripheral vascular disease is an extension of the atherosclerotic process and probably the result of microvascular disease and neuropathy found in these individuals. Clinical features include an absence of pulses, coolness in one extreme but not in the other and in its worst form gangrene or slow healing skin ulceration which may ultimately lead to systemic infection and even amputation.

Diabetic complications. Refractive changes are usually associated with poor diabetic control. Diabetics also develop senile type of cataracts early in age and a type of glaucoma which is relatively resistant to treatment. The most common ocular complications, however, is diabetic retinopathy which usually appears after 15-20 years and may occur in upto 80% of diabetics.. Proliferative retinopathy which is characterized by neovascularization, though much rarer, is the most important cause of new blindness in diabetics. Since hypertension, smoking, uremia and hyperglycemia predispose diabetics to more rapid progression of retinopathy, special efforts should be made to treat these disorders vigorously.

Nephropathy. Nephrotic syndrome and azotemia are the major causes of death in Type-I diabetics. Approximately 40% Type-I diabetics who survive for 40 years have some evidence of renal disease.

Neuropathy. Neuropathy presents as a peripheral neuritis or autonomic insufficiency. Symptomatic peripheral neuropathy may occur in 25% diabetics and is characterized by paraesthesia and pain in the lower extremities, which may be mild or severe and unrelenting, decreased vibration sense, decreased ankle and knee jerks and decreased conduction velocity. Autonomic neuropathy may present as gastroparesis with a feeling of fullness and nausea, urinary retention, impotence in males, rarely postural hypotension and diarrhoea.

Management.

There are three important components of the management of diabetes:

(*i*) Dietary control.
(*ii*) Drugs.
(*iii*) Exercise.

These components interact with each other and the total control is interdependent to the extent that no assessment and modification of one can be made without considering the effect of other two.

Dietary control. Diet plays a primary and crucial role in the theapy of all diabetics. The goals of diabetic diet are:

(*i*) To provide adequate calories for maintaining normal growth and development of young diabetics and an ideal body weight in other diabetic patients. For the obese Type-II diabetics this generally means a calorie restricted diet.

(*ii*) To provide adequate amount of carbohydrates for exogenously administered insulin in Type-I diabetics. Regularly scheduled meals and snacks at desired intervals which provide consistent amount of carbohydrates, proteins and fats are essential for the prevention of hypoglycemic reactions in response to insulin in the Type-I diabetes.

(*iii*) To minimize acute fluctuations in blood glucose levels through the restriction of simple sugars like glucose, sucrose and lactose.

(*iv*) To minimize dietary contributes to cardiovascular disease by restricting the intake of saturated fats to 10% of the total calories and advising the patients to reduce their salt (sodium) intake.

(*v*) To provide adequate proteins to the extent of 12-20% of total calorie intake and assure adequate growth and nutrition. Protein contents may be liberalized for pregnant women and children and restricted in patients with uremia or hepatic encephalopathy.

Artificial sweetners. The use of saccharin has been banned in most of the countries since it has been linked to bladder cancer in rats. Moderate use of caloric sweetner like fructose, xylitol, mannitol and sorbitol will have little effect on diabetic control as they produce less postprandial hyperglycemia as compared to glucose. Nevertheless, they have no value in low calorie diets. A new synthetic noncaloric sweetner aspartame which has no unpleasant aftertaste may become the artificial sweetner of choice in near future.

Fibre. Diets containing high fibre are recommended on the basis that they slow the absorption of carbohydrates and produce minimum fluctuations in the postprandial blood glucose levels.

Alcohol. Small amounts of alcoholic beverages may not produce any harm to a diabetic but their caloric contribution to the diet must be considered and taken into account.

Exercise. Moderate, regular exercise is highly recommended for non-insulin dependent diabetics and encouraged in insulin dependent diabetics if special precautions are taken like 30-40 min. after injection of insulin and relatively soon after a meal. There may be a need to increase the caloric intake and/or decrease the dose of insulin in such patients.

Drugs. The use of insulin along with diet is crucial to the survival of Type-I, insuln dependent diabetics. Insulin also plays a major role in the management of Type-II diabetics when their symptoms are controlled with diet alone or together with oral hypoglycemic agents. It is also used in type-II diabetics during the periods of intercurrent illness or stress (e.g. surgery or pregnancy). The use of oral sulphonylureas is reserved for the treatment of symptomatic Type-II diabetics whose symptoms cannot be controlled with diet and exercise alone. The biguanides phenformin and metformin are used only for those rare Type-II diabetics who are allergic to sulphonylureas, cannot use insulin due to allergy and mental or physical disability, cannot be controlled on diet and who have no predisposing factors to the development of lactic acidosis.

Goals of therapy. As there is no absolute cure for diabetes at present, most diabetologists agree on defining some overall goals of the therapy. They include.

(*i*) Keeping the patient free of symptoms relating to hyperglycemia or hypoglycemia.

(*ii*) Maintain the patient as close to euglycemia as possible without exposing him/her to undue risk of hypoglycemia. This would slow the progression of chronic complications associated with diabetes.

(*iii*) Try to attain normal growth and development in children.

(*iv*) Try to educate the patient about his/her disease, its treatment and compliance of therapeutic measures. Diabetic patient's knowledge and understanding of disease has a tremendous positive impact on the diabetic control.

BLINDNESS

Blindness can be defined as continuing inability to see with one or both the eyes. It may arise from injury or disease that affects any of the structures or substances that light passes through on its way to the retina, the light-sensitive tissue that lines the back and sides of the eye, or the causes of the blindness may lie in injuries or disease of the retina itself, of the optic nerve or of the visual centres of the brain.

WHO has proposed a uniform criterion and defined blindness as the visual acuity of less than 3/60 (Snellen) or its equivalent in the better eye or field of vision is 20° or less in the better eye. This, in the absence of appropriate vision charts is indicated by the inability of a person to count fingers in day light at a distance of 3 meters.

A number of infectious diseases including venereal diseases can cause blindness. Untreated gonorrhoea and syphilis in pregnant woman can cause imperfect development of the infant's eyes with resultant blindness. Other infective diseases that can cause blindness include, trachoma, leprosy, tuberculosis, meningitis, measles, diphtheria and scarlet fever. Onchocerciasis or infestation with the round worm occasionally results in blindness if the worms invade the eyes. Certain non-infective systemic diseases may also cause blindness. Diabetes mellitus may damage the retina or cause cataracts (opacity of the crystalline lens) which prevent light from reaching the retina. Atherosclerosis by blocking the blood supply causes atrophy of retinal tissue and the optic nerve. Diseases springing from nutritional deficiencies may cause blindness by making the cornea, the normally transparent section of the globe in front of the pupil and iris, soft and cloudy. Diseases of the eye itself that may bring blindness include cataract (opacity of he crystalline lens) and glaucoma which is characterized by an increase in intraocular pressure and produces its effect through the pressure on optic nerve. Table-9.2 summarizes the important causes of blindness in India.

Table 9.2 Important Causes of Blindness in India

Cataract	:	55%
Infections of the eye	:	15%
Trachoma	:	5%
Malnutrition (Vitamin A Deficiency	:	2%
Glaucoma	:	0.8%
Injuries	:	1.2%
Others (Diabetes, atherosclerosis, hypertension, tumours & congenital disorders etc.)	:	21%

Epidemiological factors.

1. **Age.** About 30 percent of the blind in India lose their eyesight before they reach the age of 20 years. Malnutrition (Vitamin A deficiency), infection of the eye, ophthalmia neonatorum, injuries, trachoma and conjunctivitis are important causes of blindness in children. In the elderly, cataract, glaucoma, diabetes and hypertension etc. lead to blindness. Accidents and injuries can occur in all age groups.
2. **Sex.** A higher prevalence of blindness is reported in females than in males in India which may be due to a higher incidence of trachoma, conjunctivitis and cataracts in females.
3. **Occupation.** People working in factories, workshops, cottage industries are more prone to blindness as they are constantly exposed to dust, airborne particles, gases, fumes and radiation etc.
4. **Social class.** Blindness is more prevalent in the lower classes as

compared to the well-to-do and affluent classes. The basic factors like ignorance, poverty, low standard of personal and community hygiene etc. have been associated with the diseases of eye and blindness.

Eye Health Care.

There are 9 million blind people in India, of which 85% are curable. Another 45 million individuals are visually impaired. Such abnormalities create a huge economic and social burden on the nation. This situation has led to the emergence of a comprehensive eye-health care concept which comprises of.

1. **Primary eye care**. The eye care component has been added to the primary health care system and this has gained world-wide acceptance. The promotion and protection of eye health, together with on the spot treatment for the commonest eye diseases are its important features.
2. **Epidemiological approach.** This approach involves studies at the population level. It focuses on the measurement of incidence, prevalence of diseases and their risk factors. The local epidemiological situation will determine the action required.
3. **The team approach**. As the number of eye specialists are not enough to take care of all eye-related problems, the auxillary health personnel are involved in Eye Health Care. They include village health guides, ophthalmic assistants, medical social workers and the voluntary agencies.
4. **Establishment of national programmes.** An important development with regard to the prevention of blindness has been the establishment of National Programme for Control of Blindness. This programme was launched by the Ministry of Health and Family Welfare, Government of India in 1976 and it is to be completed in a period of 20 years. The prevalence of blindness in India is estimated at 1.5% for the whole country and the goal of this National Programme is to reduce the blindness in the country to 0.3% by 2000 AD.

Prevention of Blindness.

It has now been recognised that blindness can be prevented to a great extent by improving nutrition, treating cases of infectious diseases, controlling the organisms which cause infection and by improving safety conditions at working places, on roads and even at home. The measures taken for the prevention of blindness can be summarized as under.

(*a*) **Initial assessment of prevalence.** It is important to first assess the magnitude, geographic distribution and causes of blindness within the country or a particular region, by conducting the prevalence surveys. This information is essential for setting priorities and for the development of appropriate intervention programmes.

(*b*) **Methods of prevention.**

(*i*) **Primary eye care.** A number of ophthalmic conditions like acute conjunctivitis, trachoma, xerophthalmia and ophthalmia neonatorum can be treated and/or prevented by trained primary health workers, medical social workers/village health guides at grass root level as they are the first to make contact with the community. They are provided with essential drugs like sulphacetamide, tetracycline, vitamin A capsules, eye bandages and shields etc. for this purpose. They are trained and instructed to refer the difficult and serious cases like corneal ulcers, penetrating foreign bodies and painful eye conditions to the nearest public health centres or a hospital. They also promote personal hygiene, sanitation, good dietary habits and safety methods for the welfare of the community.

(*ii*) **Secondary care.** Methods of secondary care include the precise management of common blinding conditions like cataract, glaucoma and ocular trauma etc. This is provided at the PHCs and district hospitals where qualified eye specialists and required facilities for treating these diseases are available. The introduction of mobile eye clinics and eye camps for cataract surgery have significantly contributed in the prevention of blindness in our villages and talukas.

(*iii*) **Tertiary care.** This provides sophisticated eye care such as retinal detachment surgery, corneal grafting and other complex forms of management not available in secondary centres. Such services are established in the medical colleges and leading medical institutions. Eye Banks have also been established at such centres which have provided eye sight to many after corneal grafting. The Government of India have established the National Institute for the Blind at Dehradun to work out new approaches and strategies for solving the problems of the blind. The other high level exclusive ophthalmic institutions include the Shankar Netralaya, Madras, Arvind Eye Hospital, Madurai, L.V. Prasad Eye Hospital, Hyderabad, Eye Hospital & Research Institute, Sitapur and Dr. Nagpal's Eye Academy, Ahmedabad etc.

(*c*) **Specific Eye Care Programmes.**

(*i*) **Trachoma control.** Endemic trachoma and infections associated with it are a major cause of blindness in many developing countries including India. Mass compaign with topical tetracycline and the improvement of socio-economic conditions have gradually reduced the incidence and severity of trachoma and associated conjunctival infections.

(*ii*) **Eye Care at school level.** School children can be easily screened and treated for defects like refractive errors, squint, amblyopia and trachoma etc. They can be taught to practice the principles of good posture, proper lighting when they read or write, avoidance of glare and adequate distance and angle between the books and the eyes. Publishers of text books should be encouraged and advised to use suitable letters types.

(*iii*) **Prophylaxis with Vitamin A.** Government of India under the Vitamin A distribution scheme provides 2,00,000 units of Vitamin A given orally at 6 monthly interval to children between 1-6 years. This helps a great deal in the control of xerophthalmia.

(*iv*) **Occupational eye care services.** The measures taken to prevent eye hazard in the industries are extremely important. Education on the prevention of any damage to the eye and the use of protective devices and proper illumination is very essential in many industries.

National and International Agencies:

The National Association for the Blind, a voluntary organization has been active in looking after the welfare of the blind throughout the country. The Royal Commonwealth Society for the Blind has also been working in this field. WHO has brought together various voluntary organizations associated with the welfare services to the blind to build a new agency, called the "International Agency for the Prevention of Blindness". This agency's primary objective is to prevent blindness. The goal of W.H.O. and the International Agency for Prevention of Blindness is to eliminate 50 per cent of the World's avoidable blindness by the year 2000.

HYPERTENSION

Hypertension is the most common adult medical problem in the industrial world. The World Health Organization estimates that 8-18% of adults have blood pressure greater than 95 torr diastolic and/or 160 torr systolic. Once the hypertension develops, it tends to be self perpetuating via amplifying mechanisms mediated by secondary structural changes in blood vessels, heart and kidney. These adaptive structural changes amplify and perpetuate hypertension by increasing systemic vascular resistance, enhancing cardiac output and impairing renal sodium and water excretion. In general, it can be stated that the greater the elevation in blood pressure, the greater the risk of morbidity and mortality due to cardiovascular and renovascular diseases. The following arbitrary stratification of hypertension by diastolic blood pressure has become conventional.

Mild	:	90-104 torr
Moderate	:	105-114 torr
Severe	:	115 torr or greater.

Epidemiology: The incidence depends on age, race and gender. Blacks at any age have twice the incidence of hypertension as Caucasians. Hypertension is slightly more common in males than in females. Individuals with family history of hypertension are at considerably greater risk of developing high blood pressure and its complications suggesting a genetic transmission of the disease. Other factors strongly associated with high blood pressure are obesity and excessive salt ingestion.

Etiology: Known or secondary causes can be identified in about 6-10% of those with hypertension. These secondary causes of hypertension are listed in the Table 9.3.

Table 9.3: Causes of Secondary Hypertension

I	Renal Disease
	a) Renoparenchymal disease
	b) Renovascular disease.
II	Coarctation of the aorta
III	Primary aldosteronism.
IV	Cushing's Syndrome.
V	Pheochromocytoma.
VI	Iatrogenic Hypertension.
	a) Oral Contraceptives.
	b) Anorectics.
	c) Alcohol
	d) Corticosteroids.

Secondary hypertension is usually curable. The majority of individuals with hypertension present with essential or primary hypertension (90-94% cases) which has no established cause.

The etiology of essential hypertension is probably multifactorial and may involve a number of abnormalities in physiological regulatory systems. The pressure receptors in the cardiovascularsystem i.e., baroreceptors may become reset at a higher pressure in response to chronic stress, overactivity of the sympathetic nervous system or heredity. The kidneys may retain too much of salt and water in response to altered reflexes which tend to maintain abnormal intravascular fluid volumes. Approximately 30% patients of hypertension are salt sensitive and their B.P. falls significantly with the restriction of dietary salt intake.

Pathophysiology: Arterial blood pressure is a highly integrated and complex system regulated by a number of variables. It allows blood pressure to remain within a relatively constant range despite changes in posture and wide variations in the demand for blood. Blood pressure is dependent on both cardiac output (CO) and peripheral resistance (PR). Mean arterial pressure (MAP) equals cardiac output (CO) times total peripheral resistance (TPR).

$$MAP = CO \times TPR$$

Cardiac output is in turn defined as the volume of blood in litres pumped by the heart per minute. Its a function of both stroke volume (SV) and heart rate (HR). Thus

$$MAP = SV \times HR \times TPR$$

If any of these factors are increased, an elevation of BP will result.However, in the chronic stage hypertension appears to be principally a disease of increased peripheral resistance resulting in the elevation of both systolic and diastolic blood pressure.

A variety of humoral changes have also been implicated in essential hypertension; among the most important of these are the renin-angiotensin system, antidiuretic hormone, prostaglandins and the kallikrein/kinin system. The renin-angiotensin system (RAS) has arisen from an academical interesting but obscure regulatory mechanism to an important hormonal pathway known to play a key role in the regulation of cardiovascular homeostasis and Na^+ balance in normal and hypertensive subjects. This system includes the following components and sources (Fig. 9.1.)

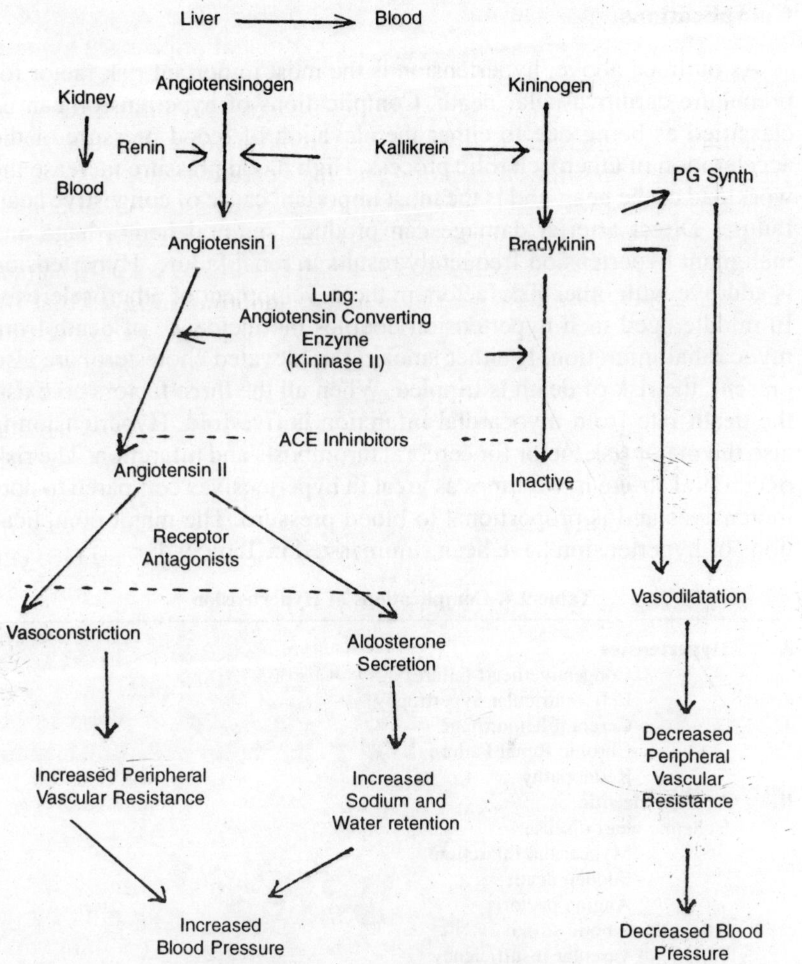

Fig. 9.1 The Renin Angiotensin System

Renin is synthesized by the kidneys and secreted into the circulation where it cleaves the decapeptide angiotensin I from angiotensinogen until it is cleared by the liver. Angiotensin I is converted to the octapeptide angiotensin II by angiotensin converting enzyme (ACE), an enzyme found in high concentrations in the pulmonary vascular bed. The active hormone of the RAS is angiotensin II, the actions of which are thought to be mediated by specific receptors located on various target organs (e.g. adrenal cortex, kidney, arterioles, and sympathetic nerve endings).

Complications:

As outlined above, hypertension is the most important risk factor for premature cardiovascular death. Complications of hypertension can be classified as being due to either the elevation of blood pressure or the acceleration of atherosclerotic process. High blood pressure increase the workload of the heart and is the most important cause of congestive heart failure. Direct arterial damage can produce cerebral hemorrhage and malignant hypertension frequently results in renal failure. Hypertension is additive with other risk factors in the development of atherosclerosis. In middle aged men hypertension doubles the incidence of death from myocardial infarction. If either smoking or elevated cholesterol are also present, the risk of death is trippled. When all the three factors co-exist, the death rate from myocardial infarction is five fold. Hypertension is also the major risk factor for cerebral thrombosis and infarction. The risk of cerebral stroke is 4-5 times as great in hypertensives compared to normotensives and is proportional to blood pressure. The major complications of hypertension have been summarized in Table 9.4.

Table 9.4. Complications of Hypertension

A. Hypertensive
- Congestive heart failure.
- Left ventricular hypertrophy
- Cerebral hemorrhage
- Chronic Renal Failure
- Retinopathy

B. Arteriosclerotic
- Ischemic heart disease
  - Myocardial infarction
  - Sudden death
  - Angina pectoris
- Atherothrombotic stroke
- Peripheral vascular insufficiency
- Aortic aneurism

Clinical Presentation:

Hypertension is usually an asymptomatic disease unless the B.P. is very high. Elevated blood pressure may be an incidental finding during routine physical examination. The diagnosis of hypertension is based on documentation of increased blood pressure on several independent readings, unless target-organ damage is already present. The signs and symptoms of primary hypertension are secondary to target organ damage. For example retinopathy causes scotomas, blurred vision and may finally lead to blindness. In severe hypertension CNS symptoms like lethargy, confusion, increased neuromuscular irritability, convulsions and coma may be present. Damage to heart results in angina pectoris or the signs and symptoms of congestive heart failure and myocardial infarction may also appear. Occipital headaches occurring in the morning may also be associated with severe hypertension.

Management

The main objective of treating systemic arterial hypertension is to reduce the risk of complications and to improve patient survival. The benefits of treatment have to be watched against its inconvenience and the possibility that the agents used may themselves have potentially harmful effects. In most instances, the discovery of hypertension commits the patient to a lifetime of supervision and treatment. It is important to treat the whole patient and not just the blood pressure. The following general guidelines can be followed for most of the mild, moderate and severe hypertensive patients.

(*a*) Before diagnosis of hypertension is made, blood pressure should be measured a number of times and on separate occasions in order to obtain accurate and reliable readings.

(*b*) Non-pharmacological measures such as weight reduction of overweight, restriction of salt and alcohol intake, and increased exercise should be used by all hypertensive patients whether taking drugs or not. Cessation of smoking is also highly recommended.

(*c*) Drug treatment should be instigated at diastolic blood pressures above 100 mm Hg. The period of blood pressure monitoring before drug treatment is used,should, however, be shorter when pressures are higher or there is evidence of target organ damage.

(*d*) The role of diuretics and betablockers as first line therapy is well defined. They are the only two drug groups with which beneficial/long term effects on morbidity and mortality have been demonstrated.

(*e*) ACE inhibitors, calcium channel blockers, and alpha blockers, are all effective antihypertensives. They should be judiciously used when diuretics and betablockers are not effective, poorly tolerated or contraindicated.

(*f*) Drug therapy should be tailored to the individual patient with regard to any co-existing disease. When all clinical factors are equal, drug costs should be taken into account. Thiazide diuretics and betablockers are cheaper than other drugs.

Prognosis and role of pharmacist:

To work effectively in the area of hypertension, pharmacists must understand the disease and the rationale for the adopted therapeutic regimen. Some of the important areas which should be understood include: How should B.P. be measured? What are the criteria to define hypertension? Which patients should be treated? Which drugs or combinations should be used? In addition skills in improving compliance are needed to sustain long term therapy.

ANGINA PECTORIS

Angina pectoris, a clinical syndrome characterized by chest pain due to transient myocardial ischemia, results when the metabolic demands of the heart for oxygen exceed the ability of diseased coronary arteries to supply adequate blood flow to the myocardium.

Angina pectoris is classified according to its frequency, severity and precipitating event.

The classical type is often referred to as **stable angina**. This is the typical angina in which discomfort is precipitated by physical activity or emotional disturbances and is relieved by rest.

Unstable angina describes a syndrome of attacks of recent onset or of increasing frequency, severity or occurring with less exercise or rest and a decrease in responsiveness to treatment. Myocardial infarction and arrhythmias are more likely to develop during periods of unstable angina.

Nocturnal angina occurs during sleep and may be associated with either dreams and rapid eye movement (REM) sleep or increased venous return in a patient with congestive heart failure.

Prinzmetal angina is atypical angina. It occurs while the patient is at rest, is associated with ventricular arrhythmias and is thought to be due to coronary artery spasm and is less responsive to the usual forms of medical treatment.

Signs and symptoms:

Angina pectoris is a manifestation of coronary artery disease, which is a clinical syndrome that results from transient myocardial ischaemia but with no evidence of permanent damage.

The patients with angina pectoris usually describe the chest discomfort as heaviness, pressure, tightness or squeezing. The patient usually will not use the word 'pain' and may ascribe his symptoms to indigestion. The substernal discomfort may radiate to the left arm, throat, jaw, shoulder, back or abdomen. The discomfort typically is precipitated by exercise, and also but less often by eating, emotional upset, exposure to cold and cigarette smoking. It is relieved by rest. The episodes usually last longer than 1 minute but no longer than 30 minutes. The physical examination of these patients may be normal between attacks. The diagnosis of angina is made from the history. Evidence of ischaemia on ECG stress testing is inversion of T waves and depression of the ST segment. Angiography and a therapeutic response to nitroglycerin may be helpful in establishing the diagnosis.

Pathogenesis:

The most common cause of angina pectoris is coronary atherosclerotic heart disease, a pathological condition of the coronary arteries characterized by atheromatous lesions which thicken and harden vessel walls. These lesions narrow the coronary vessel wall lumen and reduce blood flow to the myocardium. Although the atherosclerotic coronary arteries usually provide adequate blood flow during rest or moderate activily, stenotic arteries cannot supply the extra oxygenated blood required by the heart during exercise or other types of stress. This imbalance in the demand and supply leads to myocardial ischemia and chest pain. Progression of atherosclerotic lesions causing complete occlusion of blood flow can lead to further complications.

Prognosis and Risk Factors:

The general prognosis of angina pectoris patients after diagnosis has been shown to be progression to a fatal cardiovascular complication within 10 years. Mortality rates for specific types of angina, however, vary considerably. On the basis of coronary angiography, more diffuse disease is associated with poorer survival. The five year mortality rates for single, double and tripple vessel disease have been assessed as 7%, 35% and 45% respectively.

A number of risk factors associated with the development of angina have been identified. Among the major risk factors which may contribute to the development of angina are hypercholesterolemia, hypertension, cigarette smoking, diabetes mellitus and certain electrocardiographic abnormalities.Anxiety, severe psychological stress and the so called Type-A behaviour (hard driving, competitive and over-ambitious) may also be implicated in the genesis of angina as important risk factors. Modification of some of these risk factors may at times retard the development of angina, it is obvious that many of these factors cannot always be easily changed.

Management:

Management of angina pectoris involves three phases: a proper assessment of the severity of symptoms and the likely extent of the disease; the use of measures to control symptoms; and treatment which will improve life expectancy. The assessment of the severity of disease is precisely achieved by electrocardiography, myocardial perfusion scanning using radioactive thallium in conjunction with exercise testing and by coronary arteriography. Control of symptoms should be achieved by avoiding walking after meals, particularly in the cold or against the wind and by avoiding severe unaccustomed exertion. They should be encouraged and supported in their endeavours to stop smoking and lose weight, hyperlipedemia if present be controlled by dietary measures or adequate drug treatment, lastly, the drug treatment has to be applied to control symptoms and improve the quality and expectancy of life. There are three principal groups of drugs which help to relieve or prevent the symptoms of angina: nitrates, beta-adrenoceptor antagonists and calcium channel blockers. Although each of these groups can be shown to be superior to placebo in treating symptoms of angina, there is little convincing evidence that one group is more effective than another. The present trend is to start with sublingual nitroglycerin, to progress to a beta-blocker unless there are contraindications and then to add nifedipine or a long acting nitrate such as isosorbide dinitrate. The ultimate aim of achieving excellent control of angina with minimal side effects and the simplest possible tablet regimen is unlikely to be reached without trial and error.

Goals of therapy:

The goals in the management of angina pectoris are: to relieve symptoms, to improve the quality of life, to prevent complications such as sudden death, myocardial infarction and arrhythmias and to increase life expectancy.

CONGESTIVE HEART FAILURE

The clinical syndrome of congestive heart failure (CHF) results when the left, right or both ventricles fail to pump sufficient blood to meet the body's needs. There is a clear correlation between the incidence of CHF and both sex and age. It is considered to be a disease of the elderly and is more common in males than in famales. By the sixth decade, the incidence among men is five times that of the fourth decade. It is thus apparent that as the size of the geriatric population increases, CHF is bound to become a more frequently encountered clinical entity. Unfortunately, in spite of the treatment which is considered rational and clinically effective, the long term prognosis of patients with congestive heart failure is extremely poor. In the Framington study 60% of men and 40% of women died within 5 years of the diagnosis of CHF. These figures are approximately 7 times higher than the average annual death rates for persons without CHF.

Etiology : The most common etiological factors involved in the genesis of CHF are essential hypertension, coronary artery disease and rheumatic heart disease. Pulmonary embolism, hyperthyroidism, persistent cardiac arrhythmias and myocardiopathies, although less common, may also play an etiological role in the development of CHF. Hypertension appears to be the most important of these factors. In the Framington study, 75% of patients who developed CHF had prior histories of hypertension. The risk of developing CHF in hypertensive patients was 6 times that of patients with normal blood pressures. Coronary artery disease precede the development of CHF in 38% patients of Framington study group. However, the majority of these had concomitant hypertension.

Types of Heart Failure :

There are two major types of heart failure. **High output failure :** This occurs when the heart is unable to pump enough blood to meet the metabolic demands to the tissues. For example in hyperthyroid patients metabolic demands are greater than normal. Similarly in severely anemic patients tissues require a greater volume of blood to supply normal metabolic needs. **Low output failure :** It is the more common of the two types. It occurs when the heart is unable to pump all of the blood with which it has been presented. Whereas a normal ejection fraction (EF), percent of the ventricular volume expelled during systole) is greater than 60%, a person with serious CHF may have EF as low as 20 to 30%. Increased cardiac workload and impaired myocardial contractility are other important factors which contribute to the development of CHF.

Pathogenesis :

As the heart begins to fail, several complex compensatory mechanisms are activated by the body in order to maintain cardiac output and oxygenation of vital organs. These include cardiac (vantricular) dilatation, cardiac hypertrophy, increased sympathetic tone and sodium and water retention. A clear idea about these compensatory mechanisms is essential for understanding the signs and symptoms of congestive heart failure.

Cardiac dilatation results when the ventricles are not able to pump the entire volume of blood which they are presented. This leads to a gradual accumulation of a residual amount of blood in the ventricles. Consequently the end diastolic volume increases, myocardial fibres are stretched and the ventricles become dilated. As cardiac dilatation progresses beyond a certain point, the cardiac output starts declining. Cardiac hypertrophy is a long term adaptation to an increased diastolic volume and represents an absolute increase in myocardial muscle mass. A diminished cardiac output results in decreased tissue perfusion which in turn causes a reflex activation of the sympathetic autonomic nervous system. Both the decreased cardiac output of congestive heart failure and the vasoconstriction secondary to increased sympathetic tone produce a decrease in renal blood flow. This in turn sets off a complex chain of events leading to sodium and water retention and eventually increased blood volume. The decreased renal perfusion leads to the release of renin by the kidneys which in turn increases angiotensin formation. Angiotensin through its vasoconstrictor effect may further decrease the glomerular filtration rate and also stimulate the adrenals to secrete aldosterone which increases sodium reabsorption in the distal tubule.

Management :

Management of congestive heart failure consists of the correction of underlying disease states (e.g. hypertension), bed rest, sodium restricted diet, diuretics and cardiac glycosides. In the recent years vasodilators and in some instances inotropic agents have been used to manage congestive heart failure unresponsive to traditional therapy. The ultimate goal of therapy is to abolish disabling symptoms and improve the quality of patient's life. However, none of the aforementioned measures are curative and despite the best possible treatment, the five year survival of congestive heart failure patients is not prolonged.

Bed rest: Bed rest and consequent reduction in physical activity decrease the metabolic demands of the failing heart and minimize gravitational forces which contribute to the formation of oedema. Renal blood flow is also increased in the prone position, resulting in diuresis and eventual mobilization of oedema fluid.

Sodium-restricted diet: A diet low in sodium is usually given to decrease blood volume and to offset abnormal retention of sodium by the kidney. Unless the kidney's ability to excrete sodium is severely compromised, it is possible to achieve normal balance by restricting salt intake to match excretion.

Diuretics: Diuretic therapy is generally required in the treatment of advanced congestive heart failure, or when salt restriction alone is not enough to control volume overload. By enhancing renal excretion of sodium and water, diuretics diminish vascular volume, thus relieving ventricular and pulmonary congestion and decreasing peripheral edema.

Digitalis: Digitalis has two major pharmacologic actions on the heart. The first and most important in the treatment of congestive heart failure is that of increasing the force of contraction of both the normal and abnormal heart i.e., the positive inotropic effect. The second is the decrease in conduction velocity and prolongation of the refractory period of the A.V. node. This AV node blocking effect prolongs the PR interval and forms the rationale for its use in atrial arrhythmias. Since digitalis increases the force of contraction of the failing heart, cardiac output is increased and the compensatory mechanisms are reversed. End distolic volume is decreased, heart size is reduced and elevated venous pressure and pulmonary congestion are relieved. As tissue perfusion improves, sympathetic tone is lowered towards normal levels resulting in a diuresis and a drop in heart rate. Because it improves the primary defect which leads to the development of CHF, digitalis represents a rational choice in the pharmacotherapy of this disease. However, coupled with the inotropic effect of digitalis is a propensity to increase the automaticity and irritability and decrease the refractory period of the atrial and ventricular myocardium, which predisposes the patient to a multitude of ectopic beats and arrhythmias. Enough care and adequate preventive measures have to be taken in the management of CHF to avoid these undue toxic effects of digitalis.

Vasodilators: Drugs such as hydralazine, nitroprusside, nifedipine and prazosin are potent arterial dilating agents that can provide symptomatic relief in CHF by decreasing arterial impedence to left ventricular outflow (afterload). Nitroprusside, nitrates and prazosin also have venous dilating properties that decrease left ventricular congestion (preload). Their exact role in the management of CHF is yet to be established. At present they are primarily reserved for patients with far advanced CHF which is refractory to diuretics and digitalis.

Captopril is another promising drug which may have a role in the therapy of CHF. By inhibiting the formation of angiotensin-II, it has both afterload reducing properties (by blocking angiotensin mediated vasoconstriction) and volume reducing potential by inhibiting activation of aldosterone.

Newer inotropic agents: Currently cardiac glycosides derived from digitalis are the only orally available inotropic agents. A concern over their potential for toxicity points to the need for the identification of useful alternatives. Intravenously administered sympathomimetic amines such as dopamine and dobutamine are now frequently used in acute cardiac emergencies such as following myocardial infarction or cardiac arrest. Intravenous amrinone is a non-sympathomimetic inotropic agent undergoing clinical trials.

MYOCARDIAL INFARCTION

Acute myocardial infarction occurs primarily in patients with significant coronary artery stenosis secondary to atherosclerosis. The myocardial necrosis occurs due to acute obstruction of a coronary artery which results in occlusion of the blood flow to the dependent myocardial tissue. The exact pathogenesis of coronary artery occlusion is not well understood. The possible causes of obstruction include: coronary artery thrombosis, rupture of an atherosclerotic plague resulting in haemorrhage into the coronary artery, platelet aggregates adhering to the endothelium of atherosclerotic arteries and the spasm of coronary artery. Regardless of the etiology of occlusion there is critical imbalance between coronary blood supply and myocardial demand resulting in the ischemic changes in the myocardial tissue. These ischemic changes are reversible if blood supply returns to the tissue. However, if hypoxia persists irreversible cell necrosis occurs resulting in the myocardial infarction.

In its mildest forms the infarction may be unrecognized or silent and is diagnosed only by electrocardiographic evidence but at the other extreme there may be permanent severe disability or sudden death which may be due to ventricular fibrillation or asystole and usually occurs within the first hour of the onset of illness. If the patient survives this most critical stage, the liability to dangerous arrhythmias remains but diminishes as each hour passes by. The development of cardiac failure reflects the extent of myocardial damage and is the major cause of death in those who survive the first few hours of infarction.

Clinical features:

The cardinal symptom of myocardial infarction is pain but breathlessness, syncope, vomiting and extreme tiredness are common. The pain occurs at the same sites as for angina but it is usually more severe and lasts longer. In very serious cases pain is one of the most severe which can be explained and the patient's expression and pallor may vividly convey the seriousness of the situation.

Complications:

Arrhythmias are the most frequent complications of myocardial infarction. In most cases they are mild. Various degrees of heart block are also frequent. Ventricular fibrillation occurs in about 5-10% of hospitalized patients. It is also the major cause of death in many patients before their reaching the hospital. Acute circulatory failure is another important complication of myocardial infarction which reflects extensive myocardial damage and indicates a bad prognosis. In its presence all other complications are more likely to occur.

Management:

The essential components of the management of acute myocardial infraction include the following:

Pain relief: Opiate analgesia is most effective in reducing the pain of myocardial infraction. It is best achieved by morphine 10 mg plus cyclizine 50 mg, administered intravenously.

Ventricular fibrillation:

The earlier a patient with acute myocardial infraction is brought within the reach of a defibrillator, the better would be the prognosis.

Acute coronary thrombolysis:

Coronary thrombolysis is important for restoring the coronary patency, preserving the left ventricular function and thus improving the chances of survival. The most widely used thrombolytic agent is streptokinase 15,00,000 units given as slow i.v. infusion in 100 ml. of saline over the period of an hour. Other agents used for their thrombolytic effect include human tissue plasminogen activator (ateplase), anticoagulants like heparin or warfarin and aspirin.

Prognosis: In about 25% of all cases of myocardial infarction death occurs within few minutes without medical care. Half the deaths from myocardial infarction occur within 2 hours after the onset of symptoms and about 75% within 24 hours. About 40% of patient affected with myocardial infarction die within a month. Old age, stress and social isolation are associated with a higher mortality. Those who survive an acute attack may live upto 20 years depending on the proper treatment and care.

Prevention of coronary disease:

There is conclusive evidence that morbidity and mortality from coronary artery disease can be reduced by following the general measures outlined below:

1. Stop smoking.
2. Undertake regular exercise.
3. Maintain body weight within desirable range.
4. Dietary components be mixed including fruits, vegetables, dairy products and meat.
5. Not more than 30% of the caloric intake should be from fats.
6. Do not consume more than 30 g of alcohol in a day.

EPILEPSY

Epilepsy has plagued mankind for centuries. It has been recognized for at least 2400 years. It was known as a "sacred disease" or "falling sickness" in the ancient time and identified with supernatural forces.

The modern era of understanding epilepsy began with the writings and observations of Jackson and Gowers in the late 19th century. The introduction of bromides and phenobarbitone in the early 20'th century provided physicians with the means of treating this disorder.Our understanding of the neurophysiology of epilepsy was further enhanced by the introduction of electroencephalography by Berger in 1930s which resulted in the development of a large number of potent and specific drugs for various seizure types and the basis for rational therapy and patient monitoring.

Today, epilepsy is not considered a simple disease but is viewed as a symptom of disturbed electrical activity in the brain caused by a variety of disorders. It is not a single syndrome of similar symptoms but is a general name given to the wider range of symptoms that reflect the manifold functions of the brain in a pathologically disturbed manner. It is collection of many different types of seizures that vary widely in severity, appearance, cause, consequence and management.Epilepsy implies a periodic recurrence of seizures with or without convulsions.

A seizure results from an excessive discharge of neurons and is characterized by changes in electrical activity as measured by the electroencephalogram (EEG).In addition, there may be disturbances in consciousness, sensory systems, motor systems, subjective well being and objective behaviour. A seizure is episodic, is generally brief, has a beginning and an end, may produce post seizure impairment and is involuntary. A convulsion implies a violent involuntary contraction or series of contractions of the voluntary muscles.

Classification of seizures:

The terminology associated with epileptic seizures has been revised and developed by the International League Against Epilepsy. Using this scheme the seizures are classified as partial, generalized and unclassified. However, the older terminology is still commonly used and is simple to understand and hence it is being elaborated and described here.

Generalized tonic-clonic (grand mal) seizures are the most common type. The patient initially loses consciousness and falls. The onset of tonic muscle spasms is often accompanied by a cry which results from air being forced through the larynx. Following the tonic phase, there is a period of generalized, bilateral repetitive clonic movements. Incontinence of urine occurs during these seizures. Upon cessation of clonic movements, the patient will regain consciousness but remain confused and lethargic for some time. Grand mal seizures may be preceded by premonitory symptoms known as aura in some patients.

Absence (petit mal) seizures occur primarily in children and usually disappear at puberty, although the patient may develop a second type of seizure. Absence seizures are characterized by brief loss of consciousness which may be accompanied by mild clonic facial movements but the patient does not fall. The patient is unaware of his surroundings and will have no memory of events occurring during the seizures. Consciousness returns rapidly and there is no post attack confusion.

Atonic or akinetic seizures: Also known as "drop attacks", they are generally uncommon but frequently seen in the mentally retarded patients. Sometimes they are associated with myoclonic seizures and characterized by severe, rapid muscular contraction. There is sudden loss of consciousness and muscle tone and the patient suffers dramatic falls. Patients in sitting posture may violently slump forward. Attacks are of brief duration but there is frequent morbidity from uncontrolled falls.

Elementary partial (focal motor or sensory) seizures: They are localized to a single cerebral hemisphere, usually are of brief duration and there is no loss of consciousness. Variety of motor and sensory manifestations are common. A single limb may twitch or sometimes abnormal sensory experiences like unusual smell occur.

Complex partial (psychomotor or temporal lobe) seizures: They result from spread of abnormal focal discharges to the other cerebral hemisphere. Consciousness is impaired and the patient may show complex but inappropriate behaviour such as lip smacking, tearing of clothes and wandering aimlessly. There are often brief periods of post attack confusion.

Status epilepticus: It is a serious complication of grand mal seizures characterized by continuous seizure activity where one seizure is immediately followed by another without the patient regaining consciousness between attacks. It is always a medical emergency and requires immediate hospitalization and treatment. In those afflicted, irreversible cortical, cerebellar, frontal or temporal damage may occur due to anoxia. Status generally develops in epileptics who neglect therapy or after rapid cessation of therapy while changing from one medication to another.

Drug Therapy of Epilepsy:

Epilepsy is treated almost exclusively with pharmacotherapy. Educating patients regarding medications and at times utilization and interpretation of serum drug concentrations are essential to patient care.

The prime objective of anticonvulsant drug therapy is to reduce seizure frequency and severity, without producing undue adverse effects such as sedation and impaired activity. Complete seizure control may not always be possible. It may however be achieved in about 70-80% of patients by removing the underlying cause, increasing the seizure threshold or by preventing the synchronous spread of impulses using optimal anticonvulsant therapy. Control of seizures allows normalization of patients life styles and prevents physical harm associated with seizures. The following practical considerations are important in the management of epileptic patients.

1. Wherever possible the factors known to reduce the seizures such as fever, edema, hypoglycemia or specific drugs should be corrected by specific means.
2. The drug(s) must be selected on a rational basis depending on the seizure type. Generally, the drugs effective in the management of major motor seizures may also be effective in the treatment of focal seizures but they have little value in the management of petit mal, akinetic or myoclonic seizures. Similarly the drugs

effective in petit mal epilepsy are of some value in akinetic and myoclonic seizures but are not useful in major motor or focal seizures.

3. Initial treatment should be started with one drug only, gradually increasing the dose until seizures are controlled. It may however be discontinued if toxicity develops or a second drug may be added to the regimen.
4. The addition of second drug should be based on the blood levels of the first drug. Additional drugs must be added one at a time and increased gradually. Rational combinations comprise of the concomitant use of anticonvulsants with different mechanism of action.
5. Any changes in the therapeutic regimen should be accomplished slowly so that the possible beneficial effect can be properly evaluated. Increasing doses too fast may produce toxic effects while decreasing the doses too fast may lead to withdrawal seizures.
6. Anticonvulsant therapy is highly individualized and it must be closely monitored. The patient's age, sex and history contribute to the proper selection of his/her therapeutic regimen.
7. Strict compliance is the most important factor in the management of epilepsy. Medication must be taken on a regular daily basis and should never be stopped without professional advice.

The major anticonvulsant drugs used in the treatment of different types of seizures have been summarized in the table 9.5 in accordance with the preference for each category.

Table 9.5 Major anticonvulsants useful in various epileptic seizures

	Grand mal	Petit mal	Psychomotor	Status
First choice	Phenytoin	Ethosuximide	Primidone	Diazepam
	Phenobarbitone	Valproate		
Second choice	Carbamazepine	Clonazepam	Phenobarbital	Phenytoin
	Primidone	Methosuximide	Phenytoin	Phenobarbitone
	Valproate	Clonazepam	Carbamazepine	Phenobarbitone

MANAGEMENT OF PAIN

Human beings have always known and sought relief from pain. In fact, the act of relieving pain is as old as the medical profession itself. In the modern era pain's impact on society is still great and pain complaints are the number one reason for which patients seek medical advice.

Pain is an unpleasant sensation disturbing a patient's comfort, thought, sleep or normal daily routine and is often symptomatic of an underying disease process. Unfortunately pain is often undertreated and pain management is greatly misunderstood.

Pain is a subjective experience and therefore it is the patient who is the only one who can describe the intensity of pain. "Pain is whatever the experiencing person says it is, existing wherever he/she says it does". Thus a patient's description of pain must be believed if clinicians wish to alleviate their patient's discomfort. A baseline description of pain can be obtained by assessing PQRST characteristics as described in the Table 9.6.

Table 9.6 PQRST Characteristics of Pain

P	Palliative, provoking or precipitating factors	These factors either make the pain better or worse. They include exertion, diet, emotions, stress, infections, antacids and posture.
Q	Quality of Pain	They describe the pain e.g. sharpness, dullness, knifelike, crushing, waxing, waning or pulsating.
R	Region or radiation of pain	Describe the site of pain, e.g., substernal region radiating to the left arm which may be secondary to angina pectoris, myocardial infarction, pleuritis, esophagitis, cholecystitis, bone fracture or muscle strain.
S	Subjective description of severity of pain	e.g., awakened at night by the pain, takes the patient's breath away. How does it compare with other pain you have experienced?
T	Temporal factors	Does the intensity of pain change with time? Day or night, relationship to meals or other activities, acute or chronic.

Acute and Chronic Pain

Acute pain is a useful physiologic process warning individuals of disease states and potentially harmful situations. Unfortunately, severe, unremitting undertreated acute pain, when it outlives its biological usefulness produces many deleterious effects such as extension of myocardial ischemia after myocardial infarction.. Under normal conditions acute pain quickly subsides as the healing process decreases the pain producing stimuli; however in some instances pain may persist for months to years leading to a chronic pain state with features quite different from those of acute pain as outlined in the Table 9.7 given below:

Table 9.7 Important Characteristics of Acute and Chronic Pain

Characteristic features	Acute pain	Chronic pain
Pain relief	Highly desirable	Highly desirable
Tolerance to and dependence on analgesics	Uncommon	Common
Psychological component	Generally not present	Often a major problem
Organic etiology	Commoon	Often not present
Environmental contributions and family influence	Small	Significant
Insomnia	Unusual	Common Complaint
Treatment goal	Cure	Rehabilitation

Chronifc pain can be divided into four subtypes:

(*a*) Pain that persists beyond the normal healing time for an acute injury.

(*b*) Pain related to chronic disease

(*c*) Pain without identifiable organic cause

(*d*) Pain that involves both chronic and acute pain associated with cancer.

Patients with chronic pain generally develop severe psychological problems caused by fear and memory of past pain. In addition chronic pain patients are more likely to develop dependence and tolerance to analgesics, suffer from disturbed sleep and they more readily react to environmental changes that can intensify the pain response. It is very important to distinguish between chronic and acute pain because of entirely different management techniques adopted to treat them.

Acute pain management

The most obvious way to relieve pain is to eliminate the underlying cause. A new, severe or frequent pain should be properly investigated by the attending physician as such patients may have serious illness which may be responsible for such pain. The table 9.8 summarizes such

Table 9.8. Important Causes of Servers Pain

Site of pain	Possible serious illness
Severe eye pain	Glaucoma or other sight defects
Severe stomach or/loin	Appendicitis or ruptured peptic ulcer
Severe pain at the back of the neck	Can induce stroke
Severe neck pain	Possibly meningitis
Severe chest pain	Angina or possibly a heart attack
Severe limb pain after injury	Indicate a break or joint tear
Raging toothache	Possibly an abscess

However, most of the patients coming to a pharmacy for painkillers will not have a serious illness and will know what their problem is. People are now being encouraged to treat their minor health problems themselves and a qualified pharmacist can help them by providing proper health education and counselling. The table 9.9 outlines the top 10 causes of pain which include both acute and chronic types of pain.

Table 9.9. Top 10 Causes of Commonly Encountered Pain

1. Headache
2. Migraine
3. Back pain
4. Period (menstrual) pain
5. Sporting injuries and muscular aches and pains
6. Rheumatic pain
7. Dental pain
8. Neuralgia
9. Cold and influenza
10. Fever.

Some people feel pain more than others do. Some never complain about their headache or aching back whereas others may wince at the slightest injury. This is because we all have different responses to pain. It is also true that some element of pain is in the mind. It is strongly linked with emotion. A physician once noted that wounded soldiers in battles sometimes felt less pain than injured civilians. The soldiers' wounds meant the end of war for them. The civilians' injuries were disastrous for them. If someone is feeling lonely or depressed, their pain can actually feel worse to them. Such patients need a sympathetic ear and adequate counselling by the physician and the pharmacist. Therapeutic interventions to treat acute pain include pharmacologic treatment, stimulation therapies and psychologic therapies.

Pharmacologic Treatment

Although pharmacologic agents to effectively treat acute pains are available they are not always appropriately used. Misunderstanding of acute pain symptoms, inadequate dose titration, fear of their adverse effects, varying dosage requirement, inadequate application of currently available therapies and nonappreciation of the complications of untreated pain contribute to ineffective and inappropriate pain management. Adherence to the basic principles of the pharmacologic treatment which have been summarized in the table 9.10 will promote rational pain control decisions.

Table 9.10. Basic Principle of the Pharmacologic Treatment of Pain

1. Identify the exact source of pain
2. Use the least potent analgesic with fewest side effects.
3. Properly titrate the dose and administer for an adequate duration.
4. Do not use analgesics on as-needed basis.
5. Recognize side effects of analgesics
6. Avoid excessive sedation of patients.
7. Adjust the route of administration to the needs of the patient.
8. Use equianalgesic doses.
9. Do not use placebo therapy to diagnose psychogenic pain.

Non-narcotic agents

Analgesia should be initiated with the weakest effective analgesic having the fewest side effects. Peripherally acting agents e.g. paracetamol, aspirin, and nonsteroidal anti-inflammatory drugs (NSAIDs) like ibuprofen etc. are generally preferred over centrally acting narcotic agents in the treatment of acute, mild to moderate pain. Patient response to mild analgesics varies with the best results evident in low grade somatic type pain e.g. headache, myalgia, neuralgia and dysmenorrhoea. Results are often poor in intense or sharp visceral pain present after surgery or with headaches of vascular origin. The choice of particular agent depends upon availability, onset and duration of action, dose range, adverse effects and cost. The commonly used non-narcotic analgesics have been summarized in the Table 9.11.

Aspirin or aspirin like compounds are the most widely used peripherally acting analgesics in the world. This is because they impart antipyretic, anti-inflammatory action as well as analgesic effects. However, problems like direct gastric irritation leading to nausea, dyspepsia, gastric burning and in higher doses association with gastric ulcers, gastrointestinal bleeding, tinnitus, hypersensitivity reactions in patients with asthma and hypoprothrombinemia have limited their extensive use now. NSAIDs have effective analgesic and anti-inflammatory properties, but generally cause fewer gastrointestinal problems than aspirin. However, particular attention must be given to the effects that NSAIDs may produce on renal function. These drugs can also cause rash, tinnitus, nausea, vomiting, a burning sensation in the oesophagus and stomach, diarrhoea, constipation and vertigo. There appears to be a great deal of variability from one patient to another in the therapeutic response seen with NSAIDs. Paracetamol is relatively free from side effects, although in overdosage it can be toxic to the liver. It can be used in cases of aspirin allergy and in patients suffering from peptic ulcer disease.

Table 9.11. Pharmacokinetics and Dosage of Commonly Used Non-narcotic Analgesics

Agent	Time to reach peak concentration (h)	Elimination Half Life (h)	Onset of Analgesic action (h)	Duration of action (h)	Usual Dosage Range (mg.)
Aspirin	0.25-2.0	0.25-0.33	0.5	3-6	325-650, 4 hourly
Paracetamol	0.5-2.0	1-4	0.5-1	3-6	325-1000, 4-6 hourly
Ibuprofen	1-2	1-2.5	0.5	4-6	200-400, 6 hourly
Naproxen	2-4	12-15	1	upto 7	250-500, 6-12 hourly
Diflunisal	2-3	8-12	1	2-3	250-750, 8-12 hourly

Narcotic agents:

Most clinicians consider the use of narcotic analgesics to be the next logical step in the management of acute pain. The pharmacological activity of narcotics depends on their affinity for opiate receptors. In usual doses, narcotic analgesics do not eliminate pain, instead, they decrease its unpleasantness. Patients report that although their pain is still present, it no longer bothers them. Narcotic analgesics share related pharamcological properties and exert their most profound effects on the CNS and gastrointestinal tract. Mood changes, sedation, respiratory depression, nausea, vomiting, decreased gastrointestinal motility, dependence and tolerance are evident in varying degrees with all agents. Consideration of efficacy and side effects profile assists in the selection of most appropriate agent. The route of administration depends on the individual patient's need. These agents have been classified and summarized in the Table 9.12.

Table 9.12. Pharmacokinetics and Dosage of Commonly Used Narcotic Analgesics

Agent	Time to reach peak conc. (h)	Half Life (h)	Onset of analgesic action (min)	Duration of analgesic action (h)	Usual equianalgesic Dose (mg)
Morphine	0.5-1	2-4	15-60	3-6	10.I.M.
Hydromorphone	0.5-1	2-4	15-30	4-6	1.5 I.M.
Levorphanol	0.5-1	12-26	30-90	4-8	2 S.C.
Meperidine	0.5-1	3-4	10-15	2-4	100 I.M.
Methadone	0.5-1	15-30	30-60	4-6	10 I.M.
Pentazocine	0.25-1	2-3	15-20	3-4	30-60 I.M.
Buprenorphine	1	2-3	15	4-8	0.3-0.6 I.M.
Fentanyl	0.5-1	1.5-6.0	7-8	1-2	0.15 I.M.

The major drawbacks and limiting factors for the use of narcotic analgesics are their undesirable effects which are mostly due to their effects on the central nervous system. They have been summarized in the follwing Table 9.13.

Table 9.13. Narcotic Analgesics: Major Adverse Effects and Their Manifestations

Adverse Effects	Manifestations
Mood changes	Dysphoria, euphoria
Somnolence	Lethargy, drowsiness, apathy, inability to concentrate.
Stimulation of CTZ	Nausea, vomiting
Respiratory depression	Decreased respiratory rate
Interference with hypothalamic function	Increase in ADH, decrease in gnRF, CRF, TSH, HG, LRF and FSH; disturbed temperature regulation,
Decreased gastrointestinal motility	Constipation
Increase in sphincter tone	Biliary spasm, urinary retention
Histamine relase	Urticaria, pruritis, exacerbation of asthma
Tolerance	Larger doses for same effect
Dependence	Withdrawal symptoms upon abrupt discontinuation

Combination Therapy

The combination of narcotic and non-narcotic oral analgesics often results in analgesia superior to that produced by either agent alone. Attacking pain on two fronts peripherally and centrally enhances pain relief. The use of a combination containing a full dose of opioid with a simple analgesic is logical in providing a step up the analgesic ladder for those patients whose pain has not responded to simple analgesic alone. Their use should be restricted to patients in severe pain and only when an opioid is considered particularly appropriate and necessary.

When combined therapy is required the use of two analgesics separately allows individual dosage titration of each component. Fixed ratio combinations do not facilitate this. The clinician should not be limited by the availability of commercially established fixed dose combinations. For example, the administration of round the clock paracetamol, aspirin or other NSAIDs in combination with scheduled narcotic regimens is often very effective in treatment of pain resulting from bone metastases in advanced cancer. The cost of some of the branded fixed ratio combination analgesics is very high. Cost savings can be made by administering the two analgesics separately.

It is expected that the severity of adverse effects is lessened by the use of a combination but the range of possible effects is widened by such use. Two analgesics with different mechanism of action expose the patient to other adverse effects caused by these mechanisms. This is the case with opioid combinations. The use of an opioid analgesic with paracetamol or aspirin gives rise to a range of adverse effects not seen with aspirin or paracetamol alone.

There have been particular problems with patients who have been subjected to overdosage with paracetamol-dextropropoxyphene combination. Treatment is complicated by respiratory depression and acute heart failure from the dextropropoxyphene and hepatotoxicity from paracetamol.

With so many analgesic preparations available over the counter there is distinct danger that patients may self medicate with these drugs as well as taking their prescription medication, unless specifically warned otherwise. The danger of inadvertent paracetamol and/or opioid overdosage is real as described above.

A Combination with ibuprofen:

A recent study on the beneficial effect of a new combination of ibuprofen 300 mg modified-release with codeine phosphate 20 mg normal release has been carried out in patients with osteoarthritis and compared with its individual constituents. The study led to the conclusion that the effect of this combination was surprisingly greater than the sum of the analgesic effects of ibuprofen and codeine phosphate alone. An interesting observation was that codeine alone performed worse than placebo in reducing day pain scores and reducing the number of nights disturbed by pain. The combination proved definitely better than codeine alone.

Regional Analgesia

Regional analgesia with properly administered local anaesthetics can provide complete relief of pain and block acute pain reflex responses often deleterious in acute pain. Regional analgesics relieve pain by blocking nociceptive transmission, interrupting sympathetic reflexes and preventing increased skeletal muscle activity. Although safe they readily cross the blood brain barrier, causing signs of excitation and depression, including dizziness, tinnitus, drowsiness, disorientation, muscle twitching, seizures and respiratory arrest. Cardiovascular effects include increased PR interval, increased QRS duration, decreased cardiac output, decreased blood pressure and asystole with toxic lidocaine levels. The methods employed for producing regional analgesia need skillful technical manipulation, frequent administration and highly specialized follow up procedures. The commonly used local anaesthetics used for producing regional analgesia have been summarized in the Table 9.14.

Table 9.14 Commonly Used Local Anaesthetics for Producing Regional Analgesia

Agent	Onset (min)	Duration (h)	Equivalent cocentration(%)
Esters			
Procaine	2-5	0.25-0.50	2
Tetracaine	15	2-3	0.25
Amides			
Mepivacaine	3-5	0.75-1.5	1
Bupivacaine	5	2-4	0.25
Lidocaine	0.5-1	0.5-1	1
Dibucaine	15	3-4	0.25

Stimulation Therapy

Transcutaneous electrical nerve stimulation (TENS) and electro-acupuncture have shown moderate success in managing postoperative pain. These procedures are devoid of narcotic like side effects but lack of well controlled studies have prevented the wide acceptance of these techniques in clinical use.

Psychologic Intervention

Although the cognitive, behavioral and social aspects of pain are well established, psychologic techniques for treatment of acute pain have not been widely employed. Successful psychologic techniques include relaxation training, controlled mental imagery, controlled attention or distraction, re-inforcement of appropriate actions, hypnosis and biofeedback.

Chronic Pain Management

Managing the pain of malignant diseases encompasses both acute and chronic management techniques. Thus, pharmacologic treatment and psychologic therapies already mentioned are best combined with neurosurgical methods, anesthetic procedures and supportive care measures in a multidisciplinary approach to pain relief. The goal of chronic pain management is to provide patients with enough pain amelioration to tolerate diagnostic and therapeutic manipulation and permit them to function at a level that will allow freedom of movement and action. Unfortunately one-fourth of patients with cancer die without significant relief of pain. Pharmacologic management is the mainstay of therapy and the objective is to prevent the patient from experiencing constant fluctuation between severe pain and pain relief. This is most effectively accomplished by around the clock administration schedules which inhibit serum analgesic concentrations from below the point at which patient experiences the suffering of pain. As needed (p.r.n.) schedules are employed in conjunction with around the clock regimens and are used only when patients experience breakthrough pain. The non-narcotic agents are used as first line drugs, with NSAIDs being specially effective in treating bone pain. The choice of narcotic agent in such cases remains controversial but it should be based on patient acceptance, analgesic effectiveness, and pharmacodynamic, pharmacokinetic and adverse effects profiles.

Anesthetic and neurosurgical approaches have proved successful in all vitiating pain but require special expertise and are usually reserved for patients who are refractory to conventional analgesics.

Psychologic and Supportive Care:

Psychologic techniques e.g. relaxation training and controlled mental imagery are very helpful in treating the pain experienced in malignant diseases, and prove specially effective in conjunction with pharmacologic therapy. Supportive care in and outside the hospital is one of the cancer patients' greatest allies not only in coping with pain but also in accepting the disease.

RHEUMATOID ABTHRITIS

Rheumatoid arthritis is the commonest form of chronic inflammatory joint disease, of unknown etiology for which there is no known cure. It is an auto-immune disease and although it is systemic, it manifests itself primarily in the joints and related structures. The goals of therapy are to reduce pain and inflammation of the involved joints and preserve joint function. Some forms of drug therapy may also delay the progression of the disease. Patients who carefully follow a well thought out program of rest, exercise, heat treatment and drug therapy will find their disease significantly less disabling than do untreated patients.

Rheumatoid arthritis occurs throughout the world and in all ethnic groups. Although the incidence and course of the disease are not influenced significantly by climate or altitude, patients tend to feel better in warm and dry climates. The disease starts most commonly between the third and fifth decades but the age of onset follows a normal distribution curve and no age group is exempted. Women are affected 3 times more frequently than men. There is probably a genetic predisposition towards rheumatoid arthritis. It is generally exacerbated by emotional trauma. Exacerbations and remissions occur throughout the course of this disease which tends to be progressive.

The goals of therapy are to reduce pain and inflammation of the involved joints and preserve joint function and prevention of deformity. In addition some forms of drug therapy may delay the progression of the disease.

Clinical Features

The small joints of the hands and feet are most frequently affected and generally there is symmetry of joint involvements. Knees, shoulders, hips, elbows and ankles are frequently affected. Joints usually become warm, swollen and tender. Their involvement is frequently preceded by complaints of fatigability, loss of appetite and weight and occasional fever. Muscular pain and prolonged morning stiffness are common and the affected joints tend to become progressively worse. Limitation of movements and physical disability occur as joint pain, swelling and tenderness become worse. Weakness of muscle develops and atrophy ensures. Weakness of grip strength is prominent feature and walking becomes difficult if lower extremities are involved. Symptoms are much worse upon arising in the morning and may be limited to this period. Morning stiffness is a reliable index of disease activity.

Management:

As the aetiology of rheumatoid arthritis is unknown, treatment is empirically directed towards-

1. relief of symptoms i.e. reduction of pain and inflammation and prevention of any deformity of joints.
2. suppression of active and progressive disease.
3. conservation and restoration of function in the affected joints.

Patient education, counselling and continuing medical support are usually required for successful management while physical rehabilitation, reconstructive surgery and environmental adaptation also assume great importance when advancing joint damage and deformities are associated with functional impairment.

Physical rest, therapy with anti-inflammatory drugs and exercises form the most effective treatment for the exacerbations of rheumatoid disease. Heat treatments also provide considerable relief. The inflammatory process requires higher than normal temperatures within the joint space, thus the external application of heat, which increases blood flow to the joint and thereby cools it, reduces inflammation and pain. Rest is important to minimize excessive strain on the already inflamed joints. Admission to hospital becomes necessary for a minority of patients when widespread polyarthritis associated with signs of constitutional disturbance and there has been no response to rest at home and optimal doses of non-steroidal anti-inflammatory drugs (NSAIDs). The rest from physical and emotional stress produced by few weeks of stay in hospital, usually induces a marked remission of symptoms without recourse to strict bed rest.

Drug therapy:

The drug therapy of rheumatoid arthritis has received an extraordinary amount of attention worldwide. The chronic discomforting and disabling nature of the disease and the severe pain associated with it, has created a tremendous demand for its effective treatment leading to a highly competitive market for anti-arthritic drugs and medications.

Nonsteroidal anti-inflammatory drugs are the mainstay of therapy for active inflammatory arthritis in optimal anti-inflammatory doses. They may be very effective in relieving the pain and stiffness but they do not alter the course of the disease and the margin between effective and toxic doses is often small. Inhibition of prostaglandin synthetase is the major pharmacological action of all the NSAIDs but the consequent reduction in the cytoprotective effect of endogenous prostanoids on gastric mucosa makes them all liable to cause gastrointestinal side effects such as dyspepsia, ulceration and haemorrhage. Upper gastrointestinal haemorrhage and duodenal ulceration are the most frequent and serious adverse effects of NSAIDs. Other side effects include fluid retention, rashes, interstitial nephritis, occasional hepatotoxicity and rarely asthma and anaphylaxis. Treatment with these drugs should be avoided in patients with peptic ulceration. The overall risk of an individual developing a life threatening gastrointestinal side effect following treatment with an NSAID is approximately 1 in 10,000. The currently used NSAIDs have been summarized in Table 9.15.

Patients who fail to get adequate relief of their inflammation or who show evidence of disease progression while taking NSAIDs are the candidates for more aggressive treatment. The slow acting antirheumatic drugs such as gold salts, hydroxychloroquine and penicillamine are usually added to an NSAID. These drugs characteristically have 2 to 6 months delay between the initiation of treatment and the onset of action. They are also more toxic and require frequent monitoring to avoid serious complications.

Corticosterids are reserved for short term management of patients with severe limitation of their daily activities while waiting for a therapeutic response to a slow acting antirheumatic drug or for patients who fail to respond to all other forms of treatments.

Table 9.15. Commonly Used Non-sterial Anti-inflammatory Drugs (NSAIDs)

Drugs	Usual Doses
Carboxylic acids	
Salicylic acids	
Aspirin	600-900 mg four hourly
Diflusinal	500 mg twice daily
Anthranilic acids	
Mefenamic acid	500 mg four times daily
Propionic acids	
Naproxen	500 mg twice daily
Ibuprofen	400-800 mg four times daily
Ketoprofen	100 mg thrice daily
Flurbiprofen	100 mg thrice daily
Acetic acids	
Diclophenac	50 mg thrice daily
Naphthyl alkanones	
Nabumetone	1000 mg daily
Heterocyclic acetic acids	
Tolmetin	400 mg four times daily
Indole acetic acids	
Indomethacin	25-50 mg thrice daily
Sulindac	200 mg twice daily
Enolic acids	
Phenylbutazone	100 mg thrice daily
Oxyphenbutazone	100 mg thrice daily
Oxicams	
Piroxicam	20 mg daily

Conclusion:

Rheumatoid arthritis is a chronic, progressive and disabling disease for which there is no cure. However, well formulated therapy combined with rest and exercise can prevent or reduce the crippling which might otherwise occur. Pharmacists should be well acquainted with the pathophysiology and clinical features of rheumatoid arthritis which afflicts upto 3% of the population in any country, and have a thorough knowledge about the actions, uses and adverse effects of antirheumatic drugs so that they can be actively involved in the counselling of patients and rationale use of drugs.

GOUT

The disease gout is due to a disorder of uric acid metabolism. It is manifested by hyperuricema, acute or chronic recurrent arthritis and deposits of monosodium urate crystals. Gout is the clinical diagnosis and hyperuricemia a biochemical feature. These two terms are neither synonymous nor they are interchangeable.

Gout describes a number of disorders in which monosodium urate crystals from hyperuricemic body fluids give rise to inflammatory arthritis at different sites. Hyperuricemia is necessary but not a sufficient prerequisite for clinical manifestations of gout.

Incidence

Gout is primarily a disease of middle aged men. It seldom occurs during childhood or prior to the onset of puberty and women rarely manifest this disease before menopause. Asymptomatic hyperuricemia is 10 times more common. Serum uric acid levels are higher in urban than in rural communities and are positively correlated with intelligence, social class, weight, hemoglobin, serum proteins and a high protein diet, diabetes and atherosclerosis. These correlations have however been found inconsistent and at times contradictory. Various genetic and environmental factors lead to hyperuricemia and gout by decreasing the excretion of uric acid and/or increasing its production.

Clinical features

Clinically, gout is characterized by urate trophaceous deposits and periodic attacks of acute joint pain. The joint of great toe is the site of first attack of acute gouty arthritis in about 70% of patients, the ankle, the knee, the small joints of hands, the wrist and the elbow follow in decreasing order of frequency. The onset may be insidious or explosively sudden often waking the patient from sleep. The affected joint is hot, red and swollen with shiny overlying skin and dilated veins: it is excruciatingly painful and tender. Very acute attacks are often accompanied by fever, leucocytosis and a raised ESR and are occasionally preceded with an aura of subjective changes such as anorexia, nausea, malaise or change in mood and joint discomfort.

Management

NSAIDs are the drugs of choice. The treatment should start as early as possible in adequate doses. Salicylates and diuretics should be avoided during the acute attack. Indomenthacin (50 mg. 6 hourly) or naproxen (250 mg. 8 hourly) are given until acute attack subsides.

Prevention

Prologned treatment with drugs which lower the serum urate level should be considered following the resolution of the acute attack in patients with : a) recurrent attack of gout, (b) evidence of chronic gouty arthritis or tophi (c) accompanying renal disease and (d) gout and marked hyperuricemia.

Allopurinol: It is the drug of choice for long term prophylaxis as compliance with it is easier and the incidence of side effects is low. It lowers the serum urate by inhibiting xanthine oxidase which is responsible for the conversion of xanthine and hypoxanthine to uric acid. Treatment is commenced with 300 mg. once daily and the dose is gradually adjusted between 300-900 mg. daily to bring the sodium urate level within the normal range.

Uricosuric drugs: They are very effective in lowering the serum urate level, reducing the frequency of acute attacks of gout and decreasing the size of the tophi. Probenecid (0.5-1 g twice daily) or sulphinpyrazone (100 mg thrice daily) are usually used. Salicylates must be avoided as they antagonize the uricosuric effects of these drugs.

Diet: Excessive intake of purines and over indulgence in alcohol should be avoided. Gradual weight loss is encouraged in obese patients which is associated with fall in serum urate level.

PEPTIC ULCER

Etiology and Incidence:

A peptic ulcer can be defined as an acute or chronic ulceration of the digestive tract occurring in areas which is accessible to gastric secretions. Although all ulcerating lesions of the gastroduodenal area have traditionally been labelled as peptic ulcers, these lesions differ in anatomical location, etiology, clinical presentation and genetic relationships. They all share a common abnormality i.e. too much acid and pepsin activity for the degree of local tissue resistance. Hydrolytic and proteolytic digestion of the exposed mucosa occur followed by inflammation, necrosis and ulceration. Therapy of these disorders is directed at correction of the apparent imbalance between acid and pepsin activity and mucosal resistance. Success of the therapy is measured in terms of symptom control, ulcer healing and prevention of complications and recurrence.

Peptic ulcer disease is characteristic to man and occurs in 10-15% of the population. Duodenal ulcers are upto 10 times more prevalent in males; and males have two to three and a half times more gastric ulcers than females. Ulcers occur most commonly between the ages of 20 to 50 years. Genetic factors also appear to affect the risk of peptic ulcer. Furthermore individuals with blood group O are 40 percent more liable to duodenal ulcers than those with other blood-groups. Other risk factors involved in the etiology of peptic ulcer disease are stress, smoking, alcohol, caffeinated beverages, painkillers like aspirin and NSAIDs, corticosteroids and reserpine.

Pathophysiology:

Duodenal Ulcer: The traditional acid-peptic theory remains valid for the duodenal ulcer. Patients with these ulcers have higher average output of hydrochloric acid than do ulcer free persons. Several. theories have been proposed to explain the complex interrelationship between acid secretion and duodenal ulcer. Patients of duodenal ulcers may have an abnormally high vagal tone; excessive humoral stimulation to gastric acid; impaired inhibition of gastric secretion or a greater capacity to secrete acid. All these theories evolve entirely around acid secretion. It is nevertheless important to realize that peptic activity may have an equally important role in duodenal ulcer pathogenesis.

Gastric Ulcers: Although some patients of gastric ulcers are hypersecretors of gastric acid, most secrete either normal or less than normal amounts. It is therefore reasonable to focus more attention on gastric mucosal resistance than on acid and pepsin in this type of ulcer. Gastric ulcer may result from poor gastric emptying which leads to the stasis of gastric contents. This is followed by gastritis which lowers mucosal resistance to minimal amounts of acid and pepsin. The gastric mucosa has the capacity to prevent the penetration of normal concentrations of acid, however, when acid concentrations are increased, the mucosal barrier is broken and hydrogen ions penetrate the stomach wall resulting in gastric mucosal damage. Pyloric sphincter dysfunction may also contribute to the pathogenesis of gastric ulcers by allowing reflux of duodenal contents into the stomach. The resultant bile, bile salts, and urea reaching the stomach will cause a break in the gastric mucosa even at low concentrations of acid, permitting the back diffusion of hydrogen ions. The acid damage to mucosa and acid-pepsin lead to ulceration.

Helicobacter pylori: More recently the involvement of the organism Helicobacter pylori in the etiology of peptic ulcer disease has been the subject of much research interest. A strong consistent association between H. pylori infection and peptic ulcer disease is now well established. It has now led to significant changes in the treatment of peptic ulcers which are resistant to conventional therapy. It is now possible to stop the natural history of the disease by administering a suitable antimicrobial agent and eliminating H. pylori infection present alongside the ulcer.

Clinical Presentation:

The patients of peptic ulcer disease usually complain of recurrent episodes of abdominal pain over a period of several years. The pain may be nonspecific but it is usually described as gnawing or burning in the epigastric region, reaching maximum intensity just prior to meals. The pain is readily relieved by food, antacids or vomiting. The pain may at times awaken the patient from sleep but it is unusual to experience such pain on awakening in the morning. Approximately 10% patients of peptic ulcer suffer from its complications like hematemesis, gastrointestinal bleeding, perforation or obstruction. Peptic ulcer are chronic in nature and they are characterized by remission and exacerbation of symptoms over 20-30 years.

Management:

The aims of the treatment are to relieve symptoms, prevent complications and induce ulcer healing in the short term and to prevent relapse in the long term. While the majority of ulcers heal in 4-6 weeks of treatment, the prevention of relapse can be achieved only with maintenance treatment for years.

General measures: Patient must be strongly discouraged from cigarette smoking as it is wellknown to exacerbate the course of peptic ulcer disease. Drugs like aspirin, NSAIDs and corticosteroids should be avoided as they produce injurious effect on the gastric mucosa.

Treatment: The discovery of H_2-receptor antagonists have revolutionized the treatment of peptic ulcer. Their therapeutic effect is due to the inhibition of gastric acid and pepsin secretion by the stomach. The other drugs now available for the treatment of peptic ulcers are known to produce their beneficial effect by different mechanisms. While all the currently available drugs satisfactorily relieve symptoms and induce ulcer healing, none of them alter the nature history of the disease. The recommended doses of the drugs for the treatment of peptic ulcer and their side effects have been summarized in the Table 9.16 given below.

Table 9.16 Drugs used in the treatment of peptic ulcer disease

Drugs	Dosage schedule for Short term management	Maintenance therapy	Side effects
Cimetidine	800 mg at night or 400 mg b.d.	400 mg at night	Microsomal enzyme inhibition, delay in elimination of drugs like warfarin &phenytoin, confusion, gynecomastia
Ranitidine	300 mg at night or 150 mg b.d.	150 mg at night	Confusion
Nizatidine	300 mg at night or 150 mg b.d.	150 mg at night	Sweating, urticaria somnolece
Famotidne	40 mg at night or 20 mg b.d.	20 mg at night	Headache, dizziess, dry mouth
Roxatidine	300 mg at night or 150 mg b.d.	150 mg at night	
Pirenzepine	50 mg b.d.	Not recommended	Dry mouth, blurred vision
Bismuth chelate (De Nol)	240 mg b.d.	Not recommended	Blackens tongue, teeth, feces
Sucralfate	2 g b.d.	Not recommended	Reduces absorption of war farin, phenytoin, digoxin tetracycline
Misoprostol	200 µg q.i.d.	Not recommended	Diarrhoea, abortifacient
Omeprazole	20 mg once daily	Not recommennded	Delays elimination of diazeparn, phenytoin, warfarin, induces hypergastrinemia
Carbenoxolone	100 mg two or three times daily	Not required	Mineralocorticoid effects hypertension, edema

Antacids are prescribed principally for symptomatic relief. The dose varies with the preparation used. Not suitable for prolonged use due to the incidence of adverse effects.

10
FIRST AID

Emergency treatment in shock, snake bites, burns, poisoning, heart diseases, fractures and resuscitation methods. Elements of minor surgery and dressings.

EMERGENCY TREATMENT IN SHOCK

Shock, acute circulatory failure or low output state are terms used to describe a clinical syndrome of hypotension, peripheral vasoconstriction, oliguria and often impairment of consciousness. The basic cause is an inadequate cardiac output with compensatory vasoconstriction and renal and cerebral hypoperfusion.

Onset of shock may be sudden or gradual. The skin is cold, pale, sweaty and in advanced cases there may be peripheral cyanosis or gangrene. The systolic blood pressure is usually low, often less than 100 mm. Hg. Consciousness may be preserved but frequently there is confusion and irritability.

If the treatment is not prompt and effective, systemic consequences may ensue. Oliguria may progress to tubular necrosis. A rising plasma potassium concentration and progressive acidosis both from renal failure and ischemic necrosis of skeletal muscles may cause cardiac arrhythmias, which may eventually be intractable. Even after the recovery, permanent cerebral damage or loss of peripheral tissues may be inevitable.

Successful treatment of shock is absolutely dependent on identification of the cause and this requires a meticulous assessment of the history and physical signs and efficient use of investigation. While this is being done, the patient must be protected from fuss, unnecessary disturbance and hypothermia. The anxiety and pain should be controlled using small intravenous dose of morphine if necessary. Oxygen should be administered by face mask. A catheter should be inserted to monitor urine output and great care should be taken to protect the ischemic skin from damage.

Shock can be divided into six main categories which have been summarized in Table 10.1. At any given time, one type of shock may take on the characteristics and sequelae of another.

Table 10.1. Classification of different types of shock and their etiological factors

1. Hypovolemic shock:
   (a) Loss of blood due to hemorrhage etc.
   (b) Loss of plasma due to burns.
   (c) Loss of fluid due to diarrhoea, vomiting, diabetes mellitus, diabetes insipidus, overuse of diuretics.
2. Caridogenic shock
   (a) Myocardial infarction.
   (b) Heart failure with low cardiac output.
   (c) Arrhythmias.
3. Septic shock:
   (a) Gram negative septicemia.
   (b) Gram positive septicemia.
4. Obstruction to blood flow:
   (a) Pericardial tamponade.
   (b) Pulmonary embolism.
   (c) Dissecting aneurysm of the aorta.
5. Neuogenic shock:
   (a) Drug-induced:
   Directly toxic drugs: Daunorubicin, Adriamycin. Due to overdosage: Beta blockers, calcium channel antagonists, Disopyramide, Salicylates. Tricyclic antidepressants.
   Spinal Anesthesia.
   (b) Spinal Cord injury.
6. Others:
   (a) Anaphylactic shock
   (b) Hypoglycemia, Myxedema, Addison's Disease.

Management

The immediate objective of the emergency treatment in shock is to restore and maintain cardiac output at a satisfactory level until the cause of circulatory failure can be identified and specifically treated or allowed to resolve.

(a) **Fluid replacement :** It is the primary therapeutic consideration in the patients of hypovolemic shock because early complete correction of hypovolemia prevents the later complications of shock. This can be achieved by the intravenous administration of crystalloids, or colloids and is followed by whole blood transfusion to restore the hematocrit to at least 30%.

(b) **Drugs :** In case of cardiogenic shock vasodilation and inotropic agents are used for the control of shocked state depending on the other vital parameters. The purpose óf vasodilation therapy is to decrease pulmonary venous congestion and to improve cardiac output. Glyceryltrinitrate has been successfully used intravenously for producing effective venodilatation and dopamine, dobutamine and isoproterenol have been used as inotropic agents.

Acute pulmonary edema:

This is an important feature of circulatory failure caused by left sided heart problems. The three initial steps in its management are :

1. Morphine to alleviate breathlessness and reverse peripheral vasoconstriction.
2. A powerful diuretic such as furosemide.
3. A high concentration of oxygen.

If these immediate measures are inadequate, an inotropic agent may be used to stimulate the heart or use more powerful vasodilator to reduce left ventricular load.

Septic shock:

Septic shock occurs when invasion by microorganisms causes circulatory insufficiency and inadequate tissue perfusion. Although gram negative organisms account for majority of the cases of septic shock, gram positive cocci, clostridia, viruses, rickettsia and fungi account for some cases.

The emergency treatment of septic shock will depend on the presenting symptoms and hemodynamic profile. In many cases volume replacement and maintenance of high cardiac output is essential to prevent further worsening of shock. Alongside, chemotherapeutic measures using appropriate antibiotics are taken to cure the septicemia which is the main cause.

Anaphylactic shock:

Systemic anaphylaxis consists of a group of very severe reactions which occur rapidly following an injection of the antigen, as in the case of a drug like penicillin or the sting of an insect. The features of anaphylactic shock include bronchospasm, laryngeal oedema with extreme dyspnoea and cyanosis and a marked fall in blood pressure. There may also be nausea, vomiting and diarrhoea. Anaphylactic shock is a potentially fatal condition if not treated promptly with adrenaline (500-1000 μg) i.m. an antihistamine (e.g. chlorpheniramine 10-12 mg slowly i.v.) followed in severely ill patients by intravenous corticosteroids (e.g. hydrocortisone 100 mg. i.v.)

SNAKE BITES

Poisonous snakes are widely distributed in most countries and serious snake bites often occur. There are three families of medically important venomous snakes. All have fangs at thc front of their mouths whereby they inject venom from the parotid glands.

1. The **Elapidae** (cobras and craits etc.) : They have short fangs and are land snakes, the venom of which produce neurotoxic features. Local tissue necrosis is characteristic feature of cobra bite.
2. The **Hydrophidae** (sea snakes) : They also have short fangs and characteristic flattened tails. The venom of sea snake is myotoxic.
3. The **Viperidae** : They have long erectile fangs. They are divided into **Viperinae** (true vipers) such as Russell's viper and Carpet viper, and **Crotalidae** (pit vipers) such as rattle snakes. The venom of the **Viperidae** is vasculo-toxic.

About 50% of people bitten by snakes suffer few or no toxic effects as very little of the venom gets injected. On the contrary if thc dose of venom is high the mortality in the absence of effective treatment is 10% within 5-20 hours of cobra bites, 10% within 15 hours for sea snakes and upto 15% within 2 days for vipers.

First aid measures: Firm pressure bandaging of the bite area and immobilization of the part substantially delays the spread of venom. Patients of snake bite are unusually apprehensive and should be reassured and sedated if necessary.

Clinical features:

Viper bite: Local swelling starts almost immediately. Early signs of systemic poisoning develop within 15 minutes of the bite include vomiting, hypotension and signs of abnormal bleeding from any site. Blister formation around the site of bite is common and spreading blisters suggest a large dose of venom and precede tissue necrosis.

Cobra bite : Local swelling seldom occurs. Vomiting, hypotension and polymorph leucocytosis suggest systemic envenomation. More specific signs of muscle weakness such as ptosis indicate severe poisoning. There is danger of respiratory paralysis. Local tissue necrosis with an offensive putrid smell is typical of cobra bites.

Sea snake bite: The early features are similar to cobra bite. More specific signs are myalgia, with the appearance of myoglobinuria. Paresis of limb may follow with respiratory paralysis within a few hours of the bite.

Treatment:

1. The site of the bite should be cleansed and then left as such otherwise risk of infection is increased. If skin necrosis occurs, sloughs should be excised with skin grafts applied as appropriate.
2. General measures including intravenous fluids should be given to support vital functions.
3. Sedatives may be administered if the patient is apprehensive.
4. Appropriate antitetanus prophylaxis should be given after assessing patients immune state.
5. Antivenoms should be given only if there is clear evidence of systemic poisoning. Tissue necrosis can be avoided or minimized if antivenom is given within 4 hours of cobra bite.
6. All antivenoms may cause severe allergic reactions which may be fatal. Adrenaline (1: 1000 solution), i.m. must be given at the first sign of anaphylaxis.

BURNS

The mortality due to extensive burns remains high despite the greater understanding of the pathophysiology of burns and improved measures to cope with burn shock. Control of infection in burns by the topical application of mafenide, silver nitrate and silver sulphadiazine leads to further decline in the mortality of patients with 30-60 percent body burns.

Individuals with minor burns may not require hospitalization and may be treated as ambulatory patients but the care of seriously burnt patients is always conducted after admission to the hospital. Upon arrival in the hospital the seriously burnt is first examined for evidence of pulmonary edema, manifestations of shock and serious concomitant injuries as they require immediate care. Thereafter the history and physical examination of the patient decide the mode of the treatment for burns.

History: The following component of patients' history are very helpful in the treatment of burns.

(a) **Nature of burns:** Nature of the agents causing burns and the environment in which burn occurred indicate the possible extent of tissue damage. Burns occurring in an automobile accident are often accompanied by other injuries. There is more likelihood of upper respiratory injury if the patient has got burnt in a closed room. Hot air and metal produce deeper injuries than those produced by hot water. Hot air and flames cause dry burns whereas hot liquids produce moist burns. The area of electric burns is smaller but the actual extent of tissue damage is more.

(b) **Duration :** Time elapsed after sustaining the burn injuries affects the development of signs and the general condition of the patient. A patient seen within half an hour after an accident may not show any sign of shock or respiratory obstruction. Even blister formation of a second degree burn may not be apparent during this period.

(c) **Previous Treatment:** In acute cases history should be taken for any previous treatment received by the patient as it may determine the future line of treatment. Also the presence of other diseases like hypertension or liver or kidney diseases can alter vital signs and values of blood and urine analysis.

(d) **Tetanus immunization:** In all patients history should be taken for the last active or passive immunization against tetanus.

Physical Examination:

The examination room should be warm and well lighted. The patient should be completely undressed and laid on a sterile sheet if the burn is extensive so that entire area of burn can be exposed. The examination of burns must be done under aseptic conditions.

Location of burns and total area involved:

The total percentage of body surface involved can be estimated by the 'rule of nines'. (Fig. 10.1)

From the figure it becomes clear that the head comprise 9% of surface area of the body, each upper extremity 9%, each lower extremity 18%, the torso 18% and the genitalia 1%. Conversion charts are available for adaptation in infants and children.

Depth of burn: Burns are classified into three important categories on the basis of their depth.

(a) **First degree burn :** It is manifested as simple erythema with redness, swelling and tenderness but usually there is no death of epithelim.

(b) **Second degree burn:** It is indicated by the presence of blisters in the area of erythema.

(c) **Third degree burn:** In third degree burn the involved skin appears to be dry; it is brown or white and is anesthetic to pinprick. When charring and clear-cut thrombosis of small vessel is present, the burn is almost always full thickness.

The majority of burns are usually mixed. The deeper burn areas are usually surrounded by zones of superficial involvement.

Degree of contamination: Contamination usually includes dirt, clothing and only local medication is applied under unsterile conditions.

Circulatory Involvement: Any deep circumferential burn of extremity can produce a constrictor effect and impair circulation distal to the site of burn. A circumferential burn around the neck or chest can adversely affect breathing and produce respiratory difficulty.

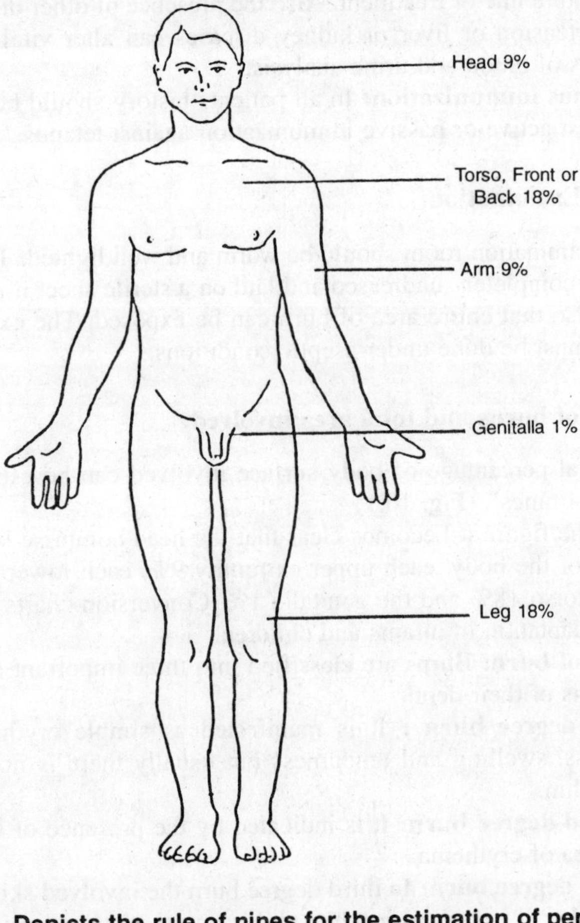

Fig. 10.1. Depicts the rule of nines for the estimation of percentage of surface area in a patient of burns.

General Examination:

Mental State: Mental state is not affected in the early stage of burns as patient remains conscious and oriented. This may not be so if there has been excessive intake of alcohol, inhalation of any toxic gas or concomitant brain damage. Such patients may need special care.

Presence of shock: Burn shock is manifested by hypotension, a rapid thready pulse, diminished sensorium, pallor, sweating and coldness of the skin in unburnt areas. The blood pressure and pulse rate are routinely monitored in the patients of burns.

Respiratory function: In the patients of burns and particularly in those who have suffered head, neck and chest burns, the respiratory function should be carefully monitored repeatedly for any evidence of congestion. The respiratory sound should be noted. Hoarseness of voice indicates respiratory obstruction. Edema, congestion and exudation in the respiratory tract take time to develop, hence periodic examination of respiratory tract function are of utmost importance.

Urinary output: It indicates kidney function and the state of hydration of the patient. In severe burn cases there is massive shift of fluid to the injured tissues leading to significant reduction in the circulating blood volume. In such patient exact recording of hourly urine output is essential. This is done by putting an indwelling catheter.

Emergency Treatment:

Ambulatory patient: Superficial burns constituting less than 5 percent of body surface and not involving lower extremities can be treated as outpatients in the emergency room.

Hospitalization: It is necessary to admit the patient in a hospital if

(a) Extensive burns involve more than 15% of body surface.
(b) There are burns of head and neck with evidence of respiratory tract involvement.
(c) Deep burns involve the lower extremity.
(d) There are late infected burns.

Prognosis:

The following factors determine the prognosis of any burn case.

Extent of burns: Burns involving less than 15 percent of total body surface are considered minor burns and carry minimal mortality. Whereas burns affecting more than 20% of total body surface are considered extensive. Burns involving 50 percent of total body surface usually have mortality of 50 percent, burns involving 75 percent of total body surface have a mortality of 90 percent and burns involving 90 percent of body surface have a mortality of 100 percent. 'Rule of nines' is used for estimating the percentage of body surface.

Depth of burns: The deeper is the destruction of skin due to severe burns, the slower would be the healing, which in turn would significantly enhance the chances of bacterial invasion of the wounds. Wound infection may be responsible for about 20% of the burn mortality.

Location of burns: Burns of the face and neck especially those infected by fire in an enclosed room are often accompanied by upper respiratory tract damage which is responsible for about 42 percent of burn deaths.

Age: The very young and the elderly, both are of greater risk to the mortality caused by burns. Children under 5 and elderly individuals over 60 years of age carry a significantly higher mortality.

Local Treatment:

(a) All burns involving more than 15 percent of total body surface should be treated in the operating room.
(b) Strict aseptic techniques must be used. Cap, mask and sterile gloves are used by all personnel in contact with the patient.
(c) The burnt area must be thoroughly cleansed with soap and water and irrigated with saline solution. All gross contaminants, dust, grease etc. should be meticulously removed. All blisters should be opened, the loose tissue thoroughly debrided and the collected serum is evacuated. The surface is first covered by a single layer of the mesh gauge impregnated with Xeroform ointment. Then comes flat, absorbing gauges of different thickness to cover the different areas of the body.

In case of extensive burns involving more than 20% of body surface the patient should be hospitalized and the type of local treatment may be decided by the surgeon-in-charge after admission. Superficial extensive burns can be treated by the closed method described above. Deep extensive burns are best treated by open method using topical antibacterial agents like mafenide, silver sulfadiazine cream or 25% silver nitrate solution.

The progress of the patient is continuously assessed till he/she is out of any donger to life.

General Treatment:

Obstruction of respiratory tract: Burns of head and neck region produce the obstruction of respiratory tract. If signs of obstruction like difficulty in breathing, retraction of intercostal space or cyanosis are present, relief is best accomplished by passing an endotracheal tube under anesthesia.

Tetanus prophylaxis: All burn injuries, irrespective of site, depth or total area involved are considered as open wounds and hence tetanus prophylaxis is mandatory and should be given to all patients before leaving the emergency room.

Antibiotics: For ambulatory patients systemic antibiotics are not necessary. In patients with extensive burns the physician may decide for a suitable antibiotic treatment on an individual basis.

Analgesics: Patients with extensive burns occasionally require treatment with analgesic drug for the relief of pain. A suitable analgesic is generally administered by intravenous route as shock impaired circulation can delay absorption of a drug given by other parenteral routes.

Intravenous Fluids: Extensive burns can produce quantitative and qualitative alterations of the extracellular fluid which must be corrected immediately. An infusion of Ringer's lactate is started immediately in such cases and the levels of sodium, potassium, chloride, urea and carbon dioxide content of the blood are monitored.

POISONING

Acute poisoning is a common and urgent medical problem in all developed and many developing countries of the world. The cases of poisoning in young children are virtually all accidental whereas in the older age groups the great majority are intentional and self-inflicted. This chapter deals with the clinical features, diagnosis, treatment and prevention of acute poisoning.

Social Patterns: Acute poisoning is more common in females than in males. The major rise in incidence has been among patients in the second and third decades reaching levels that are now many times higher than amongst the middle aged and elderly. The increase has been particularly marked in patients of lower social class. The rate of self poisoning in males has been higher among unskilled lower social class, divorcees, unemployed alcoholics and in individuals having criminal records, debt or history of family violence.

Pattern of poisoning : Drugs have always been the most frequent agents taken by adults. More than 60% of them ingest drugs that have been prescribed for themselves or a close relative and hence the pattern of acute poisoning reflects the prescribing habits to a great extent. The major groups of drugs involved in acute poisoning at present are benzodiazepines, tricyclic and related antidepressants, analgesics, non-steroidal anti-inflammatory drugs and opiate analogues. Apart from these drugs certain insecticides, barbiturates and mushrooms are often involved in poisoning. In our country the consumption of illicit liquor also leads to a number of deaths and blindness due to methanol poisoning.

Clinical features: The clinical features of most of the poisoning cases are non-specific but the diagnosis is seldom in doubt as the circumstantial evidence is often strong and many patients or their relatives give a clear history of it. Difficulties do arise particularly when such information is not available and the patient is unconscious. Many drugs in overdose produce complex neurological features of a non-specific type and so the state of pupils, abnormalities of eye movements, nystagmus and changes in limb reflexes may not be significant enough to indicate any definite diagnosis. The clinical features of some of the commonly involved drugs have been listed in Table 10.2.

Table 10.2 Clinical features of some drugs andchemicals commonly involved in poisoning

Clinical features	Possible drug or poison ingested/ inhaled/absorbed
Vomiting	Opiates and related analogues
Pinpoint pupils	Cholinesterase inhibitors (insecticides)
Depressed Respiration	Dextropropoxyphene
Dilated pupils, Distension of bladder, Absence of bowel sounds, Cardiac arrhythmias,	Tricyclic antidepressants
Sweating, Tinnitus, Deafness and Hyperventilation	Salicylates
Buccal corrosive burns	Strong acids, alkalis, phenol, cresol
Characteristic smell	Alcohol, volatile hydrocarbons, solvents
Hypothermia	Chlorpromazine, Barbiturates
Skin blisters	Barbiturates, Tricyclic antidepressants

Identification:

The conclusive identification of any drug involved in a case of poisoning is obtained following the toxicological analysis of urine, gastric aspirate or plasma and simple rapid screening methods are available for about 90% of common poisoning.

General principles of treatment :

Treatment in the majority of cases is dependent on the application of basic but good quality modern intensive therapy on a background of careful clinical assessment, coupled with the sound knowledge about the toxicology of the poison involved. Patients with significant poisoning should be regarded as genuine medical emergencies. Specific antidotes are available for about 2% of acute poisoning which have been listed in Table 10.3. Some of these produce significant side effects and hence they should be used only if the patient has serious and possibly life threatening poisoning.

Prevention of absorption: Patients with poisoning due to inhalation of toxic gases must be removed to fresh air as quickly as possible. The rescuers should not expose themselves to toxic gases without care for their own safety and if necessary use appropriate breathing apparatus. When a liquid or solid poison capable of cutaneous absorption is in contact with the patient's clothes, these must be removed and any poison on the skin washed off carefully with soap and water. When the poison has been swallowed measures to limit further absorption of ingested poisons include the following:

Table 10.3 Poisons and their specific antidotes

Poisons	Antidotes
Cholinesterase inhibitors (Organophosphorus insecticides)	Pralidoxime Olidoxime Atropine
Cyanide	Dicobalt edetate Sodium nitrite Sodium thiosulphate
Gold, Mercury	Dimercaprol
Arsenic, Copper, Zinc	Penicillamine
Iron	Desferrioxamine
Lead	Sodium calcium edetate
Opiates and analogues	Naloxone
Paracetamol	Methionine N-acetylcysteine
Thallium	Prussian Blue
Methanol	Ethanol

Oral adsorbents: The role of these substances of which activated charcoal is the safest is debatable. However, activated charcoal administered with water can be effectively used when emesis and gastric aspiration and lavage are contraindicated and also as an adjunct to these procedures. In the case of emesis, the vomiting should be over before charcoal is given. The effective ratio of charcoal to estimated amount of poison to be adsorbed is of the order of 10.1. It is therefore most useful when the poison ingested is toxic in small doses such as tricyclic antidepressants.

Activated charcoal is an effective nonspecific adsorbent of a wide variety of drugs and chemicals. Activated charcoal is fully effective when it is administered as a fine powder of small particle size thus having a large surface area and is of vegetable origin having very low mineral contents. It must be stored in tightly sealed glass or metal container as prolonged exposure to vapors of the atmosphere will decrease its adsorptive capacity.

Induction of emesis : The oral administration of Syrup of Ipecacuanha has become very popular in the treatment of poisoned patients as a means of effective gastric emptying. It should, however be used only in conscious patients within four hours of ingestion of a potentially toxic does of a poison. It is not to be used in poisoning with petroleum distillates as vomiting of these carries a high risk of aspiration into lungs. It should also not be used following the ingestion of corrosive substances. The effective dosage regimen is 15 ml in children and 30 ml in adults. This should be followed by 200 ml of water. The dosage should be repeated after 20 min if emesis has not occurred.

Gastric aspiration and lavage : The indications and contraindications for gastric aspiration and lavage are same as those for induction of emesis with some exceptions:

(1) Gastric aspiration and lavage is indicated in unconscious patients irrespective of the time after the ingestion of a toxic dose.
(2) The procedure should only be done in the patients after endotracheal intubation.
(3) When corrosive poisons have been ingested there is substantial risk of perforation of oesophagus or stomach and it is best to avoid gastric aspiration and lavage in such patients.

Other methods of elimination of poisons:

In gravely ill patients following considerable absorption of a poison, measures to enhance its elimination may be necessary. Such measures can be carried out only in hospitals as they require technical skill and special apparatus. They include forced diuresis, peritoneal dialysis, hemodialysis and hemoperfusion. The most effective of these is hemoperfusion whereby heparinized blood from the patients is passed through a column containing granules of activated charcoal coated with synthetic acrylic hydrogen or ion exchange resins. This method may be life saving for some severe poisonings such as those due to barbiturates, glutethimide, methacholine and meprobamate.

Additional supportive therapy:

Hypothermia is common in severely poisoned patients. In moderate cases the aim of treatment is to prevent further heat loss by nursing the patient covered in a blanket in a humid but warm room between 26-29°C. In severe hypothermia the inspired air may be heated by passing administered oxygen through a Water's canister or by immersing one forearm in water at 43°C in addition to above measures. Intravenous fluids should be brought to warm room temperature prior to infusion. Acid-base disturbances should be corrected and fluid and electrolyte balance achieved by appropriate replacement therapy. Epileptiform convulsions should be treated with intravenous diazepam.

Psychiatric assessment:

The management of acute poisoning patients, particularly those suffering from self-poisoning is incomplete without early and adequate psychiatric assessment and management. Ideally the psychiatrist should become involved as quickly as possible,recognize the patients who have genuine suicidal tendencies and provide them the required psychiatric help so that they recover from the trauma and do not repeat such an act again.

CARDIAC ARREST

Another disorder of the cardiovascular system which needs immediate attention and emergency treatment is cardiac arrest. Cardiac arrest is the sudden and complete loss of cardiac function. It may be due to ventricular fibrillation, asystole or electromechanical dissociation.

Ventricular fibrillation is the commonest and most easily treatable cause of sudden death. It may be due to myocardial ischemia or inappropriate electrical stimulation such as electrocution. Within seconds of the onset of ventricular fibrillation, the patient loses consciousness. Respiration ceases and death is almost certain unless treatment is started promptly. If a defibrillator is available, the immediate application of a direct current shock may store sinus rhythm within seconds. Under other circumstances it is advisable to maintain the circulation by

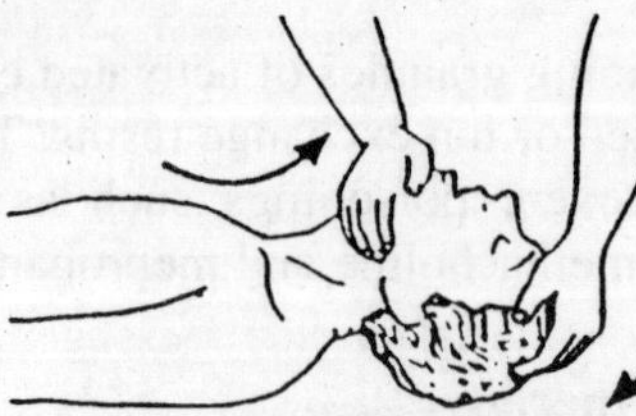

(A.) Clear the airway of vomitus
Extend the neck and raise the chin

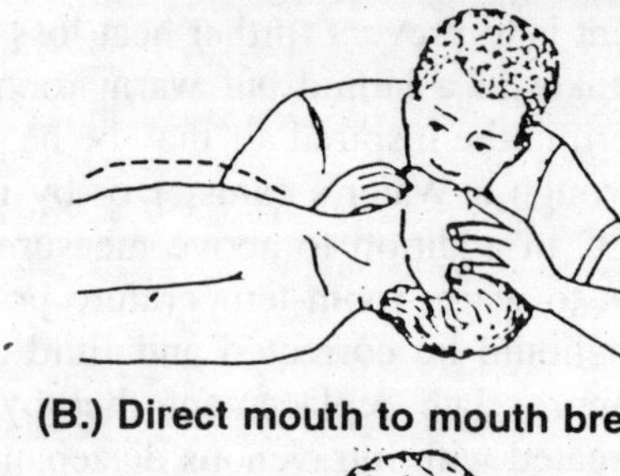

(B.) Direct mouth to mouth breathing

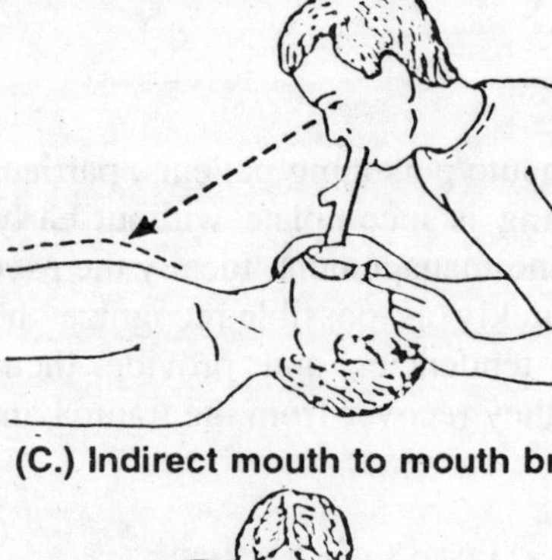

(C.) Indirect mouth to mouth breathing

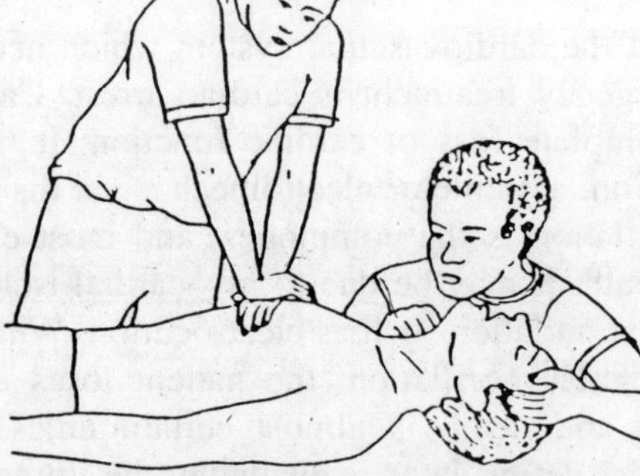

(D.) Cardiac massage

Fig. 10.2. Methods of emergency resuscitation to provide basic life support.

resuscitation procedures.

Ventricular asystole occurs when there is no electrical activity of the ventricles. It may be due to a localized failure of impulse conducting tissue or a massive ventricular damage complicating myocardial infarction. The former is amenable to cardiac massage whereas the latter is resistant to treatment.

Electromechanical dissociation occurs when there is no effective cardiac output despite the presence of normal or near normal electrical activity. It may complicate cardiac rupture or massive pulmonary embolism and is rarely amenable to treatment.

The management of cardiac arrest:

Cardiopulmonary resuscitation: Emergency measures to start cardiopulmonary resuscitation are essential because irreversible brain damage can occur unless some circulation of oxygenated blood can be achieved within two to three minutes. After confirming the diagnosis (e.g., unconscious, death-like appearance and absence of pulse), send for immediate help and deliver a sharp blow to the centre of the chest. If the heart does not start immediately as indicated by the return of the carotid or femoral pulse, start basic life support (Fig.10.2). The patient should be placed on his back on a firm surface and his legs should be elevated. Mouth to mouth, mouth to nose or mouth to airway ventilation should be used until a face mask and bag are available. Cardiac massage should be given by placing both the hands on the lower sternum (Fig. 10.2) and applying short, sharp, forceful compressions at a rate of 60 to 100 per minute. An electrocardiogram (ECG) is taken as soon as possible. When there is ventricular fibrillation, a 200 joule shock is given as soon as possible. Further manipulations can be done by expert cardiologists using defibrillator, adrenaline, lignocaine or electric shock depending upon the ECG and other parameters assessed in individual cases. In case of asystole intravenous atropine (0.6-1.2 mg) and if this fails intravenous adrenaline (1 mg) can be used to revive the patient.

Resuscitation is most likely to be successful when cardiac arrest is due to ventricular fibrillation particularly if this occurs as a result of an accident or in an uncomplicated case of myocardial infarction.

FRACTURES

Fracture denotes a broken bone which is generally caused by an offending force directly at the site of fracture or by a blow or force transferred indirectly to the breaking site, through the shaft of the bone. Even a swift muscle action is sometimes sufficient to break a bone. Fractures can be divided into the following types :

Simple fracture: It can be defined as single line of fracture without severe injury to other structures and there is no opening to the outside of the body.

Compound fracture: Compound fracture occurs when the site of break communicates with an opening in the skin.

Comminuted fracture: In comminuted fracture there are several lines of fracture crossing each other indicating that the bone has broken into several pieces.

Green-stick fracture: It is an incomplete fracture occurring only in young people and resembles the incomplete splintered break in a green stick.

Complicated fracture: It is characterized by a broken bone accompanied by other severe injuries such as torn nerves, ruptured large blood vessels and the break running into the joints or muscles.

Symptoms:

Symptoms of a fracture begin with a fall or severe injury resulting in a snap or crack, which is felt or heard by the patient, a loss of support at that point; pain at the site of injury first dull and later dull with sharp stabs, whenever the broken ends are moved. The limb bends or angles abnormally, there is often a grating that can be heard and felt by the patient and the examiner. It is due to the rubbing together of the two rough ends of the broken bones and is quite painful. In complete fracture disability results as regards the use of the bone. There is swelling of the area surrounding the fracture.

If the fracture is compound there is added danger of infection. One to three days after the accidents, the temperature rises, the pulse rate increases and the wound becomes hot, red, swollen, painful and tender. The infection if not controlled reaches the broken bone, causes destruction and absorption resulting in the loss of bone and often failure of union.

Treatment:

In all fractures delicate handling and extreme gentleness towards the patients are essential. The following steps and precautions must be taken before the physician, preferably an orthopedician is called to set the fracture or conduct other surgical manoeuvres.

1. Make the patient sit or lie in a comfortable position.
2. If a physician is not likely to be available for some time and it is necessary to move the patient, then first get the limb in its natural position by gentle movement and putting traction in the line of the broken bone. By applying traction the muscle spasm is counteracted to a considerable extent and the broken ends get approximated more nearly to their normal position and hence cause less injury.
3. Rough, jerky and injudicious handing of a fracture can aggravate the injury which may even be fatal.
4. It is often desirable to support the injured part on something soft e.g., a pillow or a quilt, maintaining if possible gentle fraction and thus preventing sagging or angulation.

Such treatment is required for all simple fractures. Before moving the patients, the bone ends must be be fixed or rendered as nearly as possible immobile. This is done by applying splints in the form of some

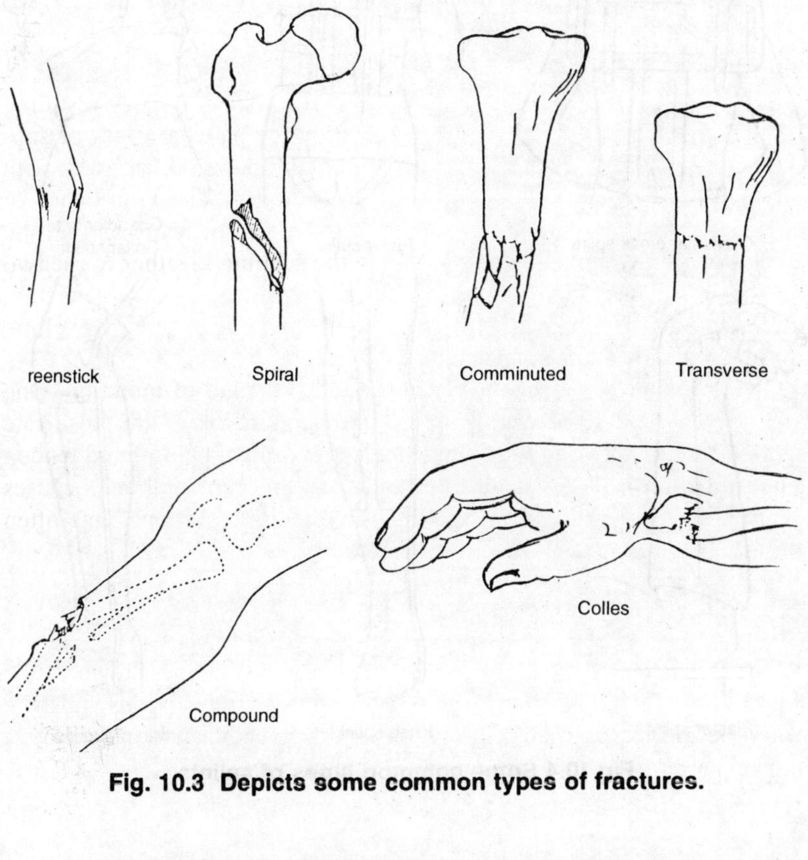

Fig. 10.3 Depicts some common types of fractures.

rigid material e.g., a wooden plank, a metal or a cardboard properly padded.

There are several requisites for splints. They must be rigid enough to hold the parts in position. They should be long enough to fix the joint above and/below the fracture. Splints should be as wide as the limb on which they are to be applied. The surface of the splints should be padded to fill the hollows and protect the bony joints. Splints should be able to increase the comfort of patients. They may be held in place by bandages, or strips of clothings. Splints should be firmly applied but they should not interfere with the circulation.

Some common types of fractures and splints have been shown in Figures 10.3 and 10.4.

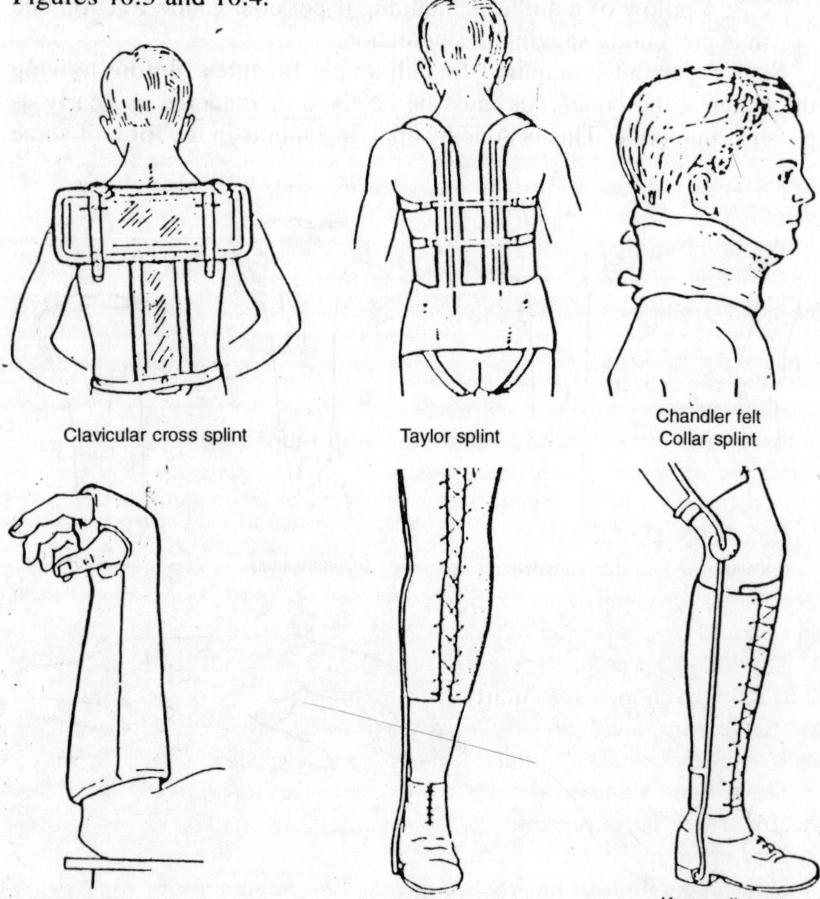

Fig.10.4 Some common types of splints

ELEMENTS OF MINOR SURGERY AND DRESSINGS

There was a time when minor surgery was confined to giving incision and draining of wounds and applying simple sutures. With the advancements of science and perfection of techniques today operations like appendicectomy, vasectomy, tubectomy and hernioplasty etc. fall into the realm of minor surgery. It is therefore important to consider various preparative procedures along with the procedures of suturing, dressing and postoperative care as the elements of minor surgery.

The preparation of a patient starts right from obtaining the consent of the patient or his close relatives for operation and anaesthesia. This is usually done by the house surgeon who also signs the form indicating that he has given the patient an explanation of what his operation will entail and who will do it. This helps to allay the patient's natural anxiety about the ordeal ahead of him.

The patient should be assured of a good night's sleep before the day of the operation. A sedative is usually given for this purpose. Routine preparation for bowel surgery usually includes an enema or colonic wash-out.

On the morning of the operation the patient should, if possible have a bath using an antiseptic soap. If the operation has to be performed on the head, trunk or lower limb,. shaving of the operative site is necessary.

The most important single point in the preparation of the patient for general anaesthesia is to ensure that the stomach is empty for at least four to six hours before the administration of an anaesthetic. This is to avoid the danger of the patient vomiting or regurgitating the stomach contents during anaesthesia when the fluid could quite easily be aspirated into the lungs.

It is usual for the patient to wear an easily removable gown. Jewellery, hair slides, pins and artificial dentures should be removed. Long hair should be confirmed by adequate covering.

The final step in the pre-operative preparation is premedication. This is usually given intramuscularly. The main purpose of premedication is to relieve pain, allay anxiety and abolish parasympathomimetic effects such as bronchial secretions, salivation and cardiac irregularities.

The patient is anaesthetized on the operating table, wheeled into the theatre where he is put into the appropriate position for his operation and the operation lights are accurately focussed on the operative site.

Skin preparation in the theatre is the final preparation of the operative side. A wide area is cleansed with the antiseptic of surgeon's choice. All antiseptis used for skin cleaning should be colored so that the area that has been cleansed can be clearly defined. All sponges used for skin cleaning should be different from those used during the operation so that they can be discarded immediately after use and not included in the count.

Swabs and Sponges:

Most of the swabs and packs used in surgery are made of cotton fibre though various synthetic materials are also available which are equally absorbent. All swabs should be disposable. They should be absorbent, nontraumatic to tissues, soft and should have no loose fibre. All swabs used for operation in the theatre should contain a radiopaque thread. Swabs for use by the anesthetists or for minor procedures like catheterization should be of different color to distinguish them from those used by the surgeons. The surgeon should ascertain by direct enquiry, before the completion of the operation, whether all swabs have been accounted for.

Sutures and ligatures:

A suture is a stitch, a length of material threaded on a needle for sewing two surfaces together. There are different types of sutures used in surgery each of them designed for a particular purpose. They can be grouped into two classes.

(a) **Interrupted sutures.** They are characterized by a suture line consisting of separate sutures, each of them tied and cut individually. This type of suture line is usually considered to be the strongest. It is suitable for tissues where the blood supply is not plentiful e.g. for anastamosis in the large bowel or for fascia which needs maximum support during healing.

(b) **Continuous Sutures.** This suture line consists of one running stitch tied at each end. It is hemostating and nonleaking. It is used for closing the peritoneum and for the anastamosis of bowel and blood vessels.

Some of the common types of skin sutures have been shown in Fig.10.5. They include:

(a) Two types of continuous sutures. They can be applied with speed.

(b) The subcuticular suture. It is invisible after insertion apart from where it is anchored at two ends. It leaves no stitch marks and the resultant scar is cosmetically perfect.

(c) Simple interrupted sutures, which canbe removed at different times, for example to drain pus from an infected area.

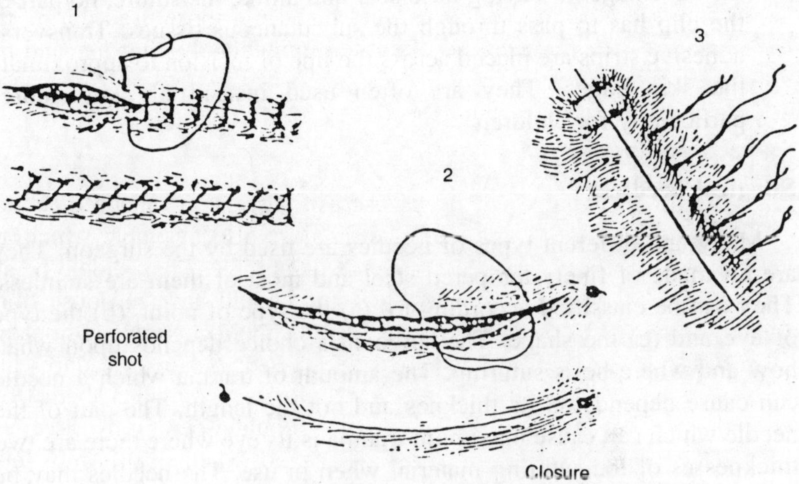

Fig. 10.5 Common types of skin sutures
1. Continuous sutures
2. Subcuticular sutures
3. Simple interrupted sutures

Ligatures:

The most common method of establishing hemostasis during surgery is by ligature. It is a length of material tied round a blood vessel, or a leash of blood vessels to prevent bleeding.

The ligatures and sutures can be classified in two groups based on the nature of material used.

1. **Absorbable:** Absorbable sutures and ligatures are generally of animal origin and they become part of the host's body after being digested by the tissues into which they are implanted during the surgical procedure. They include surgical cat gut, ribbon gut, fascia and kangaroo tendon.
2. **Nonabsorbable:** The material of nonabsorbable sutures and ligatures may be of vegetables or mineral origin, or it may be synthetically produced. They can also be left buried in the body or on the surface. If left buried, they disintegrate in time. They include silk, linen, cotton, nylon or other synthetic materials. Amongst them silk is the most commonly used. It has good tensile strength and is easy to handle. Other sutures include wire, silver and tantalum clips and michel clips. These are used to close the skin of clean wounds in the lower abdomen, breast and neck. They have

the advantage of leaving little scar and unlike the suture, no part of the clip has to pass through the subcutaneous tissues. Transverse adhesive strips are placed across the line of incision to approximate the skin edges. They are often used instead of skin sutures particularly for children.

Surgical needles:

Many and different types of needles are used by the surgeon. They are all made of finely tempered steel and most of them are stainless. They can be classified according to :(a) the type of point, (b) the type of eye and (c) the shape. The surgeons's choice depends upon what, how and where he is suturing. The amount of trauma which a needle can cause depends on its thicknes and not the length. The part of the needle which can cause maximum trauma is its eye where there are two thicknesses of the suturing material when in use. The needles may be straight or curved to different extent depending upon the site where they have to be used.

BIBLIOGRAPHY

1. Applied Therapeutics, The Clinical use of Drugs 3'rd Edition, Eds. B.S. Katcher, L.Y. Young and M.A., Koda-Kimble, Applied Therapeutics inc. Spokane, 1983.
2. Basic Pathology, Fourth Edition, S.L. Robbins and V.Kumar W.B. Saunders Company, Philadelphia, 1987.
3. Clinical Pharmacy and Therapeutics, 2'nd Edition, Eds. E.T Herfindal and J.H. Hirschman, Williams and Wilkins, Baltimore, 1979.
4. Cooper and Gunn's Tutorial Pharamcy, Ed. S.J. Carter, CBS Publishers and Distributors, New Delhi, 1986.
5. Davidson's Principles and Practice of Medicine, 16th Edition, Eds. C.R.W. Edwards, I.A. D. Bouchier, Churchill Livingstone, Edinburgh, 1991.
6. Microbiology, 5th Edition, M.J. Pelczar Jr., E.C.S. Chain, N.R. Kreig, McGraw Hill Book Company, Singapore, 1986.
7. Pharmaceutical Microbiology, Third Edition, W.B. Hugo and A.D. Russel, Blackwell Scientific Publications, Oxford, 1983.
8. Pharmacotherapy, A Pathophysiological Approach, Eds. J.T. Dipiro, R.L. Talbert, P.E. Hayes, G.C. Yees and L.M. Posey, Elsevier, New York, 1989.
9. Remington's Pharmaceutical Sciencs, 18th Edition, Ed. A.R. Gennaro, Mack Publishing Company, Easton, Pennsylvania, 1990.
10. Textbook of Preventive and Social Medicine, Twelth Edition, J.E. Park and K. Park M/s BanaraSsidas Bhanot Publishers, Jabalpur, 1989.

GLOSSARY

Acidosis: Decreased pH of the blood and body tissue resulting from accumulation of acid or depletion of alkaline reserve.

Addison's disease: A disease due to decreased functioning of adrenal glands and characterised by bronze-like skin pigmentation, progressive anemia, low blood pressure, diarrhoea and digestive disturbances.

Adenocarcinoma: Progressive overgrowth of epithelial cells of glandular tissues resulting in tumour.

Abhesion: The property of remaining in close proximity.

Algae: A plant family which is either unicellular or multicellular; not differentiated into root, stem & leaves and mostly containing chlorophyll e.g. sea weeds.

Alkalosis: A pathological condition resulting from accumulation of base or from loss of acid and characterized by increase in pH.

Ambulatory: Related to or adapted to walking.

Amplitude: Wideness or breadth of range or extent.

Anaphylaxis: An unusual or exaggerated allergic reaction of an organism to foreign protein or other substances resulting from the release of histamine, serotonin and other vasoactive substances.

Anastomosis: A communication between two vessels by collateral channels.

Anemia: A condition in which blood is deficient in quantity, in red cells or in hemoglobin and which is marked by pallor, weakness and irregular heart action.

Aneurism: A sac formed by the dilatation of the wall of an artery, a vein, or the heart.

Anorexia: Lack or loss of appetite for food.

Anorexigenic: An agent that diminishes the appetite.

Antenatal: Occurring or formed before birth.

Anthrax: An infectious disease caused by Bacillus anthracis commonly found in oxen, sheep, goats etc. but spread to human.

Apnea: Cessation of breathing, asphyxia.

Appendicectomy: Surgical removal of vermiform appendix.

Arthritis: A disorder characterised by inflammatory lesions at the joints.

Asphyxia: A condition due to lack of oxygen in inspired air resulting in impending or actual cessation of apparent life.

Aspiration pneumonia: Pneumonia due to entrance of food or other foreign matter into the respiratory passages.

Assimilation: Anabolism, conversion of nutritive material into living tissue.

Asthenia: Weakness, lack or loss of strength and energy.

Asthma: A condition marked by recurrent attacks of spasmodic contraction of the bronchi.

Asystole: Cardiac standstill; absence of a heart beat.

Ataxia: Failure of muscular coordination; irregularity of muscular action.

Atelectasis: Incomplete expansion of the lungs at birth or collapse of the adult lung.

Attenuate: To render a pathogenic microorganism less virulent.

Auditory: Pertaining to the sense of hearing.

Auscultation: The act of listening the sounds within the body for the purpose of diagnosis.

Beriberi: A disease caused by deficiency of thiamine (Vitamin B_1) and characterised by polyneuritis, cardiac pathology and edema.

Bilirubin: A bile pigment; a breakdown product of heme and heme pigments, like cytochrome.

Biodegradable: Susceptible to biological degradation by enzymes, bacteria etc.

Biopsy: Removal and examination, usually microscopic, of a tissue from the living body.

Blepharospasm: Tonic spasm of the orbicularis oculi muscle, producing closure of eyelids.

Blister: A large circumscribed elevation of the epidermis containing serous liquid.

Botulism: A type of food poisoning produced by the growth of Clostridium botulinum.

Bronchiectasis: Chronic dilatation of one or more bronchi.

Bronchiolitis: Inflammation of the bronchioles.

Bronchopneumonia: Inflammation of the lungs, usually beginning in the terminal bronchioles.

Brucellosis: A generalized infection caused by species of Brucella, primarily involving the reticuloendothelial system.

Buzzing: humming sound; confused low sound.

Cacophony: harsh discordant sound.

Candidiasis: Infection caused by fungi of the genus candida, commonly involving skin, oral mucosa, respiratory tract and vagina.

Carcinogenicity: Ability to produce cancer.

Cardiomyopathy: A general term designating primary myocardial disease.

Caseating: A from of necrosis changing the tissue into a dry amorphous mass resembling cheese.

Catarrh: Inflammation of a mucous membrane with a free discharge.

Catheter: Tube inserted into body-cavity to drain or enter fluid.

Cellulitis: Inflammation of the soft or connective tissue in which watery exudate spreads into interstitial and tissue spaces leading to ulceration and abscess.

Cervical lymphadenopathy: Any disease of the lymphnodes of cervical region.

Chagas Disease: Infection by Trypanosoma cruzi spread by blood sucking bugs. It is characterised by an erythematous nodule and by regional lymphadenopathy.

Cheilosis: Fissuring & dry soiling of the vermilion surface of the lips and angles of the mouth; a characteristic of riboflavin deficiency.

Chest percussion: Striking the chest with short, sharp blows as an aid in diagnosing the condition of the underlying parts by the sound obtained.

Chicken pox: A highly contagious disease caused by the Herpes zoster virus.

Cholecystitis: Inflammation of the gall bladder.

Cholera: An acute infectious disease caused by Vibrio cholera, characterised by severe diarrhea, vomiting, extreme fluid and electrolyte depletion and muscle cramps.

Cholestasis: Stoppage or suppression of bile flow.

Chyle: The milky fluid from food in intestine absorbed by the lacteals and passed into veins by the thoracic duct.

Chylous ascites: The presence of chyle in the peritoneal cavity due to blockage or disease of thoracic duct.

Chyluria: The presence of chyle in urine, giving it milky appearance.

Cirrhosis: Interstitial inflammation of an organ, particularly the liver.

Clammy: damp and sticky.

Coagulation: The process of clot formation.

Colostrum: The thin, yellow, milky fluid secreted by the mammary gland a few days before or after parturition.

Coma: Prolonged deep unconsciousness from which patient cannot be aroused even by powerful stimulus.

Combustible: Capable of rapid oxidation with emission of heat.

Commensal: An organism living on or within another but not causing injury to the host.

Congenital: Existing at, and usually before birth.

Conjunctivitis: Inflammation of the delicate membrane lining the eyelids and covering the eyeballs.

Constipation: Infrequent or difficult evacuation of faces.

Contagious: A disease capable of getting spread from person-to-person.

Convulsion: An involuntary contraction or series of contractions of the voluntary muscle.

Corrosive: An agent destructive to the texture or substance of the tissues.

Coryza: Profuse discharge from the mucous membrane of the nose.

Cramps: Painful sudden involuntary muscular contractions.

Cyanosis: Blue discoloration of skins and mucous membrane due to excessive concentration of reduced hemoglobin in the blood.

Cyst: A closed epithelium lined sac or cavity (2) A stage in life cycle of certain parasite where they are covered with protective layer.

Cystitis: Inflammation of the urinary bladder.

Cystoscope: An instrument for visual examination of the urinary bladder.

Debride: To remove foreign material or dead tissue from or nearby the traumatic or infected tissue.

Debridement: Act of debriding.

Defecation: Evacuation of fecal material from the rectum.

Deglutition: The act of swallowing.

Delirium: A disordered state of mind; wildly excited mood marked by illusions, delusions, hallucinations, restlessness and incoherence.

Delusion: False belief or impression about external reality and firmly maintained even when there is strong proof or evidence against it.

Dementia: Organic loss of intellectual function.

Dengue: An infectious viral disease of tropical areas spread by mosquito and marked by severe pain in the head, eyes, muscles and joints, sorethroat, skin eruptions and painful swelling of parts.

Desquamation: The shedding of epithelial elements, chiefly of the skin, in scales or sheets.

Diarrhoea: Abnormal frequency and liquidity of fecal discharges. Excessive evacuation of too fluid feces.

Diphtheria: An acute infection caused by Corynebacterium diptheriae and its toxin and marked by fever, pain and inflammation of mucus membranes of nose, throat and larynx.

Dorsal: Pertaining to the back.

Dysentery: Inflammation of the intestine characterised by abdominal pain, frequent stools containing blood and mucus.

Dyspnea: Labored or difficult breathing.

Dysuria: Painful or difficult urination.

Ecological: Concerning the environmental factors which affect life of organisms.

Ectopic: Arising from an abnormal site or tissue.

Eczema: A superficial inflammation of the skin, marked by initial redness, itching, minute papules and vesicles, oozing , crusting and scaling.

Elephantiasis: A chronic disease due to infection with Burgia malayi or Wuchereria bancrofti spread by bites of infective mosquitoes marked by inflammation and obstruction of lymphatics and hypertrophy of the skin and subcutaneous tissues, chiefly affecting the legs and external genitals.

Embolism: Sudden blockage of artery by a mobile clot or foreign material.

Encephalitis: Inflammation of the brain.

Endotracheal: Within the trachea.

Enteritis: Inflammation of the small intestine.

Enterovirus: Viruses infecting the gastrointestinal tract and discharged in feces. They include poliovirus, coxsackie viruses and echoviruses.

Eosinophilia: Abnormal increase of eosinophilic leucocytes in the blood.

Epidemic: A disease attacking many people in a region at the same time; widely diffused and rapidly spreading.

Epididymitis: Inflammation of the epididymis.

Epistaxis: Bleeding from the nose.

Erectile: Tissues containing large venous spaces with which arteries communicate directly as in the penis and clitoris.

Erythema: Reddening of the skin due to capillary constriction.

Etiology: Science that deals with the causes of disease.

Expectoration: Coughing up and spitting out materials from the lungs, bronchi and trachea.

Fang: Root of a tooth; canine tooth especially of dog, cat etc. or the envenomed tooth of a serpent.

Fauces: The passage between the throat and pharynx.

Febrile: Characterized by fever.

Fermentation: Anaerobic enzymatic conversion of organic compounds to simpler ones.

Fibrosis: The formation of fibrous tissue.

Filariasis: The infection caused by nematode worms-W. bancrofti, B. malayi and B. timorii-transmitted to man by bites of infected mosquitoes and marked by inflammation & obstruction of lymphatics.

Flatulence: excessive gas formation in the stomach or intestine.

Flocculation: a colloid phenomena in which the disperse phase separates like a tuft of wool.

Fluorescent: Capable of emitting light of a wavelength longer than that of absorbed light.

Fluorosis: Condition due to ingestion of excessive amounts of fluorine causing defective bones and teeth.

Fowl: Domestic cock or hen as kept for eggs and flesh; bird.

Fremitus: Vibration perceptible on palpation.

Frenum: A restraining structure of part.

Fulminant: that occurring suddenly with great intensity.

Fungoides: Resembling a fungus or mushrooms.

Gasgangrene: An anaerobic bacterial infection of muscles and subcutaneous tissue, filling it with gas along with blockage of blood supply to that part.

Gastroenteritis: Inflammation of the stomach and small intestine.

Generic: denoting a drug name not protected by a trademark, usually describing its chemical structure.

Genome: The complete set of hereditary factors as contained in the haploid assortment of chromosome.

Giardiasis: An infectious disease of the intestinal tract caused by flagellate protozoa G.lambia causing intermittent diarrhoea and malabsorption.

Glomerulonephritis: Nephritis with inflammation of the capillary loops in the renal glomeruli.

GNP: Gross National Product.

Goiter: Enlargement of the thyroid gland causing a swelling in the front part of the neck.

Gonococcemia: the presence of gonococci in the blood.

Gonorrhoea: Infection with Neisseria gonorrhoeae, a sexually transmitted disease marked with inflammation of urethra, pain and puslike discharge in males, and commonly asymptomatic in females but may show symptoms like inflammation of ovary uterine tubes and peritoneum.

Granuloma: A tumor like mass or granulation tissue due to a chronic inflammatory process associated with infectious disease or invasion by a foreign body.

Gravel: Fairly coarse concretions of mineral salts, as from the kidney or bladder, of smaller size than the so called stones.

Guineaworm disease: A vector borne parasitic disease caused by nematode Dracunculus medinensis.

Gummas: A soft, gummy tumour such as that occurring in tertiary syphilis.

Hallucination: a sense perception that is actually not present.

Hayfever: A seasonal form of allergic rhinitis with acute conjunctivitis, lacrimation, itching, swelling of nasal mucosa caused by specific allergen (e.g. Pollen grains).

Helminth: A parasitic worm.

Hematuria: Presence of blood in urine.

Hemodialysis: Purification of blood by removing certain elements by virtue of difference in rates of their diffusion through a semipermeable membrane.

Hemolysis: Liberation of hemoglobin due to lysis of red blood cells.

Hemoperfusion: Passage of blood through an extracorporeal adsorptive system to remove compounds of larger molecular size than can be removed by hemodialysis.

Hemophilia: A hereditary deficiency of a blood coagulation factor leading to hemorrhagic tendencies.

Hemoptysis: The spitting of blood or of blood-strained sputum.

Hemorrhagic: Tendency to bleed from the blood vessels.

Hepatitis: Inflammation of the liver.

Hepatomegaly: Enlargement of the liver.

Hereditary: That which is genetically transmitted from parent to offspring.

Hernioplasty: A operation to repair the protrusion of internal part of organ through aperture in enclosing membrane.

Heterozygous: Two or more alternative forms of genes at same locus, expressing a unit character, are different.

Histoplasmosis: Infection with Histoplasma capsulatum usually asymptomatic but may cause acute pneumonia, over-growth of reticuloendothelial cells, anemia, escape of fluid into joints, and red nodules.

Holistic: The concept of man as a functioning whole.

Homozygous: Two or more alternative forms of genes at same locus, expressing a unit character, are same.

Humus: Organic constituent of soil formed by decomposition of plant.

Hyperemic: having excessive blood in a part.

Hypernatremia: An excess of sodium in the blood.

Hypersensitivity: A state in which body reacts with an exaggerated immune response to a foreign agent.

Hypoplasia: Incomplete or under development of an organ or tissue.

Illumination: The process of rendering a subject capable to resist and overcome infection.

Impervious: Impenetrable.

Impetigo: Contagious skin due to streptococcal or staphylococcal or skin infection marked by vesicles which rupture to form yellow crusts.

Impounding: Collecting in reservoir.

Incipient: beginning, in early stage.

Incubation: (1) Providing proper conditions for growth and development for bacteria, tissue culture or premature infant. (2) A stage from entry of pathogen upto appearance of clinical symptoms (3) Development of the embryo in the eggs of oviparous animal.

Infarction: Formation of Localized area of ischemic necrosis produced by arterial or venous occlusion.

Infirmity: Weakness as from disease or oldage.

Influenza: An acute viral infection of the respiratory tract with inflammation of the nasal mucosa, pharynx and conjunctiva, headache and severe myalgia.

Innocuous: Harmless

Inoculation: Introduction of microorganisms, infective material, serum or other substances into tissues of living organisms, or culture media.

Inotropic: affecting the force of muscular contraction.

Insidious: proceeding unnoticed but harmfully.

Interstitial: pertaining to small space or gaps of a tissue.

Intertrigous: Pertaining to superficial dermatitis in the folded surfaces such as creases in the neck, folds of armpit or groin.

Intravascular: Within the blood vessels.

Ischaemic: The body part deficient in blood supply due to functional or actual obstruction of blood vessels.

Jaundice: Hyperbilirubinemia and bile pigment deposition in the skin, sclera, and mucous membranes resulting in yellow appearance of the patient.

Juvenile: Pertaining to youth or childhood.

Juvenile delinquency: Criminal and antisocial conduct by a minor (child)

Keratinization: Process of formation and deposition of scleroprotein (keratin) in the epidermis, hair, nails, enamels etc.

Ketosis: Accumulation of large amount of ketone bodies in tissues and body fluids.

Kwashiorkor: a syndrome due to severe protein deficiency which includes symptoms like retarded growth, changes in skin and hair pigment, edema and pathologic changes in liver.

Larvae: Insects in the stage between egg and pupa where they are structurally and functionally quite different from manure insects.

Larvivorous: Feeding on or consuming larvae.

Laryngitis: Inflammation of the larynx.

Lassa fever: A highly fatal, acute febrile disease caused by extremely virulent arenavirus occurring in West Africa.

Leprosy: A chronic surface infection by Mycobacterium leprae and characterised by the production of granulomatous lesions of the skin, mucous membranes and peripheral nervous system.

Leptospirosis: Any infectious disease due to leptospira, manifested by the lymphocytic meningitis, nephritis and hepatitis.

Lesions: Any pathological or traumatic discontinuity of tissue or loss of function of a part.

Leucopenia: Reduction of the number of leukocytes in the blood, the count being 5000 or less per cubic millimeter of blood.

Leukemia: Progressive disease of blood forming organs with abnormal accumulation of white corpuscles and its precursors in blood and bone marrow.

Lupoid reactions: Pertaining to lupus vulgaris, the most common and severe form of tuberculosis of the skin.

Lupus erythematosus: A chronic connective tissue disease manifested in two main types (a) **discoid lupus erythematosus:** superficial inflammation of skin in form of red macules forming typical butterfly pattern over the bridge of nose and cheeks, but other areas may be involved. (b) **Systemic lupus erythematosus:** It includes mild to severe skin eruptions, arthralgia, arthritis, leukopenia, anemia, visceral lesions, neurologic manifestations, lymphadenopathy and fever as main constitutional symptoms.

Lymphadenitis: Inflammation of the lymph nodes.

Lymphadenopathy: Disease of the lymph node.

Lymphangitis: Inflammation of the lymphatic vessel

Macrophage: Highly phagocytic cells derived from monocytes, found in walls of blood vessels or loose connective tissue, usually immobile but become actively mobile when stimulated by inflammation.

Macular: Pertaining to or characterised by the presence of maculae.

Maculae: Discolored spots on the skin alongwith small circumscribed elevation.

Malaise: Vague feeling of bodily discomfort.

Malaria: An infectious disease caused by protozoa of genus plasmodium which are parasitic in red blood cells and are transmitted mainly by female anopheles mosquitoes.

Malnutrition: Any disorder of nutrition either due to imbalance or insufficient diet or defective utlisation.

Marasmus: A type of protein-calorie malnutrition occurring in infants and characterised by growth retardation, wasting of subcutaneous fats and muscles.

Mastication: Process of chewing food for swallowing & digestion.

Maternal: Pertaining to the mother.

Measles: Rubeola, A highly contagious viral disease of primarily respiratory tract. Typical maculopapular spots appear on the skin preceded by symptoms like coryza, conjunctivitis, myalgia, malaise, fever.

Melanin: A dark amorphous pigment present in skin, hair, choroid coat of the eye & substantia nigra of the brain. Produced by oxidation products of tyrosine and dihydroxy phenyl compounds.

Meningitis: Inflammation of the meninges (membranes covering the brain & spinal cord.

Mite: Minute animals of arthropod family of order Acarina-transparent or semi-transparent causing various skin irritations.

Mitochondria: Small spherical to rod shaped cell organelles synthesising mainly ATP for cell functioning.

Morbidity: The condition of being diseased.

Morphology: The science of the forms & structure of organism; organ or part.

Mortuary: Building where dead bodies can be kept for some time.

Mumps: An acute contagious paramyxovirus disease seen mainly in childhood. It chiefly affects parotid salivary gland but can also affect the meninges and testes.

Mutagenicity: the property of inducing permanent transmissible genetic changes.

Myalgia: Pain in muscles.

Mycosis: any fungal disease.

Myocarditis: Inflammation of the myocardium.

Myoglobinuria: Excrection of myoglobin, a oxygen transporting pigment of muscle resembling a single subunit of hemoglobin.

Myotoxic: toxic to muscles.

Myxedema: Dry, waxy, swelling with abnormal deposits of mucin in the skin and other tissues, usually found in thyroid deficiency.

Nasopharyngeal: Pertaining to the pharynx above the soft palate.

Nausea: Referred unpleasant sensation to abdomen with a tendency to vomit.

Necrosis: Localized death of tissue caused by progressive enzymatic degradation.

Necrotic: that part which has undergone necrosis.

Necrotizing: causing necrosis.

Neonate: A newborn infant.

Nephritis: Inflammation of the kidney.

Neurotic: 1. Pertaining to nervous system. 2. A nervous person in whom emotions predominate over reasons.

Nocturnal: done or active in the night.

Nystagmus: Involuntary, rapid-movement of the eye ball.

Oliguria: Decreased urine secretion in relation to fluid intake.

Oncologist: Expert in the study of tumor.

Ophthalmia Neonatorum: Inflammation of the eyes in neonates (within 10 days of life) characterised by acute conjunctivitis with discharge of pus.

Optimum: Most favourable conditions.

Orchitis: Inflammation of the testes.

Osteomalacia: Softening of the bones resulting from vitamin D deficiency.

Osteomyelitis: Inflammation of the bone due to pus forming infection.

Osteoporosis: Abnormal reduction in density of bone.

Otitis media: Inflammation of the middle ear.

Ova: an egg, the female reproductive cell which after fertilization by sperm is capable to develop into new organism of same species.

Ovarian: Pertaining to ovary (female reproductive organ producing ova).

Palatable: Pleasant to taste or agreeable to the mind.

Palatal palsy: Paralysis of the partition separating the nasal & oral cavities.

Pallor: Paleness, as of the skin.

Pandemic: Diseases having world wide distribution.

Panencephalitis: Encephalitis resulting in parenchymatous lesions of white and gray matter simultaneously.

Pannus: (*i*) Superficial vascularization of cornea with infiltration of granulation tissue. (*ii*) Exudate overlying the inflamed synovial cells on the inside of a joint (*iii*) the subcutaneous fat.

Papule: a small, circumscribed, superficial solid elevation of the skin.

Parasthenia: A condition leading the organic tissue to function at abnormal intervals.

Paresis: Partial paralysis.

Paroxysmal. Recurrent sudden intensification of symptoms.

Pasteurization: Heating of liquids at moderate temperature (60°C) for definite period so as to kill pathogenic microorganisms.

Pathogen: Any disease producing microorganism.

Pathogenesis: The development of morbid conditions or of disease.

Pathology: The science which studies the structural and functional changes of the tissues due to disease.

Paediatric: The branch of medicine concerned with treatment of children and their development and care.

Pediculosis: Infestation with the lice of family pediculidae

Pellicle: A thin skin or film, such as a thin film on the surface of a liquid.

Percussion: Forcible striking of body with sharp blows, for the purpose of diagnosis of the conditions of the underlying parts by the sound obtained.

Perinatal: Relating to the period just before and after the birth.

Perineum: The region between the thighs, in males between scrotum and anus and in females between vulva and anus.

Peripheral neuritis: Inflammation of the peripheral nerves.

Peristalsis: Wave of contraction passing along the alimentary canal for variable distances.

Peritonitis: Inflammation of the serous membrane lining the walls of the abdominal and pelvic cavities and that enclosing the viscera.

Pernicious anemia: Anemia due to vitamin B_{12} deficiency caused by reduced secretion of intrinsic factor by gastric mucosa, which is necessary for absorption of vitamin B_{12} from intestine to blood.

Pesticide: Substance for destroying harmful insects.

Phagocytosis: The process of engulfing of microorganism or other cells and foreign particles by a phagocyte (engulfing cell).

Pheromone: A substance secreted by an organism outside the body whose smell is capable to induce specific behaviour in the other organism.

Phlebitis; Inflammation of a vein.

Photophobia: Fear or aversion to light, visual intolerance to light.

Placenta: An organ joining mother to her developing fetus helping in transport of substances from mother's blood to the fetus and also capable of secreting hormones.

Plague: Acute infectious disease caused by Yersinia pestis and transmitted to man from rats by rat flea bites and characterised by fever, vomiting, diarrhoea, swelling of lymph nodes (Bubonic plague), pneumonia (pneumonic or pulmonic plague) and presence of the microorganism in blood (septicemic plague).

Pleocytosis: Presence of abnormally high number of cells in cerebrospinal fluid.

Pneumonia: Inflammation of lung making it hard, and releasing fluid.

Polio: Poliomyelitis

Poliomyelitis: An acute viral disease causing fever, sore throat, headache, vomiting, back and neck stiffness and in few cases paralysing one or more limbs.

Polyneuritis: Inflammation of many nerves simultaneously.

Porphyria: Increased formation and excretion of iron or magnesium free cyclic tetrapyrole derivatives (porphyrins) universally found as respiratory pigments in protoplasm of any cell.

Prenatal: Before birth.

Prodromal: Symptoms that are indicative of onset of disease.

Prolapse: Downward displacement of part of organ in abdomen or other body cavities.

Promiscuous: Having casual sex relation with many people.

Promiscuity: tendency for casual sex relation with many people.

Prophylactic: Anything done to prevent the causation of disease.

Prosthesis: Artificial substitute for a missing body part e.g. artificial arms, leg, eye etc.

Proximate: Nearest to a reference point.

Psychologist: Expert in dealing with the mind and mental processes especially in relation to human behaviour.

Psychosis: Severe mental derangement involving whole personality and loss of contact with reality.

Psychotic: Person exhibiting psychosis.

Ptosis: (*i*) Downward displacement of an organ or a part (*ii*) Paralytic hanging down of eyelids.

Puerperium: The period of confinement after child birth.

Puerperal: Pertaining to a woman who has just given birth to a child.

Pupae: Premature insects in the second stage of development between the larva and the imago.

Purulent: That forming or having pus.

Pustular: Skin having a small, elevated circumscribed, pus-containing lesion.

Pustule: A pus-containing, elevated skin lesion.

Pyelonephritis: a bacterial infection causing inflammation of the kidney and its pelvis.

Pyrexia: fever, Increased body temperature.

Quackery: The fraudulent misrepresentation of one's ability and experience in the diagnosis and treatment of disease.

Quarantine: Restriction placed on movements of possible carriers of disease.

Q fever: A rickettsial infection, usually of respiratory tract caused by Coxiella brunetii.

Rabies: An acute viral infection of central nervous system which in final stages result in paralysis of muscles used for swallowing, hydrophobia (fear of water), maniac behaviour, respiratory paralysis and tetany etc.

Radiology: Scientific study of radiation and its use for diagnosis and treatment of disease.

Rales: Abnormal respiratory sounds indicative of a disease.

Rash: temporary eruptions of the skin.

Recrudescence: recurrence of symptoms after some time.

Refinery: Place where any substances are freed from impurities.

Refuse: Waste or rejected materials.

Regimen: prescribed course of treatment, diet, exercise etc.

Regurgitate: (*i*) Backward flow of blood through defective heart value (*ii*) Bring out the swallowed food back to mouth.

Rehabilitation: Restoration to useful activity of diseased or disabled person.

Relapse: Return of a disease after temporary ceasing.

Ribosome: A cell organelle acting as a site for protein synthesis.

Rickets: Deficiency disease of Vitamin D in infants and children resulting in abnormal bone formation causing bending and distortion of bone.

Rickettsial pox: A disease caused by Rickettsia marked with pus containing skin rash.

Rigor: a chill, inflexibility or stiffness.

Risus sardonicus: A broad smile type expression produced by spasm of facial muscle.

Salmonellosis: Infection with any organism of genus salmonella.

Sandfly fever: Fever of short duration caused by viruses transmitted by sandfly, also known as phlebotomus fever.

Sanitary: Promoting or pertaining to health.

Scab: The crust of a superficial sore.

Scabies: A contagious skin disease caused by itch mite, Saroptes scabiei causing intense itching.

Scar: A mark remaining after the healing of wound.

Scarlet fever: disease caused by group Ab-hemolytic streptococci characterised by scarlet colored rash.

Schistosomiasis: Infection with schistosomia (a genus of blood-fluke).

Sclerosing: Causing abnormal hardening of tissue.

Scrub Typhus fever: An infectious disease caused by Rickettsia tsutsugamushi spread by larvae of mites, and characterised by sudden onset of fever with a primary skin lesion and development of a rash by the 5th day.

Scurvy: Vitamin C deficiency; disease marked by anemia, spongy gums and a tendency to mucocutaneous hemorrhage.

Sedentary: of inactive habits.

Sensorium: A sensory nerve center.

Septicemia: Presence of pathogenic microorganism or their toxins in blood.

Serum sickness: A hypersensitivity following the administration of foreign serum or serum proteins, marked by urticaria, arthralgia, edema & lymph node disorders.

Sewage: Waste matter conveyed in underground drain pipe.

Silicosis: Lung disease caused by inhaling dust containing silica.

Sloughs: Necrotic tissue in prossess of separation from living tissue.

Soot: black powdery substance rising in smoke and deposited by it on surfaces.

Splenomegaly: Enlargement of spleen.

Splinter: Rough or sharp-edged or thin fragment broken or split off from some hard material (eg. bone).

Sprue: a chronic form of malabsorption syndrome.

Sterilization: Procedure for complete elimination or destruction of all living microorganism.

Stomatitis: A generalized inflammation of oral cavity.

Stomatitis (angular) Inflammation with exudation, softening and fissuring at the connecting point of two lips.

Stratum: a layer.

Stratum corneum: a horn like or horny keratin containing layer.

Stroke: a sudden and a servere attack.

Substerranean: underground.

Succulent: thick & fleshy.

Surveillance: close watch especially on suspected person.

Syphilis: a sexually transmitted disease caused by Treponema pallidium leading to many structural and cutaneous lesions.

Tamponade: (*i*) Surgical use of a pack, pad or plug of cotton or other material use to plug the nose, vagina etc. to control bleeding (*ii*) Compression of heart due to collection of blood in pericardium.

Tepid: Slightly warm.

Teratogenicity: The property of producing deformity in the developing embryo.

Terrestrial: of or on the earth (land).

Tetany: A syndrome caused by decreased concentration of calcium in blood: symptoms include sharp bending of wrist and ankle joints, muscle twitching, cramps and convulsion.

Thrombosis: Formation of aggregation of platelet, fibrin and cellular elements of blood, capable of causing obstruction to blood flow.

Tinnitus: a noise in ears, which sometimes may be heard by other than the patient.

Tortuous: Going in spiral or crooked or curved course.

Toxemia: The conditions resulting from the spread of bacterial product toxins by the blood stream.

Tracheitis: Inflammation of the trachea.

Tracheostomy: Surgical creation of an opening in the trachea through the neck.

Trachoma: Chronic infection by chlamydia trachomatous of eye mainly affecting cornea and conjunctiva.

Traction: Drawing along the long axis of a structure by exerting a pulling force.

Transmission: Spread of infection from one organism to other.

Trench fever: A self-limited rickettsial disease due to Rochalimae quintana, transmitted by the body louse, Pediculus humanus, marked by intermittent fever, generalised aches and pains, chills, sweating, vertigo, malaise and typhus-like rash.

Tubectomy: Excision of a portion of the uterine tube.,

Tularemia: An infectious disease, resembling plague especially of rodents, caused by Franciselle tublarensis. it can be transmitted by bites of flies, fleas, ticks & lice.

Typhus fever: A rickettsial infection characterised by severe headache, sustained high fever and macular or maculopapular skin lesion.

Ulcer: A local defect or excavation of the surface of an organ or tissue, which is produced by the slouging of inflammatory necrotic tissue.

Ulcerative colitis: a chronic recurrent ulceration in the colon.

Umbilical cord: Cord connecting the placenta to fetus.

Uraemia: Accumulation of products of protein metabolism in blood.

Urolithiasis: Formation of urinary calculi.

Urticaria: An allergic skin eruption by transient appearance of smooth elevated patches often associated with itching.

Vacuole: any small space or cavity in protoplasm of a cell.

Varicella form: resembling chicken pox.

Varicose: Unnatural permanent distension.

Vascular: Pertaining to blood vessel.

Vascularization: Natural or surgically induced development of vessels in a tissue.

Vasculitis: Inflammation of a vessel.

Vasculotoxic: Pertaining to or causing deleterious effect on vessels of the body.

Vasectomy: Surgical removal of vas deferens or a portion of it, to induce infertility.

Vector: a carrier, especially the animal (usually an arthropod e.g., flies, mosquitoes etc.) which transfers an infective agent from one host to other.

Vesicular: Composed of small bladder or sac containing liquid as on the skin.

Vibrations: (*i*) Oscillation (*ii*) shaking of the body as therapeutic measure (*iii*) a form of massage.

Virulence: Degree of disease causing capacity of a microorganism.

Vocal fremitus: perception of vibrations caused by speaking by placing hand or stethoscope on chest.

Volar: Indicating the surface of fore arm with palm on top side.

Weeds: Plants of no use and growing to the damage of a crop.

Whooping Cough: An infection caused by Bordetella pertussis characterised by inflammation of mucous membrane of respiratory tract with free discharge and peculiar paroxysms of cough.

Xerophthalmia: A Vitmin A deficiency disorder causing dryness of the conjunctiva and cornea.

Yaws : An infectious disease of children caused by spirochete Treponema pertenue usually found in tropical areas and characterised by granulomatous initial lesions at the site of implantation of the organism followed by development of granulomatous papulses distributed over the body and finally syphilis type of lesions and destructive bone lesion.

Yellow fever: An acute viral infection spread by mosquito bites and marked by fever, jaundice and albuminuria (excretion of albumin in urine).

INDEX